trim
healthy
mama
plan

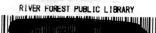
trim
healthy
mama
plan

THE EASY-DOES-IT APPROACH TO
VIBRANT HEALTH AND A SLIM WAISTLINE

Pear' n

12/15

Published in the United States by Harmony Books, an imprint of the Crown Publishing Group,
a division of Penguin Random House LLC, New York.
www.crownpublishing.com

Harmony Books is a registered trademark, and the Circle colophon
is a trademark of Penguin Random House LLC.

Library of Congress Cataloging-in-Publication Data is available upon request.

ISBN 978-1-101-90263-9
eBook ISBN 978-1-101-90264-6

Printed in the United States of America

Cover photograph by Kris D'Amico Photography

1   3   5   7   9   8   6   4   2

First Edition

We dedicate this book to our families—our husbands and
children who put up with us so patiently while
we poured our guts into this project.

"I'll take you out on a special day when this book is done."

"We'll go camping when this book is done."

"We'll make time for fun stuff when this book is done."

They heard lines like these every day and took them with a smile even
though completing what was supposed to be a little ... but grew into
a medium-size book took much longer than we expected.

"Can you change the baby's diaper while
I am writing the end of this chapter?"

"Honey ... can you go grocery shopping for me
because there's just no way I can fit it in?"

They all stepped up to the plate and worked hard to keep
our homes running "kinda" smoothly. The sweetest part was
their loving understanding when we became less than sane
burning the candles at both ends with hours of research
and writing marathons together. We love you guys!!!!

contents

introduction

Food freedom! Are you ready for it?

What a comfort when the realization hits: Discovering your trim and healthy self does not have to feel like a brutal sprint you must endure. It can be a relaxing, lifelong journey you'll actually enjoy. There are no number goals to be met by a certain time. No self-scolding if weight doesn't come off according to someone else's patterns. No scale obsession. No strict portion sizes to adhere to. Good riddance to all of that! You don't need it.

The key to finding and maintaining "your trim" for life is not mustering up more self-control. It's not found in obsessively measuring portions and counting bites. Our own willpower fails most of us in the end. The key is finding a simple, slimming way of eating—a way of eating you would actually prefer, day in and day out, over your old way of eating. Once you start enjoying your healthy, slimming foods so much that you feel sorry for everybody else who is not eating like you, that's when you know you've found the answer—you've got the recipe for lifelong success right there, baby!

Our motto: Treat yourself to goal, then keep on treating for life.

It wasn't our Creator's plan for it to be a miserable, almost impossible feat to have a trim figure after the age of twenty-five and a couple pregnancies under your belt. It just takes some understanding. Gain the right knowledge and you'll never look at your plate of food in the same way. Your body will begin the mystifying Trim Healthy Mama shrink!

This is the gentle and fun road to trim and healthy. It is not just for crunchy health food types. You don't have to be an exercise fanatic to make this work. Whether you love to cook from scratch with the purest of ingredients or you can barely boil water, come as you are.

THE CRAZY STORY

Once upon a time (well, three years ago to be more exact), something incredible happened. We self-published a book about how we had found our way out of the maze of diet fads, food fear, and miserable food bondage. We shared the concept of Food Freedom: a way of eating that is naturally slimming, healthy, and so indulgent and tasty that it makes you look like an idiot because you can't stop trying to force it onto your friends and family. Shamelessly, you don't care about your new dorky reputation because you want others to experience this freedom, too.

We knew nothing about book publishing, blogging, or marketing so we thought we might give away (force) some copies of the book on friends and neighbors and possibly sell a few on a homemade website. We were compelled to throw this lifeline of hope out there since it had revolutionized our own lives.

Somehow, the message caught on.

The Trim and Healthy versus skinny and deprived approach to eating resonated deep in diet-weary souls. Mamas shared the message with other Mamas and our ridiculous-looking homemade website started humming with hundreds, then thousands, then tens of thousands of orders. Soon, families, women's groups, churches, and entire communities ditched the diet fads with us and the Food Freedom movement was born.

Gotta confess, we felt special for maybe a minute or two but then quickly realized the spread of Trim Healthy Mama was not due to any genius writing skills on our part. Our readers were the reason this message became a movement. They caught the bug and would not stay quiet.

We're not doctors, certified nutritionists, or dieticians wearing sterile white coats. We are stay-at-home Mamas with stains on our T-shirts; crazy, chaotic lives; and eighteen children between us. We are *homeperts* not experts, but amazingly women all over the globe gave us a little bit of baby-step belief. Those seeds of faith grew into huge life transformations. That way-too-big, 640-page book, written by diet guru nobodies, became a *New York Times* bestseller without a cent spent on advertising—spelling mistakes and all! (Spelling *piza* instead of *pizza*, among other errors, is a tad unprofessional—blush.)

It would be impossible to get tired of reading all the messages, Facebook posts, and e-mails that stream in daily from people who half expect their scale to go up due to the decadent food they get to thrive on on the plan. There's often a lot of disbelief at first:

Chocolate? Coffee and cream? Butter? Pancakes? Muffins? Ice cream? *You mean I get to eat all that and the scale moves down? Where's the catch?*

We can almost hear the laughter in their messages to us, "It's working!"

Hope.

It zings out of their words.

And we laugh, and sometimes cry tears of joy, right along with them. Because we know the feeling—we remember well that first glimpse of food peace and freedom. The constant confusion about what to eat for both health and weight began to fade into the past.

Ahem . . . scuze us while we clear our throats for a second before coming clean. Okay, we admit it, not *all* our fan mail has been perfectly rosy. We were flooded with daily messages asking us to write a smaller book, one that teaches the plan in a more concise manner, one that a guy might actually want to pick up and read; and some even asked us to nix all our (awesome) sisterly chitchat.

THE NERVE!!!! Nah, we actually get it: Even (riveting) chitchat like ours can be too much at times.

We also heard from thousands of people who took our book to office supply stores and *(GASP!)* had it cut up. They separated the recipe section from the plan itself because they found the enormous book much too cumbersome to have in the kitchen—and they were serious about making our recipes.

"Give us the plan—keep it simple. Give us a cookbook—keep it separate." We heard those two requests over and over.

So here you have it, a much smaller, more concise book that teaches you the basics of the plan in a simple way. This book is a mere pipsqueak in size compared with the first Goliath of a book, as we don't want you spending your hard-earned money chopping this one up. *Trim Healthy Mama Plan: Keep It Simple, Keep It Sane* also includes lots of tips to help you get started, along with menu ideas for your unique situation. We also have new information we've been burning to share for the last year or so. For this reason we couldn't get 'er done in one hundred pages or less, but we think you'll agree you'd rather be fully informed than have a speedy read.

Is this book one a guy will want to read? Honestly? Jury's out on that one: Our own husbands never read our first book despite loving all our THM foods and we doubt they'll read this one, either. While thousands of men have lost weight and gained health the Trim Healthy way (including our own guys), we are women who write to women, that's our thang. But we did include one chapter for men. Hopefully the male species won't need to read too much more than that one small chapter to get the gist of what this is all about. And don't ask too much from us; we did our best to suppress most of our (enchanting) chitchat but we couldn't help letting a few exchanges slide.

The companion cookbook, the *Trim Healthy Mama Cookbook,* is chock-full of new recipes along with some of our most popular recipes. It includes lots of beautiful color pictures to inspire you to get cooking. The recipes are easy, fast, tasty, and family friendly, and we've also included many recipes for people who are sensitive to gluten or dairy. If your budget is tight and purchasing the cookbook is too much of a stretch, don't fret, there are hundreds of free Trim Healthy Mama recipes on Pinterest, on hundreds of blogger sites, and on our own Facebook fan page and website. Ask for the cookbook for your birthday or Christmas or reserve it at your library, but in the meantime there's no reason you can't get started without it. In fact, while new recipes are fun and tasty, you don't actually need them to do this plan. Once you understand the principles you can simply tweak your own family's favorite meals to make them Trim Healthy Mama friendly or come up with your own simple ideas.

THE PLACE CALLED DONE

While we were blown away at the response to the Trim Healthy Mama message, once that surprise wore off we began to realize—no wonder!—Mamas relate to being stuck in an awful place called "done." That place where you throw your hands up because you have had enough of the fads, enough of the seesawing of weight loss and weight gain. It is a huge relief to know there is a way out. For too long we had been stuck there ourselves.

If the Trim Healthy Mama approach is new to you, perhaps you're currently in your own state of done. You are tired of hearing all the conflicting and confusing noise about what to eat and are doing your darnedest to avoid all the diet nonsense that keeps cycling around. You're so "done," you'd rather tune it all out, thank you very much.

Hanging out in Doneville has its downsides but the alternatives are even less appealing. Like us, you've been on so many different food fads that you're gun-shy about dramatically changing your eating habits once again. You've tried the diets that leave you hungry, leave out food groups, leave out calories, leave you out of pocket, leave out the rest of the family, and worst of all, leave out practicality and basic common sense.

You're so "done" trying to do better and discouraged that it has to be so difficult that you're almost willing to live with extra pounds and health issues rather than try another weight-loss plan.

Just hearing the words *new diet* makes you do an inward grimace. Roll eyes. Been there done that—no thanks! Yet the headlines and advertisements continue to scream ridiculous promises: HOW TO LOSE TEN POUNDS IN TEN DAYS, or DROP TWENTY-FIVE POUNDS IN YOUR FIRST MONTH ON A DOCTOR-APPROVED PLAN!

THE TRIM HEALTHY MAMA GUARANTEE

Here's our promise to you: We guarantee zero pounds lost in the first month!

Yep!

Are we nuts for making this claim? What *is* nuts is the same old dietary boot camp approach that is continually pushed on us Mamas. Nuts is doing something miserable and unsustainable just so you can force a new low number on the scale by a certain date.

In your first few weeks on Trim Healthy Mama, you will probably lose a lot more than zero pounds (most people do), but if you don't lose any weight in the first month that is perfectly fine. Why allow a number to rob your joy? There is no need to throw in the towel or feel like a failure if the scale doesn't move much at first. Some people don't lose weight initially because their bodies have some healing to do after all the metabolism-destroying diets they've been on. And hey, it takes a little while to learn to live a lifestyle versus a strict diet. Others don't lose weight because weight is not the issue; they want to do this plan for blood-sugar stability and health rather than a number on the scale. Others are doing this plan to nourish a healthy pregnancy, and weight loss is not the goal during this time.

We'll be the first to admit there are lots of diets that will whip weight off you in a much speedier fashion than with the Trim Healthy Mama approach. If speed is all you are looking for, you are reading the wrong book. The first two words of this book are "Food Freedom." Keep them in mind. You can boot-camp your way to drop quick pounds; but if it is just more misery, then how is that going to work out for your future? It's not. Nuff said.

Deep down we all know diets tied to promises and guarantees like these are not sustainable. They ask things of you that are too difficult to keep up when life hits hard—and life always does. Your instincts whisper a sane caution. Why go back down those rabbit holes? You're maxed out already. How to find the time? How to make it work with the family? How to afford it? Most of us with families cannot wave a magic wand that transforms our budget to cover "organic only." Don't they get it? There is no way you can slip a full hour or two of exercise into your day, or spend precious time juicing several pounds of carrots, or give up meat or dairy or coffee or the occasional glass of wine. Might as well just stay here in Doneville, thanks. It's starting to feel real comfortable.

But the danger of being "done" is that it is stagnant. It's like a vehicle stopped on the side of the highway. That vehicle will only rust and deteriorate if it doesn't get back on the road. The previous direction may have been the wrong way, but skidding to a halt and remaining in one precarious place is not going to fix anything. Stopping has to be the initiation of a new direction, the beginning of a turnaround.

WHICH DIRECTION?

Mustering enough faith to try again, to "do better," can be scary. We get that. It is especially scary when you have your suspicions that nobody actually knows what "better" is supposed to be. There are so many conflicting "betters." Sure, fewer potato chips, drive-thru burgers, or sodas is a good start, but what do you replace those with?

Rabbit food? Meal replacement shakes? Little boxes of microwaved "mini me" diet food? Shudder!

Should you go paleo and eat like a caveman?

Should you cut out meat altogether or eat mostly meat?

Should you shun carbs or load up on them? Shun fats or load up on them?

How about just eating healthy? Sounds sensible enough. Hmm, but what does that really mean? To make sure not one GMO food ever touches your lips? To shop only at your organic food market? Sure, let's avoid genetically modified foods when we can; but is it really possible to live in that kind of bubble and stay sane? Ever heard of anyone sick with anxiety over food purity? Yup, it happened to us!

Truth be told, many people eat a whole lot better than a sodas-and-fries diet yet still have major issues with weight and health. They steer away from toxins and chemicals, not a whole lot of junk food for them. What gives? Why does consuming healthy, homemade food make some of us as overweight as when we eat fast food, and why do health problems remain?

If you cut to the chase, which diet is really the right way to eat? "Do" versus "done" can be a real dilemma. We'd spent our lives searching for the optimum diet and only harmed our health in the process following fad after fad. We were desperate and determined to find a solid footing in the churning sea of dietary confusion. But we had to sift through all the nonsense before we finally found the truths.

For instance, the low-fat diet dogma tells us to cut out fats, especially saturated fats like butter and red meat. Don't eat too many eggs, its champions warn. These foods will lead to high cholesterol, heart attacks, and weight gain. A diet based on nourishing whole grains and only lean forms of proteins is the way to health. Eat lots of fruits and vegetables, maybe throw in a little fish or chicken breast here and there—but too much red meat will kill ya!

The high-fat people? Their books and websites inform us that low-fat was for the eighties! Eat all the fat you want, including butter, red meat, and eggs. You'll only be healthier. Run away from grains, though.

The confusion only gets thicker when you take into consideration the argument from the "whole foods only" people. They urge us to keep foods as close to their original state as possible. Eat both fats and carbs and never worry about a calorie as long as your foods are pure, organic, and unadulterated. Anything unprocessed or organic is king in the whole-foods kitchen.

Wait, there's the other side of that argument: The low-calorie folk must have their say. Purity of food does not matter nearly as much as calories do. Eat whatever the heck style you want, just make sure your calories stay low (or count your points). Calories in, calories out—that's the most important foundation for weight and overall health, they insist. *Hmm . . . sure about that? How's that supposed to work during the challenging seasons of nursing and pregnancy? Low-calorie = sadly lacking milk supply and not enough nourishment for growing baby.*

What about plant-based diets? Many vegetarians and vegans don't worry about calories as much as the evils of meat. Their experts tell us to forgo meat and, if possible, all dairy to cleanse and alkalize the body.

The low-carb camp speaks up. They still blame carbs for sickness and obesity. But of course there is a backlash to that camp, too. A growing number of people who've been too low-carb for too long are gaining a strong voice in the dietary arena. Their thyroid and adrenal hormones are shot, in part from lack of healthy carbohydrates, and many are demanding answers.

Stop . . . ENOUGH!!!! How is any of this sane?

If your brain is about to explode, we were right there with you.

PATHWAY OF TRUTH

Have you ever felt like throwing a tantrum (stomping included) and yelling, "FOR ONCE AND FOR ALL . . . WHO'S RIGHT? SOMEBODY TELL ME! BECAUSE I AM SO DONE TRYING TO FIGURE THIS ALL OUT!!! I'M DONE! DONE! DONE. IN FACT, I'M SO DONE TRYING, ONLY TO FAIL, THAT I DON'T CARE ANYMORE. SOMEBODY GIVE ME A DONUT, NOW!"

Good thing most of us have never literally thrown this fit in public. If this frustration has been a silent anguish for you, though, you're not alone.

It wasn't until we both reached this place called "done"—until all our extreme diet efforts essentially became "undone"—that a new path of truth emerged. Instead of looking to the next guru, we looked to the Bible. Who could know better than our Creator? Thankfully the Bible holds sound advice, simple advice. So simple it is profound.

We were finally able to drop so many fears, hang-ups, and anxieties over what is and what isn't good for us when we searched the scriptures for answers. It is restful to lean on a plan founded in biblical truths because man-made ideas will always conflict, confuse, rise up as fads, drop down as passé, then constantly recycle.

While people of all religions and beliefs have embraced the principles of this plan—and we welcome them all—we based Trim Healthy Mama on biblical truths. God designed all the food groups for our health, so why nix any of them? (And trust us, we've nixed many of them over the years.) His ways are wiser than any new diet book, any study, or any Internet advice that doesn't line up with His word. Every diet has studies for backup. There has to be something more reliable than those. It took us decades to learn and to finally trust our Creator on this subject, but when we did— Ahhh! Peace. Nothing like that feeling!

FITTING PUZZLE PIECES

It occurred to us: What if some of these opposing diet theories contain certain necessary pieces of the puzzle even if they don't have the whole picture? Instead of choosing sides and bashing other diets, why can't we treasure the best premises each of these offers? None of these diets would be so well known if some aspect of them was not effective, at least in the short term.

Why pitch a battered tent in just one dietary camp when we can build a wonderful dream home smack dab in the middle of all these arguments instead? Yes, a dream home—a place where you actually want to live! Eating foods that you actually want to eat. Foods that make you grin!

We can glean from the truths but reject the extremes. The parts that conflict with God's word are out for us! The parts that are not doable for busy lives are out! The parts that are just plain ridiculous … get 'em outta here! Hey … just because your blood type is O doesn't mean you have to eat three and a half baby carrots at three thirty in the afternoon, lest your body get out of balance and you have to eat four and a half edamame beans at four thirty. Good grief! It shouldn't be that complicated.

Once you put all the pieces of the puzzle together, the big picture is beautiful, doable, and "oh so tasty"! Think of a tapestry. You won't see the full design by looking at only one colored spool of thread before weaving. But weave many different colored spools together and you have a colorful masterpiece.

YOU DON'T HAVE TO BE A CERTAIN TYPE!

We might be sisters but we are not twinsies when it comes to eating styles. Even though the core premise of the way we eat is the same, we don't see eye to eye on everything. Trim Healthy Mama is based on whole foods but some of us Mamas take this food purity premise further than others. Our plan embraces those who prefer to cook from scratch and shun anything less than absolute food purity. Thankfully it also throws arms wide open to Mamas who have no desire to spend lots of time in the kitchen and who couldn't care less if there is a slightly suspect, not quite perfectly natural ingredient in a couple of store-bought food items. Welcome, everyone! We don't have to be cookie cutters of one another! And yes, we can learn from one another rather than debate the issues. We's going to be who we's going to be!

Serene is much more of a "food purist" while Pearl is yet to reform her ways as a "shortcut queen." The plan works incredibly for both of us but we implement it in slightly different ways. Serene's kitchen is full of kefir grains, kombucha mushrooms, sprouting grains, and giant stockpots filled with bones releasing their nutrients. Pearl made sourdough bread once and vowed to never try it again. Big flop! She doesn't mind buying sprouted bread from the grocery store or using a convenience, packaged item or two here and there. Serene never cheats on off-plan foods. Pearl does now and then. If you ever see the word *microwave* mentioned in a recipe, that will be Pearl's suggestion; Serene will be running from the radiation and offering her purist friends alternatives—after she has given Pearl a lecture!

YOUR OWN UNIQUE JOURNEY

Don't sell yourself short by relying on someone else to do your dietary thinking for you. We are going to clearly explain the plan here in as short a fashion as is possible but this is not Trim Healthy Mama for dummies. You're not going to be denied whole food groups. You will eat carbs and fats and proteins; we'll just show you how to enjoy them in a way that allows you to stay healthy, trim, and happy. Once you understand these principles, you'll be set for a lifetime and you'll be making your own wise nutritional decisions. We could give you a week's worth of specific weight-loss meals with exact portion sizes and basically say, "Eat this; you will lose weight." Or there are the thirty- to ninety-day plans—you know the ones. We'd control your dietary life for one to three months and then leave you to your own devices after that. But that's all just more of the same and it only leads to more "done."

You need to make this plan your own if this is to be a forever solution, and that means you have to think—at first.

Trim Healthy Mama is not made up of a bunch of rules and lists. It does have some guidelines—like fueling your body by eating every three to four hours throughout the day, knowing which foods to eat together and which to eat separately—but it cannot be fully understood if it's stripped down to just numbers and a Top Ten of "Foods You Must Avoid." There is not "only one way" to make it work. We want you to understand the spirit of freedom behind it and the "whys." Then it will click and you'll find your own groove.

As a unique person, you require different amounts of food than the person to your left or right. You have different tastes, health issues, family challenges, schedules, abilities in the kitchen; and you burn fat at different rates than others do. A lifetime approach to trim and healthy requires an understanding that our bodies will all react differently and the word *healthy* in this plan is every bit as important as the word *trim*. We're going to take a pass on those conventional diet book formulas and lead you through the particulars, the struggles, and all the baby-stepping questions.

If you are a nursing or pregnant Mama, yes, you can absolutely eat the Trim Healthy way but your needs will be different from those of a woman beyond that stage of life. Throw another gender into a set program and that muddles things even further. Asking a six-foot-two man to eat the same amounts as a five-foot-two woman doesn't even make sense.

Maybe you have hormone issues—polycystic ovary syndrome (PCOS), thyroid issues, or hormone decline due to menopause.

Are you gluten-free or do you have multiple food allergies?

Perhaps you are feeding a large family and your budget is extremely tight.

Or maybe you are a businessman or businesswoman and cannot avoid eating out frequently.

How could a week's worth of rigid meals and measured portions meet all of these variant needs? Short answer: They can't. Diets that force-feed you that sort of rigidity are only more fraudulent dead ends, and we refuse to be part of them.

READY?

Let's do this! Don't be afraid of failing. We have adopted the seal's policy of "no Mama left behind." (But if you're the rare man who reads this book, "no man left behind" fits, too.) If you stink at diets—well, that is excellent. Most people doing this along with you stink at diets, too. Many of us also stink at exercising; that's okay. You may not have the energy for exercise when you first start. But slowly . . . as your health and energy levels improve . . . you'll want to do some sort of exercise to let off that energy steam. And then we'll tell you to chill out and stop exercising so much! Overexercising is not allowed. Settle down, girl!

Please just relax and read this book through before you begin tossing junk food out of your cupboard! Don't go buying a whole bunch of special ingredients you're not quite ready for. You can do this plan with everyday, inexpensive food from your grocery store and then, as you learn about other helpful ingredients, you can choose to incorporate them slowly—or not at all. Special ingredients are fun but they are not "must haves." Take this one chapter at a time, giving yourself time to digest the information. Release that tension rising inside you that's concerned with all the changes you are going to have to make and how overwhelmed that is going to make you feel. Nope, that's your meanie voice. We're going to train you not to listen to that voice. Tune in to the kind and gentle voice—the one that says you don't have to get this down perfectly on your first day. You are going to make mistakes. No biggie. You've got a lifetime to get this right.

This lifestyle is forgiving. You'll get up when you mess up, dust yourself off, and jump right back into the journey. Guilt, shame, and self-loathing are not on plan! Here's another important THM mantra: "You are always only three hours away from your next slimming meal."

All you need to start your journey is an open mind and a willingness to shed bad habits. But this is very attainable when you replace those old bad habits with new ones that are fun and easy. Your new food choices will have nothing in common with doldrums and deprivation. You'll learn to build up your body and your immune system in the yummiest of ways with ample protein at every meal. You will eat fats in luscious quantities; you will also eat carbs. Meat, dairy, veggies, beans, gentle grains, fruit, and oh so many treats are all on plan. If you have allergies or sensitivities to any of the foods, that is not a deal breaker. You'll still be able to enjoy plenty of yummy, health-giving foods doing the plan your own way.

So get yourself a cup of joe, find a spot to read (even if you have to lock yourself in the bathroom to get some peace), and let's begin!

PART ONE

the
basics

chapter 1
GETTING TO KNOW YOU

Trim Healthy Mama is designed for sanity—a truly family-friendly, doable LIFE-TIME plan. This part of your life that has always felt beyond your control can now be manageable. You sit in the driver's seat. You can use the Trim Healthy Mama principles to lose, gain, or sustain weight while optimizing your health.

Whether you are running after multiple children or postmenopausal, nursing or pregnant, or even a single, young woman, welcome to the THM sisterhood, where the word *Mama* applies to women of all ages and stages. The powerful knowledge you'll gain provides you with the ability to drive this THM vehicle yet be able to change gears for the different stages of your life. The core of the plan is simple, no rocket science involved. Yes, there is a learning curve, but once you start practicing the principles it'll become second nature after a while.

The Trim Healthy Mama plan is deeply nourishing. Even the most demanding times of a woman's life, such as pregnancy, can be supported nutritionally without the worry of unneeded pounds. The plan can also meet the needs of other times in life when hormone imbalances or metabolic challenges can seem like fog in your headlights. You will learn to tweak the core plan to make it work for your specific season or situation.

We know. You want to jump into the nitty-gritty of the plan right now. That's coming—we promise. Right next door in Chapter 2, "The Basics" (page 16). Hey... stop! Caught ya jumping ahead to try to find the menus! Oh, and this book starts at the introduction—skipped it? Tut Tut. We'll wait while you go get that read.

First, we're going to have some fun in this chapter by getting to know you a little so we can all find some common ground despite our wonderful differences. We're also going to give you a couple of Serene-and-Pearl-style biology lessons. Gotta learn the "whys," remember? Hang in here with us chapter by chapter so you can gain the knowledge you need to make this a lifelong, sustainable approach.

COME IN . . . GRAB A SEAT!

Welcome to a little get-to-know-you therapy session at an IDA meeting—short for Imbalanced Diets Anonymous. (No, there is no such thing, but maybe there should be.) The meeting opens and new members are asked to share a little about themselves. You might find you have some things in common with one or two of these IDA members.

Whole Grain Jane (and Brown Bread Fred)

Jane stands up and clears her throat. "Hi, I'm Whole Grain Jane." She pats the hand of the man sitting next to her. "And this is my husband, Brown Bread Fred." (Fred doesn't look thrilled to be here.) "We have five children whom we homeschool. I'm doing my best trying to raise a healthy family. I grind my own flour, bake my own bread and muffins made from whole-grain spelt flour. My girls and I make those a lot but we use applesauce in place of oil because we are trying to cut down on fats. We've been trying meatless Mondays at home, using lots of rice and beans to get enough protein."

Jane glances down at her husband. "Which is not going over too well with Fred and our teenage son. Oh—and I love my homemade granola. I sweeten it with honey, of course; we stopped using white sugar several years ago." Jane's face turns downcast. "I'm doing all my doctor has advised me to do diet-wise, yet I—oh, I'll just say it—I can't zip up my size twelve capris anymore." Jane looks at her husband and whispers, "Do you want to share?"

He obviously does not.

Jane continues. "Our doctor advised Fred to lay off whole eggs and cut out red meat a few years back as his cholesterol is too high. He is now on medication for that. Dr. Fatfear also advised him to drop thirty pounds, but he is finding that challenging, right, Fred?"

Fred nods, looks wistfully at the exit sign. "I fix Fred whole-grain cereal with skim milk most mornings, or whole-wheat toast with peanut butter . . . but so far nothing has really helped. Could be that Fred enjoys my oatmeal raisin cookies a little too often—but they're made with honey, of course. Not sure what is going on with us, must be aging." Jane takes her seat to a round of smattered applause and a look of relief from Fred.

There are some "Hi, Janes" from the circle of IDA members as the next new member gets ready to share.

Drive Thru Sue (and Fast Food Dude)

Sue's turn. She shyly asks if she can just share while sitting down, she's not comfortable with public speaking. The circle erupts in encouragement: "Just as you are, Sue!"

"You can do it, Sue!"

"That's why we're here, Sue. Bare your heart. Take your time!"

"I'm Sue. I'm twenty-nine; the big three-o is right around the corner. Married, two children, first just started second grade, the other is in preschool. My husband is not here today. He has never had to worry about his weight a day in his life and he eats circles around me."

"Not fair!" someone yells in good-natured support.

Sue takes a deep breath. "But I brought my brother with me—Fast Food Dude. We both have some issues, as you can see." She chuckles and holds up her Big Gulp full of pop. Dude does the same with a shy smile but lets his sister continue. "And it's not just the two of us; there are a lot of weight and health issues in our family tree."

Sue pauses to find the right words. "I'm completely confused by which diet I should do but I've been ignoring the red flags too long and it's past time. I used to skip meals in high school and college, and that worked back then, but as you can see"—Sue reddens uncomfortably—"it's not working now. I haven't even climbed on the scale this year because . . . well, it's far too depressing. I joined Pound Trackers some years ago, lost some but gained it all back. Counting points all day is not my thing, that I do know. I was miserable."

Sue chokes a little on her words and glances at her brother. "Our father passed away from complications from Type 2 diabetes three years ago. He was in his early sixties. My doctor recently told me that I could end up like him if I don't lose this weight. It's affecting every part of my life but my doctor's most concerned about my blood sugar. I have to take pills to help control my blood-sugar numbers and I'm not even thirty yet." Sue takes a long pause, trying to gain composure, and wipes her eyes.

"We're all here for you, Sue," someone from the circle encourages.

Sue finds her voice. "I look at my children and my heart squeezes. I want to be there for them. No, I want more than that. I want the energy to be able to toss them the ball, push them on a swing, or chase them at the park without being winded."

Sue pauses, then continues with more strength. "Somehow, I want to stop this weight from climbing but more important, I want to be healthy. I don't want my children to go through the heartache of losing a parent too early like I did."

Sue wipes her eyes, chuckles a little. "I'm not much of a cook. Guess I'm an expert at ordering pizza or making mac and cheese from a box. But I want more for my kids. I want to get healthy for me and pass it along to them so this family cycle can finally be broken. I dragged my brother here with me because we need to support each other in this."

Sue gets a long hug from the woman sitting next to her, who then gets up to introduce herself.

Farm Fresh Tess (and Organic Only Tony)

Tess lets go of Sue with a final pat on her arm, wipes her eyes with a tissue, and introduces herself and her husband, Organic Only Tony. She shares that they are living their dream on thirty acres. They raise grass-fed cows and goats for meat and milk, gather eggs from their free-range hens, and grow a big, four-season garden. Tess doesn't trust most grocery stores because she can't see what goes into the food.

Tess is in her forties. She has a lot of bubbling energy and begins to chuckle a little as she takes out some notes that she has prepared. "Have to remind myself on what to say or I'll forget. Let's see, I choose not to dwell on my weight because I'm strong and enjoy working hard on our farm. I've never been a Skinny Minny, though. I guess if I had to say a number it would be forty pounds more than my wedding day, and I was no waif then." She smiles affectionately at Tony. "But he tells me I'm beautiful."

Tony takes the cue to stand up, putting an arm around his wife. "As pretty as the day I met her. I love my wife's cooking. She makes the best peach cobbler on the face of God's green earth with peaches we have grown from seedlings." He pats his paunch. "But as you can see, I guess her cooking doesn't like me."

Tony continues. "Middle age is tough—doc says I have a bad case of high blood pressure and along with meds for that he's making me wear a sleep apnea mask. My snoring was getting so loud Tess was unable to sleep—"

Tess interrupts. "If anyone has any snoring remedies, let me know and we'll swap e-mails. He might not be snoring now but I'm not comfortable sleeping next to him wearing that thing and I'm not accepting that he'll have to be on blood pressure medication for the rest of his life, either. Doc also says Tony has to go off salt, whole eggs, red meat, and our fresh cream and butter. He hates the bland food he has to eat now and I want my happy husband back." She folds her notes and speaks from her heart. "Tony is even considering selling the farm now. What's the point of it all if we can't enjoy the food from our own farm?" Tess shrugs, then takes her seat.

Raw Green Colleen (and Carrot Juice Bruce)

Colleen takes one last sip from a jar of green juice before she stands up.

"Hi, I'm Colleen and this is my eldest son, Carrot Juice Bruce. We are so excited to announce that Bruce and I have just finished a fourteen-day juice cleanse together. I did not force him into it. Bruce might only be nineteen, but he wants to devote his life to health and wellness. He does all the juicing for the family. We go through fifty pounds of carrots a week. As part of this juice cleanse, we ate only one-hundred-percent-raw plant food," she shares proudly.

Colleen continues. "A really exciting thing right now is that while Bruce was interning at the Raw Alive Institute over the summer, he met a colonic irrigationist who lives in our area. I had several colonics recently, so I'm feeling very cleaned out right now, which is wonderful. The irrigationist mentioned I passed several parasites." She glances at her son. "What was it she called them? Oh yes, roundworms or some such thing."

Colleen hesitates for a minute when Brown Bread Fred makes a nervous throat-clearing sound. "Sorry if that was too much information for some of you, but in this kind of setting I feel very open."

Brown Bread Fred chances another longing look at the exit.

Colleen continues. "I know people think of me as that crazy health-nut lady, but five years ago my mother was diagnosed with breast cancer, and the year after that, her sister, my aunt Dee. It was a long struggle for both of them. My mom is still here and cancer-free—knock on wood—but my aunt is not."

Farm Fresh Tess pulls out her tissues again and sniffs quietly while Colleen speaks. "I don't want to be another statistic for disease. I don't want to go through what my aunt and mother did. I don't want my children to eat the toxins and dead garbage that make up the standard diet most people live on—the very one we used to eat until my mom got sick and I started researching. Maybe my approach to food is extreme, maybe it takes hours out of my day, and maybe my husband misses the meat I used to cook him; but I don't know what else to do. Look around us—disease and obesity—it's everywhere."

Colleen sips on her green juice again because her mouth has gone dry.

"Now that this juice fast has ended, I'm more determined than ever to keep most of our food in a raw state and keep meat out of the house. When I first went vegan three years ago I dropped those twenty pounds that I didn't need and felt great. Lately I've been dragging, though. I also feel bloated a lot even though my weight is okay. Not really sure why. I think a liver cleanse is next. The colonic irrigationist mentioned that I should come in every week. This is all getting rather expensive but I just know it is worth it. It has to be.

"My protein came back low on a recent blood test so I am adding more sprouted, dehydrated seeds and nuts to my diet and trying to combat the reactive hypoglycemia I was recently diagnosed with by adding more snacks of grapes and bananas. My naturopath has me on several supplements to help me control this issue plus a bunch of other ones for other reasons." She chuckles nervously. "Feels like I'm swallowing fifty pills a day sometimes. Let me tell you, some of the supplements I'm on, I have them all on a spreadsheet here." She fumbles in her purse and lets out a joyous squeal. "Oh goodie, I have my recent blood work numbers here, too. I'll pass them around and you can all take a look . . ."

Brown Bread Fred has gone past polite visible discomfort to obvious vexation. He quickly hands off Colleen's papers to the next person without even a courteous glance. He whispers to his wife, "She better not find her roundworm in that purse. I'm not touching it."

Whole Grain Jane shushes him.

Scared of Carbs Barb (and Back to Cave Dave)

Barb realizes she needs to make her move now to keep the meeting progressing. To everyone's relief she stands up. "Thanks, Colleen. Guess it is my turn." Colleen sits down.

"I'll come right to the point. Low carb works for me. I should say, when I do it, it works. No bread, no fruit, no rice. I eat bacon and eggs every morning and I drop thirty pounds. It's great at the beginning; I mean, who doesn't love bacon, right? After a couple weeks, though, I don't want to look at bacon anymore. I get sick of eggs, meat, and protein bars and I just want to sink my teeth into a juicy apple. But what do I do? I don't eat that apple.

I drive home from work and Dairy Queen's caramel-topped chocolate shake gets the best of me."

She chuckles. "Actually, my husband, who is not here today, is always happier when I give in because I get cranky without carbs and he doesn't mind me pleasantly plump as long as I'm pleasant. But seriously, carbs terrify me! I only have to look at them and I gain back those thirty pounds within a couple months, and they bring some friends with them. My cousin here, Back to Cave Dave, has been like a coach to me over the years—although I'm sure I frustrate him a lot, because he never carb-binges. I'm serious, he could live on beef jerky alone and be deliriously happy!"

Dave stands up, a tall, wiry man who looks like a cross between a college professor and a gym rat. He clears his throat and pauses to find the right words. "The early primate intestinal system was suitable for berries and foraging, perhaps some insects. Grains, however, were not a part of paleo man's diet. I'm very concerned with the inclusion of—"

Barb nudges him. "Okay, one of Dave's hot topics. I know you could do a whole weekend seminar on paleo history, but we should let the next members have their turn." She chuckles nervously, pulls him back down to his seat, and takes her own.

Adrenal Splat Pat (and Thyroid Mess Jess)

Pat and Jess stand up together, both in their mid-forties. They share that they are friends who met online at an adrenal support forum.

Pat sighs and begins speaking first. "Where do I start? Well, I wish I could start, but my body is in stop mode. I've stopped losing weight, stopped being able to exercise—that's due to the fibromyalgia—and I've been diagnosed with sensitivities to twenty different foods. You tell me what is left to eat when you can't have gluten, dairy, eggs, soy, nuts, strawberries, nightshade vegetables, and the list goes on. I can have white rice and boiled meat, not much else."

Thyroid Mess Jess fills the silence left over from Pat's abrupt finish. "Guess it's my turn. I'm Jess, and I'm on a healing journey, not a weight-loss one. In fact, I've gained about twenty pounds on the new protocol I'm on. Even though this pushed me out of a healthy BMI, this is for the best. I need to raise my thyroid hormone levels and dieting is not going to do that. The fun part about what I'm doing right now is that I can eat chocolate ice cream most nights before bed and not have to feel guilty. My body needs sugar to soothe my agitated hormones. I really need to give my adrenals a rest. I spent too many years starving myself and denying, denying, denying. So yes, I'm gaining weight. Yes, my blood pressure and fasting blood sugar have gone back up to borderline high but my morning basal temperatures are so much better. I'm going to focus on resting my thyroid and adrenals, then figure out how to get this weight off again without destroying my health in the process. Guess I am a bit stumped on how to do that but I'll cross that bridge when I come to it."

Jess and Pat both sit down. Everyone at the IDA meeting is encouraged to get into smaller circle groups and share more deeply about themselves and their struggles. Whole Grain Jane, who has always wanted to try a juice fast, invites Raw Green Colleen to sit next to her in their group. Brown Bread Fred disappears into the men's room, intending to take his time.

COMMON GROUND

If you saw yourself in any of these characters or have had another frustrating journey of weight gain and loss, of health ups and downs, welcome to the club. Between the two of us we had most of them covered in our own bumpy diet journeys. We couldn't help poking a little fun at meetings like this and at ourselves, too, for all the different diet tangents we've been on. But if you relate to anyone at that meeting, you know it's not all a laughing manner. Hopelessness hurts. Damaged health and weight issues hurt.

As different as they are, most of these diets we've tried over the years have one thing in common: They have all vilified a certain food group or macronutrient and urged the removal of it. In order to lose weight, people usually try to give up fats or carbs or animal foods or healthy amounts of calories. Choose your misery. These extreme diets are nearly impossible to maintain.

After all, what happens when a whole food group is removed? Imbalances start. In the case of Whole Grain Jane and her hubby, Brown Bread Fred, fats are feared, so they are avoided. What takes over? Whole-grain pasta, whole-grain rice, whole-grain crackers, whole-grain bars—these become foundational foods. Lots of fresh and dried fruit as well. Even though our friends here try to steer clear of processed forms of sugar and rarely snack on candy bars, sugar is the biggest part of their diet. It's the biggest part of almost everyone's diet. And it's a problem.

We can hear the gasps of disbelief. "What do you mean? They don't even eat sugar—she said they use honey."

Your bloodstream does not care whether sugar comes from hefty servings of brown-rice pasta, honey-sweetened homemade granola, or a Snickers candy bar—the end result is sugar in the blood, known as glucose.

At first glance, Drive Thru Sue might be the most obvious member here with high sugar issues; but Farm Fresh Tess and her husband, Organic Only Tony, are not exempt despite their food purity and organic approach. Baked potato = sugar. Homemade, honey-sweetened apple pie = sugar; whole-grain mac and cheese = sugar.

While whole-grain forms of starches spike your blood sugar less than white refined forms do, it is the abundance of them in both Whole Grain Jane's and Farm Fresh Tess's diets that causes health and weight issues. Even though they have very little fat in their diet, Jane and Fred are struggling with their weight because of this deceptive problem. Any time there is excess sugar in the bloodstream it is deposited in your fat cells. It suddenly turns into fat.

Blood sugar itself (otherwise known as glucose) is not a baddie. Your brain and body require this stuff to thrive. But too much blood sugar? That is the problem that has reached epidemic proportions and is destroying the health of countless millions. But there's no need to throw up our hands in despair and give up. High blood sugar is reversible: You can start turning this problem around in your very next meal.

FAT IN SUGAR CLOTHING

We're going to stress this once again just so you get it well and good: ANY BLOOD SUGAR THAT YOUR BODY CANNOT USE WILL TURN TO FAT!

Once a fat cell receives blood sugar, a transformation takes place. Abracadabra: Sugar is not sugar anymore—it is now fat. It doesn't matter if the package the food came in said "Fat-Free" or not. Your body made that a lie.

Time for a little biology lesson to show how this happens: Think of your fat cells as wild party animals and your muscle cells as sensible librarian types. Your muscle cells use blood sugar for energy, but once they are full they very tidily close up shop and accept no more. Your fat cells, on the other hand, will party 24-7. They never turn away glucose, even if they are already stuffed with a boatload of it. They'll be like, "More blood sugar? Yeah baby, bring it on! Blood sugar in the hayouse! Partaaay!!!"

Your hormone insulin comes into play in this magic transformation of sugar to fat. Many of us are taught to think of insulin as a big bad hormone whose only intention is to fatten us up. While it does promote fat gain if levels of it are constantly too high in the body, God created this very necessary hormone to transport glucose, proteins, and fat out of your bloodstream and into your cells.

We like to think of insulin as a friendly neighborhood delivery truck. It loads up blood sugar and takes it out of your bloodstream. The first place it goes is to your muscle cells: "Beep beep—got a glucose load here for you—open up!" If you are a young person with a healthy metabolism, your cells are friendly to insulin. They'll open wide and accept glucose and then burn it up for fuel . . . wonderful. No need for the body to store any fat in that scenario.

Problems arise due to our modern diet. Very few of us can burn through all the blood sugar our modern diet consists of with carbs being such a ridiculously high part of it. Also, as we age the problem gets worse. We become more insulin resistant—ever heard that phrase? It is thrown around a lot. Insulin resistance is a rampant condition, especially if we have lived life on a high-carb/sugar diet. It just means your cells are not on friendly terms with insulin.

A case of insulin resistance goes down something like this: Insulin says, "Open up to receive blood sugar." Your cells respond by completely ignoring the request; or if they do open up to receive the load, they do it halfheartedly and accept only about half of the blood-sugar load.

On your cells' behalf, it is not really that they want to be rude; they are usually just simply too stuffed with glucose from their previous meal or snack. They truly can't fit any more in. They never get the chance to empty out and feel that natural desire for more glucose. They are sick of insulin constantly arriving at their doorstep with loads of blood sugar. "Gimme a break!" they moan.

So insulin is like, "Be like that, then; I know some folks who'll be happy to take this load and the next after this." Where does insulin go with the rest of the blood sugar? Yep, you guessed it: to your fat cells at Hip Party Central, who are only too happy to accept it. Doesn't matter if that load of blood sugar came from a so-called healthy meal of a honey and peanut butter sandwich on wheat with whole-wheat pretzels on the side and a fruit-sweetened, low-fat yogurt for dessert, or whether it came from Pepsi and a Snickers bar.

The end result is often far too similar. Your fat cells will party on and grow ever larger by accepting more and more loads of glucose while your muscle cells will retire to bed early and grow ever more insulin resistant.

DON'T THROW OUT THE CARBS WITH THE BATH WATER!

The knee-jerk response to all this is to avoid carbs like the plague. But just because many have now figured out that overdoing carbs (even so-called healthy "whole-grain carbs") is detrimental, we should not toss them out altogether and go from one extreme to another. Thyroid Mess Jess's story shows us that that approach only ends with more problems.

God didn't create carbohydrates without important purpose. The Bible depicts God's blessing on all food groups in Deuteronomy 32, where it describes God taking care of His people. He mentions the food He gave them and we can see in this beautiful passage how God depicts Himself as a caring parent, careful to leave nothing out of their diet. The passage, starting at verse 13, mentions how He gave the children of Israel "the increase of the field" (grains and greens), "honey from the rock" (glucose), "oil from the flinty rock" (fats/oils), "the fat of the ram" (meat and animal fats), "butter of kine" (butter from cows), "the milk of the sheep" (sheep's dairy products), and "the pure blood of the grape" (fruit). Grains and fruits are clearly in that verse—carbs are gifts to us! They just need to be used wisely.

So how about we stop denying ourselves important food groups in the effort to find our trim and healthiest selves. We've all had about enough, haven't we? Imbalanced diets don't work. We all know that. But not only do they not work, they also do harm. They mess with your metabolism and cause a sense of failure when you inevitably give them up when life gets in the way despite your best intentions. How about we find a sane balance again together and start fueling rather than restricting. We can fuel our bodies all the way to trim.

Join the many who are now living in this Food Freedom. Excess weight is being shed; blood-sugar numbers are coming down, blood pressure is stabilizing, inflammation is decreasing—and it is all really quite simple once you give yourself some time to apply it.

BASIC INSTINCTS

Once you understand this term *Food Freedom* you will understand the Trim Healthy Mama Plan. Food Freedom simply means you won't have to miss out—you'll celebrate foods rather than deny yourself. You won't miss out on decadent fats, but you won't miss your healthy carbs, either. In fact you must eat both of those important food fuels. You'll just do it smartly—you'll get your savvy on by learning when and how to eat fats and carbs and to make sure they are always anchored by protein. It's not complicated, it just takes a little practice.

Why do we crave fats or carbs when we're denied them? Easy: Our Creator, in His infinite design, knows we need them to thrive. Is our loving heavenly Father so cruel that He would give us these cravings from birth but then punish us for eating them with health consequences? We don't believe that for a minute.

Going without either carbs or fats always puts the body into a state of imbalance and depletion. Our bodies scream "Gimme Gimme" for good reason. The desire for these fuels is so innate that we usually end up giving up on efforts to rigidly avoid them. Sadly, that often means diving deep into the wrong types of carbs or fat.

"I'll have the double cheeseburger, medium—no, make that large fries, and add in the chocolate shake."

Sound familiar?

Maybe a damaging drive-thru run is not your thing. Some of our purist-minded Mamas have different vices. Coming off a three-day detox cleanse they may think, "Mmm, I gotta have me some homemade, honey-sweetened banana cake, made with organic, gluten-free flour, and of course pastured whipped cream on top, following my grass-fed steak and garden-grown baked potato."

While this meal might sound awfully clean and healthy to the whole-foodsy, purist mind, it causes the rise of OUTTA CONTROL blood sugar due to the combination of grains (even gluten-free grains), honey, banana, and other starches in the meal. Sure, they're all natural sources of carbs, none of them processed or containing any toxins; but added together they are a train wreck when it comes to your blood sugar. And don't forget the fats in that generous dollop of pastured cream and in the steak. Loading fats on top of carbs is simply too much fuel for most of us adults to handle. The ingredients alone in this meal might be pure and natural but there is nothing very natural about high blood sugar and an exploding waistline.

You see, finding your trim doesn't happen by eating only more healthy food and less junk food. Even healthy food can make you gain weight. Many women come to Trim Healthy Mama from food purist backgrounds, just like Farm Fresh Tess. They don't understand why their bodies hold on to pounds despite eating all organic foods and spending hours in the kitchen cooking from scratch. Once they learn to use the THM power tools of knowledge, though, it clicks! Both mind and body get it and they can still be as "from scratchy" as they want. A little bit of knowledge on how their blood sugar reacts to different foods makes all the difference.

BALANCE: YOUR NEW SANE APPROACH

As a Trim Healthy Mama you'll balance your blood sugar with protein, fats, veggies, and slow-burning carbs instead of gigantic mounds of fast carbs that are dangerous to your insulin levels.

You'll balance your food fuels by juggling fats and healthy carbs throughout your week, never getting into a fuel rut.

You'll balance your rest times with wise, safe exercise sessions that you only do when you feel ready; and they will not be so long or brutal that they'll mess up the balance of your hormones.

You'll naturally balance your calories, no counting needed, by enjoying both rich, indulgent foods and refreshing lighter fare.

You'll balance weight-loss goals and the desire for restored health with the enjoyable journey of the here and now with all its imperfections.

You'll balance determination to stay on plan with an ease of spirit that shoves away all shame when you mess up.

There is even a handshake, common-turf, respectful balance between the vastly different approaches of Drive Thru Sue and her purist friends like Farm Fresh Tess.

So let's get to it.

chapter 2

THE BASICS

"JUST TELL ME HOW THIS THING WORKS!"

That's the number-one question we hear! So, in a nutshell, here's the gist of it:

On Trim Healthy Mama you won't focus on restricting food groups or calories. You will focus on fueling your body every three to four hours.

We'll go into more details later but basically here's how fueling works:

- If you have weight to lose, you'll focus on one primary fuel at a time in your meals.
- If you don't have weight to lose and want to maintain weight (in a healthy, blood-sugar-friendly way), you'll combine fuels in what we call Tandem Fueling.

The food choices will be endless. Unless you have an allergy, all food groups are in. Meats? Yep. Fruit? Sure. Gentle grains, veggies, legumes, nuts and seeds, eggs, and butter and oils? Yes, all are on board—and let's not forget the very important "food group" of chocolate. Big Yes Indeedy to that one!

We can hear some of you asking, "Can I do the plan as a vegetarian?" Or "What if I am allergic to eggs, to grains, to coconuts?" Don't fret over these things. You'll learn the basic principles of the plan and can then make it your own. None of us does the plan exactly the same way and if we did, it would just be another boring diet. No matter your challenges, you can customize Trim Healthy Mama to fit your needs, your preferences, your challenges, and your unique family. This won't stick unless you learn to make it your own.

KNOW YOUR PRIMARY FUELS

There are two primary fuel sources that your body uses:

1. Glucose (blood sugar derived from carbohydrates)
2. Fats

Your body needs both of these primary fuels to keep chugging along. But let's make it even easier and call this dynamic duo CARBS and FATS. (It is crucial that protein be included in every meal but it is not a primary fuel for the body.) Something incredible happens when you focus on these two fuels individually rather than combined: Natural weight loss happens. Woo-hoo! For some it starts slowly; for others it whooshes off quickly and then zigzags in a gentler downward fashion; and for certain others it happens only at a turtle's pace.

The goal is better health by eating yummy, indulgent food for life. Weight loss is merely icing on the cake. Please don't get fixated on the scale, or compare your journey with anyone else's. Your trim will happen when your body considers itself ready. Allowing your body the time it needs to heal rather than obsessively cajoling it toward a certain number on the scale will help you keep your joy, your sanity, and your vitality.

Pregnant and nursing women can do a combination of both separating and combining fuels to ensure adequate weight gain for pregnancy and a great milk supply for nursing. (Read Chapter 23, "Heads Up: Pregnant and Nursing Mamas!," on page 199, for more info about how to do the plan while pregnant or nursing.)

Children can also be taught from early ages to fuel their bodies wisely and not spike their blood sugar. Children have higher metabolic needs so most of their meals will have to be tandem-fueled, where fats and carbs are combined, unless they have a severe weight problem. Including both of these fuels in most meals supplies what their rapid growth demands. Children usually have less insulin resistance so they can handle more frequent carb and fat combos on their plates than most of us adults can. This does not mean children get a free pass to eat carbs all day. It is best to ditch processed and empty carbs and starches in your children's diets—but obviously we're not shooting for perfection here. Kids can still enjoy pizza and ice cream at birthday parties. Obesity, however, is a growing problem even among children. Those with weight issues can enjoy some single-fueled meals along with tandem fueling and find healthier weights.

START FUELING!

This premise of fueling rather than restricting works because you constantly need fuel to survive. Your body will be a continual consumer of fuel as long as it is alive. If you diet restrictively and barely give yourself enough fuel for basic function (lowering calories or pulling out food groups), your body will end up opposing your efforts with adamant defiance. That results in a messed-up metabolism, imprisoned fat stores, and hormones underfed into imbalance and depletion.

Not enough fuel leads to a dead end, but so does stuffing fuel into your mouth any ol' how, any ol' time. Just because we can doesn't mean we should. If you focus on one primary fuel at a time, rather than squishing both together at every meal, you will burn through the fuel provided. After that your body must look around for something else to burn. It is given no choice but to switch directly to the task of burning your own adipose tissue. In other words your body chows down on its own body fat.

"Mmm … that scrumptious muffin top hanging over my jeans looks appetizing. I'll chomp on that for a while, then those jigglies on my thighs will hit the spot. Later on tonight my double chin will come in handy when I need more fuel!"

Sounds silly, but it is a reasonably accurate picture of what happens. You've got to burn something and with this new knowledge you can guide your body to burn its own body fat. You'll trim down because your body is finally using its padding as energy without you starving!

This idea of using fuels individually rather than combined is nothing weird or mysterious. Your body does it naturally on its own. The Trim Healthy Mama Plan just helps that natural process along a bit. Your body does not burn both fats and carbs at the same time. When you eat a meal, you must always burn the carbs in that meal first. This is so you can stay alive! Your body cannot handle a state of high blood sugar. The fat in your meal goes into storage to wait its turn to be used as fuel until blood sugar is cleared to safe zones. Remember in Chapter 1, "Getting to Know You" (page 3), how we described insulin as your friendly neighborhood delivery truck? After a meal, insulin is released to clear the blood sugar from your bloodstream and feed it to your muscle cells. Only once it has completed that task will your body get on to burning any fat from your meal.

Sadly, actual fat burning does not happen very frequently these days. The standard high-carb meals of our modern diet make burning through all that blood sugar an almost impossible task. Fat moves in for good rather than being the temporary tenant it was supposed to be.

Picture the fat from your meal, bags still packed, eagerly awaiting the journey out of its temporary storehouse—hoping to be able to shine as the fuel it was designed to be. But time passes, and your body is so busy spending all its efforts getting rid of excess blood sugar that the fat is forgotten. It unpacks its bags, turns on the TV. Resigned, it sets up house and orders drapes for the windows. You can almost hear it sigh in a dreary Eeyore voice, "Here to stay." Jeans get that slightest bit tighter.

Let's give this tragic story a much happier ending! Fat can and should be a superstar fuel for your body. You just need to give it a chance. And you're about to with THM.

SATISFYING AND ENERGIZING FUELS

The two all-important parent meals on plan are known as Satisfying (S) and Energizing (E). They utilize those primary fuels of both fats and carbs and allow each of them to shine as fuel stars for your body. We Trim Healthy Mamas love to shorten everything to acronyms. While at first this might seem like a new language, you'll quickly get the hang of it.

- S stands for "Satisfying" and focuses on the fuel of luscious, delightful fats—yes, even butter and steak!
- E stands for "Energizing" and focuses on the fuel of glucose through the safe amount of healthy carbs like gentle grains (unless you have sensitivity to them), fruits, beans, and sweet potatoes.

Both of these meal types are centered solidly around protein.

Baby Step 1: Memorize these two main meal types (S and E) and understand that S meals focus on fats while E meals focus on carbs.

Picture S and E meals as your primary caregivers: They are Mommy and Daddy, providing you with all the nutrients you need. As different as they are, both are weight-loss meals (for the majority of people who do not have extremely broken metabolism issues). These parent meals will always take care of you and even once you've reached goal weight they will still be enjoyed often to allow you to keep your trim for life.

You'll soon learn the details and the differences between S and E meals and how and when to implement them. The most important thing to know about them for now is that both are necessary. You don't eat only one or the other. The way you incorporate these meals into your life will be unique. You don't have to switch automatically from S to E, then S to E—boring! You'll find your own groove and soon (but don't skip there yet) we'll give you lots of examples on how to change up between them. You'll enjoy a wonderful variety of foods each and every week.

PROTEIN TAKES PRIORITY!

Both S and E meals are centered solidly around balanced sources of protein. E meals always contain lean protein sources. S meals can contain either lean or fatty protein sources (if an S meal contains a lean protein source like chicken breast, it will need to contain fat in some other form like butter, oils, or high-fat dairy). Protein repairs your body, steadies your blood sugar, and, blessedly, helps fill you up. Without sufficient protein, our bodies start to age at a faster rate. Our muscles, organs, bones, cartilage, skin, and the antibodies that guard against disease are all made of protein. Without enough protein, none of these can repair themselves and they decline into cellular breakdown.

If you need to lose weight, protein is the samurai sword in your weaponry against obesity. Eating protein, especially animal protein, can boost the metabolism by 25 percent. A 2011 study cited in the *Journal of Nutrition* reveals the body expends twenty-five times more energy digesting protein than it does digesting carbs, or even fat. According to this study, women on a protein-rich plan lose up to 21 percent more weight and 21 percent more belly fat than women on higher-carb plans.

Protein is crucial on the THM Plan because it causes your body to release a hormone called glucagon. This hormone has a balancing effect on insulin. Insulin is a hormone that can cause your body to go into fat-storing mode, while glucagon causes your body to go into fat-burning mode. It literally helps release fat from your cells. The perfect hormonal balance is achieved when protein anchors the meal.

Even with protein we must stress balance. We just told you that animal protein is wonderful. Is there a catch? No catch; but when many of us think of protein we immediately visualize chicken breasts, steak strips, cottage cheese, canned tuna, and egg whites. Those foods are a blessing and are absolutely on plan, but if they are your only protein sources you're still missing out.

There are some other protein-rich food sources you desperately need and you're probably missing. The amino acids they contain are the most effective at causing your body to release glucagon, which, as we mentioned, is the way your cells let go of fat. These foods have fallen out of vogue, and by shunning them we've shot ourselves in the foot. With obesity a murdering epidemic, we need to bring them back.

What are these snubbed protein sources? Chicken on the bone and chicken with skin; roast beef bone in; BPA-free canned fish with skin and bones included; and soups, stews, and chilis made from rich bone stock. All these foods are rich in the amino acids glycine and proline, but with today's prettily packaged, everything-perfect, skin-and-bones-removed meat from the grocery store, many of us are dangerously deficient in these amino acids.

Don't want to eat meat at every meal? You can supplement with clean sources of gelatin and collagen to receive a great, glucagon-releasing protein boost. Throw a scoop or two into simmering sauces, soups, coffee, tea, smoothies, and treats.

Don't get caught up in a set daily number for protein requirements. Once you start implementing the plan, your body will receive plenty of protein but in a beautiful balance with other food groups. Some meals and snacks will be extremely protein rich, others will have less, but never—NEVER—will you have any main meals devoid of protein. That is a blood-sugar-spiking and hormone-disrupting scenario.

Unless you have kidney disease, it is considered safe to consume one gram of protein per day per pound of body weight. Many studies have shown that even higher amounts are not damaging to healthy kidneys. You don't have to start to obsessively count to see if your meals add up to that number. On the plan you'll eat naturally from varied protein sources and won't have to do math equations in your head at every meal. **You'll simply pick a protein and have fats with it for an S meal or pick a protein and have healthy carbs with it for an E meal. Easy.**

Baby Step 2: At every meal always ask yourself, "Where's my protein?"

ROUND OUT YOUR PLATE WITH FUEL PULLS (FP)

You're not going to put only carbs or fats with hunks of protein on your dinner plate. Fill that plate with foods that match both S and E fuels. We call these Fuel Pull (FP) foods and you can think of them as your khaki skirt or pants: They match both S and E meals without causing an awful clash of too much fuel for your body to burn through. We call these foods Fuel Pulls because they don't offer your body ample amounts of fats or carbs but they're fantastic fillers and have incredible health benefits.

Even though Fuel Pulls are not primary sources of fuel, they are extremely important on the plan. They supply vital nutrients but also offer a natural difference in caloric load. On the Trim Healthy Mama Plan we don't have to count calories, but neither should we abuse them. Some S meals like cheese-topped steak followed by plan-approved cheesecake with a nut crust and whipped cream on top are super-dense in calories. This is not a bad thing. A meal like this has its place but if these dense foods are your constant, your balance is off kilter. Fuel Pulls ensure that your meals are not constantly heavy in calories—and they ensure you eat your veggies.

What are Fuel Pull foods? We'll get into a lot more detail later but basically, all the non-starchy veggies you want, berries, and certain lean forms of meats and dairy (if you do not have an allergy to dairy). Hold on, are you envisioning having to stuff dry salad and brittle broccoli into your mouth? Think again! Broccoli is a whole different animal when it is tossed with S fuels of melted butter, a little grated cheese, and a sprinkle of high-mineral salt (see page 157) and black pepper. You won't feel forced to eat your salad greens when they're drizzled with generous, anti-inflammatory olive oil or creamy dressing and topped with lots of other yummy fixings like bacon bits or nuts. No Spartan rabbit food for us Trim Healthy Mamas! We'll wager that you'll eat more veggies than you ever have but you'll delight in every bite!

Baby Step 3: Fill up the rest of your plate with Fuel Pulls—they match, they don't clash!

YOUR UNIQUE DIETARY NEEDS: MAINTAINING AND HELPING

Guess what? You just learned the basic principles behind the weight-loss part of this plan. And you're not even completely overwhelmed, right? Well, if you are a teensy bit frazzled finding yourself frantically thinking thoughts like, "S stands for what now?!" breathe deep. This info will settle in; give it some time. Listen to the kind voice inside your head that says "you can do this." Ignore the meanie voice that says "this is too hard," or "what's the use." You've tried and failed too many times before. Ain't nobody got time for that voice—ditch it!

But not all of us need to lose pounds. And even if you do, once you've lost your extra weight, you don't go back to the same old ways that led to the health and weight issues you so desperately wanted to overcome. The actual weight-loss stage will be the shortest part of your Trim Healthy journey. Even if you have lots to lose—even if it takes you five years—yes, it will still be the shortest part of your journey. Open your mind to the long-term vision of this plan, which is the art of lifelong healthy eating. Maintaining a healthy weight will be the greatest part of it whether that day seems incredibly far away from now or not.

This is where two more meal types come into the plan: Crossovers (XO) and S Helpers (SH). They are the friends of pregnant women, children, high-metabolism husbands (you know, those who have to eat all day just so their jeans don't fall down), and those of us who are close to or at goal weight.

It is important to know that these types of meals, while not as weight-loss inducing, are part of the plan, just as S and E meals and Fuel Pulls are. They are not "cheat meals" even if they don't cause the scale to go down. They'll both be explained in more detail, but the gist of a Crossover meal is that it is the opposite of an S or an E meal. That means that instead of separating the fuels of fats and carbs, it pairs them together in a safe, blood-sugar-friendly way and always in a protein-rich environment. Crossovers are the right way to "tandem fuel," which means to burn more than just one primary fuel in your meal. They keep weight on healthfully, so they are eaten more frequently once you have reached goal weight (along with S and E meals, too). They help ensure pregnant women gain enough pregnancy weight and have plenty of rich milk to feed babies, and they meet the high metabolic needs of growing children.

Baby Step 4: Crossovers are not cheats. They are important meals that help us maintain weight and meet the different dietary needs of more demanding stages in our lives.

So what do we have so far? S meals . . . E meals . . . Fuel Pulls . . . Crossovers. We mentioned one more—now welcome S Helpers to the stage. If you're just starting out and want to shed pounds, you probably won't be utilizing S Helpers for a while, so you won't have to spend much time figuring out this last meal type. Still, the concept is pretty easy. They are a basic S meal (one that focuses on the fuel of fats) but they add just a little bit of carbs in the form of starch or fruit. They can help people who desire weight loss but want the loss to go a bit slower. Remember, fast weight loss is not always best.

S Helper meals are great for pregnant women (especially pregnant women with gestational diabetes). They are useful for those of us who are close to goal weight or at goal weight and they are fantastic for children with weight issues, too. They can very gently and healthfully help overweight children slim down.

Baby Step 5: S Helpers are great for individuals who are closer to goal weight, pregnant or nursing women, or children who need to safely slim down.

WHY SEPARATE FUELS . . . WHY NOT JUST EAT SENSIBLY?

In a perfect world (one in which we all have super-high metabolisms and no insulin resistance) there wouldn't be a need for this separation of fuels to find a trim waistline. We'd be able to burn through our carbs in our food, then the fat in our food, and not worry about burning that third fuel of excess adipose tissue (body fat). But most of us grow up in a state very far removed from biblical times when people were not faced with the vast array of food choices we are constantly bombarded with today. The foods spoken about in the Bible, such as a hunk of rustic sourdough bread, raw goat's or sheep's milk (likely cultured, which reduced sugars), or a bit of roasted meat or fish with herbs, were far gentler on blood-sugar levels than our modern-day foods are.

Sometimes we read in the scriptures about folk eating honey or a few dates, but those forms of glucose were very much needed due to their more physically demanding lives. We ride in cars, they walked. We use a washing machine and turn on a tap for water. They beat clothes in a stream and had to haul water from a well. You get the picture. And cells that were not fed a lifetime of a too-high carb diet would have been much more insulin receptive—in direct contrast to the epidemic of insulin resistance that afflicts most of us adults now. We are not date or honey haters but there are seasons of our lives during which some foods help and some foods hinder.

We must get proactive. We cannot take a "normal approach" to food any longer because so-called normal meals these days usually result in too much weight gain for most body types. The reason, of course, is that they are shockingly full of hidden carbs and high sugars and our bodies have had enough!

Let's look at a recap of our baby-step basics; then in the next few chapters we'll look at these different fuel types in more detail so you can begin putting together a meal or two on your own real soon.

SUMMARY

1. Your two main meals are S and E. S meals focus on fats, E meals focus on carbs.

2. At every meal always ask yourself, "Where's my protein?"

3. Fill up the rest of your plate with Fuel Pulls. They match, they don't clash!

4. Crossovers are not cheats. They are important tandem-fueled meals that help us maintain weight and meet the different dietary needs of the more demanding stages in our lives like pregnancy or nursing.

5. S Helpers are great for individuals who are closer to goal weight, pregnant or nursing women, or children who need to safely slim down.

chapter 3
THE SATISFYING MEAL (S FOR SHORT)

What you'll love about this kind of meal is that it lives up to its name. It is ultra-satisfying. Come here, you creamy, drippy, succulent S meal, with all your rich, buttery goodness, and get in my tummy! That's the way we Trim Healthy Mamas look at our S meals. We're shamelessly brazen about them.

There will be many examples of S meals as you keep reading through the book, but here is a quick visual picture of what an S Evening Meal might be:

> Pot roast, slow-cooked to perfection, smothered with gravy
> Creamed cauliflower (mmm . . . many of us love this better than mashed potatoes)
> Side salad with creamy dressing or drizzled liberally with olive oil and vinegar and optional grated cheese

S meals are liberal with fats so they must have lower carbs if they are to assist in weight loss. That is the trick to get you chugging on the Trim Train. It's important to remember to keep grains and most fruits (with the exception of berries) away from S meals. You can bring carbs back in with fats more often once you are close to or at goal weight.

Think of a seesaw. S meal ratios look like this on a seesaw. Look at the difference in heights between carbs and fats. Note that when fat is higher in a meal, carbs are naturally lower. Protein sits solidly at the balancing point of the seesaw.

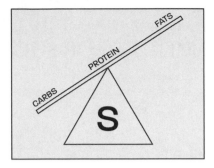

BUILD YOUR FIRST S MEAL

This can be done in three easy steps:

1. Choose your protein: lean or fatty meat or fish, such as chicken (with skin for more fat) or chicken breast without skin (for lean), whole eggs and egg whites, certain cultured dairy products (or choose from Integral Collagen, Just Gelatin, or Pristine Whey Protein—discussed in Chapter 18, "Specialty Food Stars," on page 140).
2. Add fats as desired. Even if your protein source contains fat, other fats can be added to the meal.
3. Add optional Fuel Pull foods to your plate, such as non-starchy veggies, berries, and certain forms of dairy (check out the example list of Fuel Pull foods on pages 58–60).

In practical terms this might look like the following:

Breakfast—Your protein might be 2 to 3 whole eggs fried in butter or 2 eggs with optional breakfast sausage or bacon (as natural as you can find it). You may prefer to add finely diced zucchini, spinach, or mushrooms to the pan with the frying eggs for a veggie portion instead of a meat—or have your eggs on a piece of S-friendly bread, either store-bought and plan-approved or homemade (found in the "Breads and Pizza Crusts" chapter in the *Trim Healthy Mama Cookbook*).

Lunch—Your protein might be chicken, turkey, or salmon. You can pile it on a huge bed of salad greens and top with a decadent, fat-based dressing or combine your meat with mayo, dill pickles, and celery and put it between a couple slices of one of our many S-friendly bread options.

Dinner—Your protein might be meat loaf. Add broccoli tossed with sea salt and butter and a side salad with luscious dressing. (You can always follow your meal with an on plan dessert.)

CHOOSE GOOD FATS

You might be surprised at some of the foods we suggest as "good fats." Most of us are taught that extra-virgin olive oil and avocados are the two exclusive members in the elite "good fats" group. Perhaps a few raw nuts get included from time to time but membership stops there. We're not downing olive oil and avocados, but this "good fats" group is like a popular high-school clique that looks down on the "out crowd." Liberal amounts of olive oil are on the plan—what a great way to combat inflammation in the body. But olive oil has never had to bear teasing and wear a sign on its back saying, I WILL GIVE YOU HEART DISEASE. Half an avocado on your salad is another wonderful option. But avocado hasn't had to endure the hurt of being called an artery clogger.

You're going to open your mind to making friends with the kicked-around nerd fats, the underdogs. These so-called no-no fats like egg yolks, butter, red meat, coconut oil, red palm oil, and some full-fat dairy like heavy cream and hard cheeses are going to have their day in the sun (if you don't have sensitivities to dairy)!

Many families on the plan also enjoy bacon! Nothing better than bacon and eggs to start your Saturday morning off right. Ain't nobody gonna feel sorry for themselves eating a breakfast like that! We enjoy bacon, too, but use the turkey variety due to our biblical beliefs. The choice to eat real pork bacon and other meats not deemed clean in Leviticus and Deuteronomy in the Bible is completely up to you. We can't help but squeeze in the point that God surely knew what He was talking about when He suggested in the scriptures which meats were made for our bodies to eat and which weren't. (Okay—nuff said 'bout that—don't want to start a big ol' debate.) Got a pig fattening up in your backyard? Have at it!

Saturated fats like butter and coconut oil are far too often on the naughty lists of the media and diet "dictocrats." They've been given a bad rap over the years and it is hard to shake these ingrained notions. The oils we suggest you cook with are coconut oil, butter, or red palm oil. These are the most saturated oils and therefore safest oils to heat. Most vegetable oils (like canola oil) are highly unstable when heated and can turn into trans fats. If you want to stick with the cool club and not give the nerds a fair try in your cooking, olive oil and grapeseed oil may be okay for light sautéing here and there at lower heats. We also enjoy the flavor of sesame oil for certain dishes.

Most cold-pressed oils are fine for S meals in a raw state; however, we suggest you steer clear of canola, corn, vegetable, and soybean oil. We understand, though, that soybean oil is an ingredient in most store-bought mayonnaise. Our Drive Thru Sue and mayo-loving Mamas may not care too much about this and still purchase their favorite brand of mayonnaise; and if this helps keep them on their plan, then *woot!* You can find mayonnaise made with healthier oils at health food stores, but they are a little more expensive. Hey, try making your own! It's easy.

FATTY FEARS

We spent many years as vegans, extremely skeptical of the saturated fats in butter, egg yolks, and red meat. We'd read countless books about the perils of meat and fat and they all had scientific evidence to back up their theories. It was biblical truth that finally freed us. The angel of the Lord—or what the Hebrew language depicts as Jehovah Himself (in Genesis 18)—ate both butter and red meat in the meal Abraham set before Him. Was He setting us a bad example? Of course not. Deuteronomy 14:4 says, "These are the beasts which ye shall eat; the ox, the sheep, the goat...." Hmm ... did you notice that two of those animals out of three are red meat of the fatty kind? And look at that word *shall*. It doesn't say, "Well, if you have to eat meat, which is second best to plant food, try to cut back and just eat a little fish or chicken now and then ..." No, it clearly says you SHALL.

Fully embracing scriptures like this and many others, we found, requires trust. Could we trust our Creator that He knew better than the diet gurus we had been following all those years? And asking ourselves that question gave us a quick answer: Duh, of course we could! You can still be a vegetarian Trim Healthy Mama, as we outline in Chapter 25, "Heads Up: Vegetarians!" (page 231), but one of our biggest reasons for eating a plant-based diet was fear—and that's no way to live!

Letting go of all our past food theories felt like skydiving out of an airplane: terrifying yet exhilarating. Incredibly, we soon came to learn science backs up God's word over and over again. Butter is rich in antioxidants and boasts high amounts of selenium, which shields the body from free radical damage. It is rich in iodine, which is essential to thyroid health and protective of breast and ovarian cancers. It contains a readily absorbable form of vitamin A and is an excellent form of vitamin D, which maintains strong bones and lowers the risk of heart disease and osteoporosis. If you're still having some trouble shaking the "butter is bad" theory, you may need some therapy. Try saying this a few times: "Oooh, I love me some buttah!!!"

WHAT ELSE GOES ON MY PLATE?

You've got Three Amigos that help you master S meals.

1. Non-starchy Veggies

Remember, we don't want blood sugar to be the chief fuel in an S meal. It is fat's turn to "burn, baby, burn." Aside from protein, which is the anchor of all meal types, non-starchy veggies are huge players in S meals as they have minimal effect on your blood sugar. "What's a non-starchy vegetable?" you ask. Basically any vegetable that is not a root vegetable (like a potato, sweet potato, or carrot) or a starch (such as corn). That still leaves you with literally hundreds of choices. We want you to eat plenty of non-starchy veggies—oodles of them, all scrumptiously prepared. And don't get all caught up with counting the carbs in them or limiting amounts like many low-carb diets suggest. They are low enough in carbs that they will not cause much of a rise in blood sugar even with large helpings.

Non-starchy veggies are in the Fuel Pull category. We have an example list of them in the chapter on Fuel Pulls (see page 59) for you to look at. For interest's sake, we count only net carbs on Trim Healthy Mama, which is total carbs minus fiber. Most non-starchy veggies have between two and six net carbs, with a few slightly higher and some even lower. Lettuce and other leafy greens have the lowest amounts of starch of all vegetables. They have less than one gram of carb per serving and minuscule calories. That is ridiculously low, so filling up on them makes perfect sense. Any form of tasty animal protein like chicken, beef, or salmon over a nice, BIG plate of lettuce with succulent dressing makes a quick, complete, slimming, and inexpensive meal.

Sadly, non-starchy veggies are usually overshadowed by sides like potatoes and mac and cheese—but that's about to change! Non-starchies can also accompany E meals, but when they are paired with fats in an S meal . . . "oh my."

Many conventional diets want you to eat lots of vegetables, but dry leaves and stalks are unappetizing to most of us. We have to force ourselves to be good and try to get our quota in, and some of us avoid them altogether (you know who you are). There is nothing worse than being told not only to eat more broccoli, but to eat it dry and unsavory. This goes against human taste buds, we think. But broccoli is delicious tossed with butter and sea salt, or made into a creamy casserole. Roasted veggies with coconut oil—divine! Sautéed veggies with a peanut Thai sauce—yum! Cauliflower creamed up with butter and sea salt—a great sub for mashed potatoes!

Speaking of which . . . time for your first little quiz.

Question: If you pair mashed potatoes with an S meal what happens?
Answer:
A. You get the hiccups
B. You feel the urge to scratch your left ankle
C. You have second helpings
D. No body fat will be burned

Got the answer? Not yet? Little hint then: White potatoes have lots of carbs and cause a significant rise in your blood sugar. Clicking now? Is option D starting to ding ding ding? Yep . . . you're right . . . what occurs is a serious case of tandem fueling. Your body will have to first burn through all that glucose from the potatoes before it gets around to burning any of the fat in the steak. One thing you can bank on: No body-fat burning will occur. Potatoes can be a bit rough on blood sugar so we want you to give them a little rest for a while. You'll be busy using all these other delightful veggies, so you won't feel deprived. You can eat a white potato here and there once you're at Crossover stage.

2. Nuts

Nuts are predominantly made of protein and fat with just a few carbs, so they fit into the S fuel. Unlike non-starchy veggies, however, they don't need to be used as frequently on the S meal plate. We do want you to enjoy them but we can't give license to go crazy with nuts since, unlike non-starchy veggies, they are very high in calories. Remember, while we don't count calories we don't abuse them, either, so don't make a meal out of nuts alone! Moderation is a good idea; a handful or two for a snack can be a good S option.

Got a peanut butter addiction? Don't worry. We're not going to take that good stuff away from you. Natural peanut butter without sugar is fine. Slather some on your celery or put a tablespoon or so in an S smoothie, but don't be like Little Jack Horner sitting in the corner eating it out of the jar by the spoonful! That could be in the abuse category. If you want more peanut flavor without going crazy, try pressed peanut flour. Our Trim Healthy Mama Pressed Peanut Flour is high in protein and has simply been pressed (to extract a lot of the oil). The result is a nice flour/meal texture that has less fat and fewer calories but heaps of peanutty flavor. It is awesome in smoothies or shakes, baked goods, and savory Thai sauces. Check out the recipe for Peanut Junkie Butter in our "Condiments and Extras" chapter in the *Trim Healthy Mama Cookbook*.

Speaking of nut flours—welcome to the world of Trim Healthy Baking! Nut flours will enable you to have moist muffins, cookies, and cakes that are kind to your blood sugar—even for breakfast if you want! Who makes all those rules, anyway? If we want frosted chocolate cake for breakfast or a big ol' muffin slathered with buttah—we have it! Trim Healthy Mama baked goods are high in protein, full of superfoods, topped up with chocolaty or cinnamony goodness, and keep us happy. Pressed coconut flour is another great flour option for baking, but we're most excited about our Gluten-Free Trim Healthy Mama baking flour blend. It is a combination of various pressed seed flours and other superfood goodies. The result is a wonderful texture and taste for baking. We designed the THM Baking Blend to have a lighter caloric load so you can add wonderful superfood fats like coconut oil and whole eggs to it and not abuse calories. It's a jack-of-all-trades: pancakes, muffins, cookies, brownies, cakes, biscuits, sandwich breads, and even breading for chicken and fish—it has you covered. But since we have a "no special ingredients required" policy, you can also bake with golden flax meal, which is blessedly inexpensive and easily found at almost all grocery stores. Almond flour is easy to find in stores, too, but sadly it is not so inexpensive. You can make wonderful muffins and other baked goodies with either or both of those S-friendly flours. Check out many free Trim Healthy Mama recipes using those two flours on Pinterest or make our tried-and-tested favorites from the *Trim Healthy Mama Cookbook*.

FRANKENFOODS OR SHORTCUTS?

Here's where we are a bit different in our approaches. If you take a more purist approach to eating, like Serene does, you will be satisfied with S meals by simply eating all the delicious meals you can put together with pure, whole foods only. But some of us, like Pearl and her Drive Thru Sue peeps, are not quite at that level of purism. We are all aiming for a lifelong approach here, and if food prep gets too time-consuming or involved, some Mamas start falling off the wagon. Not everyone wants to constantly have to make homemade S-friendly breads or use zucchini as noodles. We get in a hurry and want easy.

You can purchase many convenient items at your grocery store that will help you stay on plan and give you superquick options for sandwiches, burritos, pasta, and quesadillas. Some of these items are definitely not in the superfood category but are also not destructive to the plan when used in moderation. Check out the list of what Serene calls Frankenfoods and what Pearl calls shortcuts at the end of our S Foods list, where we categorize them as "Personal Choice" Items.

3. Berries

These little power-packed gems of goodness are shining stars in the world of super-foods and thankfully are low enough in sugar that you can include some in both your S and E meals. They're fantastic baked into muffins, topping a salad, mixed into Greek yogurt, topping a healthy cheesecake, or just popped into your mouth.

We could go on and on listing their benefits, but this is supposed to be a short book. Buy them fresh or frozen. Eat 'em, love 'em—that's the short of it. (Lemons and limes are also welcome in S meals but other fruits are not S-friendly.)

S FOODS LIST

S-FRIENDLY MEATS
- All meats and fish, both fatty or lean, that fit within your religious guidelines (grass-fed is best but not mandatory)

S-FRIENDLY EGGS

- Whole eggs and egg whites

S-FRIENDLY DAIRY

- Heavy cream (raw pastured is healthiest but not mandatory)
- Half-and-half for coffee
- Butter
- All cheeses, including hard cheeses and softer cheeses like cream cheese (⅓-less-fat cream cheese is just as creamy but not as heavy in calories, so is a good option)
- Sour cream
- Double-fermented kefir
- Both full-fat and reduced-fat forms of cottage cheese, ricotta cheese, feta cheese, and paneer
- Full-fat plain Greek yogurt (unstrained yogurt that is not Greek style is not S friendly)—you can sweeten with plan-approved sweeteners
- 0% fat plain Greek yogurt (a full cup of Greek yogurt can be used in an S meal as your main protein source; best to keep to a half cup if having as a dessert after a meal, due to carb content)—you can sweeten with plan-approved sweeteners at home; but lately some brands of Greek yogurt are starting to sell stevia-sweetened versions, which are fine on the plan
- Laughing Cow Creamy Light Swiss cheese wedges (these are also on the list of "Personal Choice" Items [page 38], given that they are not a usual choice for purists)

S-FRIENDLY VEGGIES

- All non-starchy veggies. This includes literally hundreds of non-starchy veggies too numerous to list. Check out the Fuel Pull Food List (page 58). Starchy vegetables are potatoes, corn, sweet potatoes, turnips, and cooked carrots—so avoid those in S meals (small amounts of cooked carrots in stir-fry recipes should be okay). Be liberal with all non-starchy veggies in S meals with the exception of tomatoes, onions, and peas. Enjoy those but don't go overboard with them; for instance; don't roast a huge onion and put it on the side of your steak. A quarter to half of a small to medium onion or half of a large tomato is fine. Limit butternut and acorn squash to half-cup amounts in S meals.

S-FRIENDLY FRUIT
- Up to 1 cup of all kinds of berries can be used in S meals but keep blueberries to ½ cup (as they have more fruit sugars). (Note: You don't have to always use a full cup of berries; ¼- to ½-cup amounts of berries are just fine in S meals and don't push carb limits as high.)
- Enjoy lemons and limes.
- Avoid other fruits (with the exception of 1 teaspoon all-fruit jelly).

S-FRIENDLY NUTS AND SEEDS
- All kinds of raw or roasted nuts (salted or unsalted; in moderation)
- All kinds of raw or roasted seeds (salted or unsalted; in moderation)
- All nut butters without sugar, such as peanut, almond, sunflower, cashew, and pumpkin (in moderation)
- All nut and seed flours, including Trim Healthy Mama Baking Blend, which is a blend of pressed nut and seed flours and other goodies like collagen and oat fiber

S-FRIENDLY CONDIMENTS
- All oils that are cold pressed (remember to cook primarily with saturated oils)
- Mayo
- Mustard
- Horseradish sauce
- All vinegars
- Salad dressings—full fat is fine (Make your own! Or, if relying on store-bought, try to buy options with a carb count of two or less, and water down before serving.)
- Nonsweet pickles
- Olives
- Nutritional yeast
- All broth or stock prepared without sugar
- Spices and seasonings (without sugar and other needless fillers)
- Unsweetened cocoa powder/cacao nibs
- Bragg Liquid Aminos/Coconut Aminos/Tamari/Soy sauce
- Ketchup (sugar-free homemade is best but small amounts of regular ketchup on a low-carb burger should not throw you off too much)

- Hot sauce (sugar-free is best)—Frank's RedHot and Texas Pete are good brands (look for one carb or less)

S-FRIENDLY GRAINS AND BEANS
- Keep these foods away from your S meals with the exception of very small garnish amounts to be used occasionally. A quarter cup of beans could fit into an S meal, but it's still best not to use grains or beans in every single S meal. Now and then is fine. You can fit one Light Rye, Fiber, or Flax Seed Wasa cracker or one Sesame Ryvita cracker into an S meal now and then, too.

S-FRIENDLY HEALTHY SPECIALTY ITEMS
- Pristine Whey Protein Powder (www.trimhealthymama.com)
- Integral Collagen (www.trimhealthymama.com)
- Just Gelatin (www.trimhealthymama.com)
- Glucomannan "Gluccie" Organic Fiber Supplement (www.trimhealthymama.com); nonorganic also available
- Plan-approved natural sweeteners (www.trimhealthymama.com); see page 103 for guidelines
- Trim Healthy Mama Baking Blend (www.trimhealthymama.com)
- Pressed Peanut Flour (www.trimhealthymama.com)
- Not-Naughty-Noodles and Not-Naughty-Rice (www.trimhealthymama.com)
- Stevia-sweetened chocolate or a square or two of 85% dark chocolate (85% chocolate does have a small amount of sugar, but when eaten in very small amounts the carbs stay low and the sugar is not significant enough to do damage for those who just want a quick, easy chocolate fix)
- 100% cacao baker's chocolate
- Unsweetened nut milks, such as almond, cashew, coconut, or flaxseed

(Check out Chapter 18, "Specialty Food Stars," on page 140, in which we give descriptions and benefits of many of the above products and tell you what to look for in other brands or seek locally if you don't want to purchase online.)

S-FRIENDLY "PERSONAL CHOICE" ITEMS

- Joseph's low-carb pita or lavash bread (not all Joseph's products fit on plan; look for four net carbs or less per serving)
- Low-carb tortillas or wraps (Olé Xtreme Wellness and Mission brands are common in grocery stores)
- Fat-free Reddi-wip (avoid light or fat-free Cool Whip due to the inclusion of high-fructose corn syrup)
- Laughing Cow Creamy Light Swiss cheese wedges
- Dreamfields pasta (limit to once a week or every other week). Assess your own reaction to this pasta. The package used to say five net carbs per serving; it no longer does due to legal language, but many Mamas (not all) find it is kind enough to blood-sugar levels due to its resistant starch to be able to be used in an S setting.

chapter 4
THE ENERGIZING MEAL (E FOR SHORT)

There are two common extremes when it comes to carbohydrates: People are addicted to them or they are terrified of them. Yes, carbs are notorious for fattening us up and causing inflammatory blood-sugar spikes, but these are situations in which carbs are distorted or abused. Healthy carbs should never be shunned because of this bad rap. That's like completely avoiding sunshine, closing yourself off in darkness, for fear of a sunburn. No way to live. Bring on the rays!

E meals will allow you to gain health, vitality, and a fired-up metabolism while eating carbs—delicious, energizing carbs—always safely anchored by protein.

Here's what an E evening meal may look like:

Moist chicken breast cooked with salsa and caramelized onions over a bed of brown rice or quinoa

Tender field greens spritzed with olive oil and drizzled generously with balsamic vinegar

Grapefruit slushie to end your meal

When enjoyed in the amounts we describe, the carbs that star in your E meals won't be Monster Meanies on your blood-sugar levels. You'll get to include fruit, sweet potatoes, beans/legumes of all kinds, and gentle whole grains in your Energizing meals. We describe these grains, such as oatmeal or quinoa, as gentle because they are not bullies to your blood sugar. Brown rice may get a little pushy at times, so if you have any form of

Type 2 diabetes or severe insulin resistance, you can choose quinoa, whole barley, or farro over brown rice. Those options are gentler on your blood sugar.

Think again of a seesaw. E meal ratios show a big difference in heights between carbs and fats. Note that when carbs are higher in a meal, fats are naturally lower. Protein sits solidly at the balancing point of the seesaw.

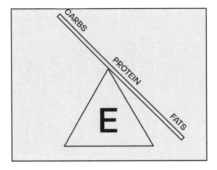

BUILD YOUR FIRST E MEAL

1. Choose your protein: lean meat or fish, low-fat dairy, or egg whites (or choose from Integral Collagen, Just Gelatin, or Pristine Whey Protein—discussed in Chapter 18, "Specialty Food Stars," on page 140).
2. Add your carb: fruit, gentle whole grains, beans/legumes, or sweet potatoes.
3. Add minimal fat (roughly one teaspoon); nuts and seeds are used only in garnish amounts.
4. Add optional Fuel Pull foods to your plate, such as non-starchy veggies and berries.

In practical terms this might look like the following:

Breakfast—Your protein might be Greek yogurt dolloped on top of a generous bowl of oatmeal with cinnamon-spiced stewed apples.

Lunch—Your protein might be lean deli meat of your choice sandwiched between two pieces of sprouted or artisan sourdough bread, either store-bought or homemade. Your sandwich might include fresh tomato slices, lettuce, onion, mustard or horseradish sauce, a little smear of mayo, or a spritz of oil and a drizzle of vinegar. Low-fat cottage cheese and a small slice of cantaloupe will be a great side option for this meal.

Dinner—Your protein might be lean ground turkey seasoned Cajun-style. You can load a sweet potato high with the meat crumbles, chopped lettuce, diced tomatoes and cucumber, Greek yogurt, hot sauce, a spritz or two of olive oil, and drizzles of vinegar.

SCARED OF CARBS?

We need to take a minute to make this crystal clear because carbs have suffered much persecution. YOU NEED CARBS—THEY ARE SLIMMING—THEY ARE HEALING! We had to yell, only because we have to be a tad cruel to be kind. We know what living in fear of carbs feels like, and it's no fun. Some of you will need tough love to shake you out of carb terror. Many coming from low-carb diets believe even a few bites of oatmeal or fruit may cause exploding weight gain.

"Watch out, Mama's about to balloon up—she ate an apple!"

This fear is unfounded. Song of Solomon 2:5 (ESV) reads, "Refresh me with apples." Just as the Bible doesn't gel with fear of fat, it also doesn't jibe with fear of carbs. Yes, there might be a bit of an uptick on the scale after a couple of healthy carb-based meals; but this is only due to your muscle cells taking in the fuel of glucose, and they do so by also pulling in fluid. This is a good and very natural function of your body. The goal when eating carbs the right way is a long-term downward trend on the scale thanks to a revved-up metabolism. Little upticks noticed from too much scale watching are not the big picture.

You must keep your body guessing if you don't want it to adapt to one type of fuel and lower its thermal burn. Long periods of eating too few carbs take the fire out of your metabolic fuel-burning ability. Carbs are important for your thyroid health. Feed your body only low-carb meals and watch what happens after a while: It will catch on. "Ahhh, I know what you are going to give me . . . more fats and protein again and again! I am so used to that now, I'm just gonna start storing whatever you feed me." The thyroid hormone T3, which your body uses for so many bodily functions—including a healthy metabolism—takes a nosedive. Give your body some glucose and watch it start to do the rumba by having to burn another fuel. Shake it up, baby!

Carbs are essential for your happiness as they elevate serotonin levels in your brain. This is an important neurotransmitter that combats the blahs. It is also a natural pain reliever. A constant low-carb state means your brain won't be releasing as much of this pleasant feeling. On the other hand, ever heard of a sugar high? That is an extremely high serotonin state caused by eating too many carbs. The bliss from the bowl of Moose Tracks ice cream feels good for a little while but inevitably results in a crash. What goes up must come down. The serotonin low makes you feel grumpy, washed out, and in need of some more sugar! Just as we must get the highs and lows of blood sugar under control, our brain chemistry relies on the balance of the fuels we give it, too. Eating the right amount of good carbs can help to balance out the extremes of skyrocketing then plummeting serotonin levels.

"Adrenal fatigue" is a common buzz phrase these days, but it is notorious for causing stubborn weight that won't let go. Take a whole fuel (like carbs) away from your body and it is going to feel pretty stressed. It will have to release the stress hormone cortisol that is notorious for fattening us up. This is only logical since our Creator designed us to burn two primary fuels. Would you fly a twin-engine plane on only one of its engines? That would be an extremely stressful situation. If we constantly offer our bodies only one kind of fuel, our adrenal glands panic. Healthy carbs (in safe amounts) sing soothing lullabies to your adrenals.

Balance must always reign. The other side of the coin is that our adrenal glands do not thrive in a high-carb state, either. Soaring blood sugar from eating too many carbs requires high levels of insulin to be released for cleanup. What happens when you have to make lots of insulin? Your body feels stressed and releases more cortisol—boo! Let's avoid these extremes. Let's learn to eat carbs the right way.

THE E-MEAL CARB LIMIT

It's so important to remember that E meals are not an excuse to gorge on carbs. Gorging on carbs will result in hazardous blood-sugar levels and weight gain (especially around the belly) whether the carbs are whole-grain or not. Keep the starchy carb portion to a palm-size serving on your plate unless you are eating beans—and you can have more of those.

Keeping grains, fruit, and sweet potatoes to palm-size portions will naturally keep you around or under forty-five grams of net carbs, which is the limit we advise. That amount gives your body glucose as fuel for energy, but it can still be burned off without too much trouble. This is how the E meal becomes a slimming sensation. Since you are not over-stuffing your cells with glucose fuel, your body will have to search for more fuel once it has devoured the easy-burn E carb. The signal is released for your body fat to come out of storage so you can keep going. Jeans get that slightest bit looser!

Fruit is a fantastic E option, but this doesn't mean you should overdo it. One apple, orange, peach, or nectarine with an E meal is wonderful; but going overboard with fruit can provide too much sugar in the body. Higher-glycemic fruits like mango, pineapple, grapes, and watermelon are best kept to one-cup servings. If you have severe insulin resistance or any pre- or full-blown Type 2 diabetes, it may be best if you steer away from the higher-glycemic fruits at first (or use only half servings of them) and stick to more medium-glycemic fruits like apples, peaches, and cherries until your blood sugars are better stabilized. Bananas are a high-sugar fruit that are too often overeaten, but it is a myth that they cannot be eaten on THM. We simply suggest sticking with half a large banana (or one small) in an E meal or snack.

We don't want you doing a bunch of carb counting because it leads only to needless obsessions and robs you of the joy in your journey. The suggested portions of starch and fruit in our E list of approved foods are already given in safe helping sizes so you won't need to think too much about it. It's no fun doing math in your head at every meal. Staying close to these safe portion boundaries of glucose fuel will keep you from the dangerous fat-storing troll that waits on the other side of the carb-limit fence. This doesn't mean you'll be hungry or your plate will look woefully meager; your carb fuel is just one part of the yummy whole picture on your plate. Just like with S meals, you'll be adding other Fuel Pull options such as non-starchy veggies and lean meat, dairy, or egg whites.

Let's compare a Trim Healthy Mama E meal to one eaten in dangerous Trollville outside the fenced safety of the limits we advise. Imagine that breakfast we mentioned earlier of a generous bowl of oatmeal with added fruit or berries and a dollop of Greek yogurt. Your blood sugar should still be within safe and healthy limits after a filling thirty- to forty-five-gram carb meal like this. Compare that to a common evening meal that contains a baked potato of around sixty carbs, a white dinner roll (or two) of around twenty-five carbs each, and a sugar-laden dessert around eighty carbs. Put the three together, as many people do, and you have well over a hundred carbs in just one meal. Now that's out of conTROLL! No wonder the epidemic of obesity is still raging.

WHERE'S THE FAT?

Fat takes a backseat in an E meal but it is not banished. You can add one little pat—a teaspoon. Okay, we know how much peanut butter we personally have been able to fit on a teaspoon in our lives; there are Guinness World Records to break on that one, right? We mean a *flat* (level) teaspoon. (Check out Chapter 10, "Just the Numbers," on page 85, if you are a numbers person and think in numbers versus visual amounts.)

This optional teaspoon of fat is added for three reasons:

1. Fat helps you absorb vital fat-soluble vitamins and minerals from your meal. A fat-free meal sounds awful and is less nutritious.
2. Fat (along with all important protein) gentles down the speed with which glucose is absorbed into your bloodstream. The gentler the rise of your blood sugar, the safer the meal (especially for those with diabetic issues).
3. It is a more balanced approach to not completely remove a full macronutrient (like fat) from a meal. Your hormones appreciate this. This little pat of fat is not enough to cause a tandem-fueling effect.

Is this teaspoon of added fat mandatory? No, especially if your protein source has a lean but still existing amount of fat, as does salmon or lean dairy (such as 1% cottage cheese). Some of the grains that we encourage, like oatmeal and quinoa, also naturally contain their own small amount of fat, so you don't have to concern yourself with always adding more.

But this also doesn't mean that if your protein source or grain does contain a little bit of fat you must deny yourself that teaspoon of oil on your salad or coconut oil to sauté your salmon. You're still likely to be in safe waters adding the small amount we advise. Here's a little practical advice to make your salads more succulent in E meals: Use an extra-virgin olive oil spritz, which coats every leaf without overdoing it. Adding a sour agent like vinegar or lemon helps to curb the rise of too-high blood sugar. It also brings more succulence to your salad, so if you do decide not to add any fat at all, then double up on the balsamic vinegar or lemon juice.

Note: Middle-chain triglyceride (MCT) oil is the lowest oil of all in calories and your body burns this sort of fat faster than any other form of fat. You can learn more about this oil in Chapter 18, "Specialty Food Stars" (page 140). Sometimes it might be okay to use two teaspoons of MCT oil in an E meal. For example, you might use one on your salad and then include one in one of our drink recipes like Beauty Milk found in the "More Drinks" chapter of the *Trim Healthy Mama Cookbook* or Healing Trimmy (in the "Hot Drinks" chapter of the *Trim Healthy Mama Cookbook*). Drinks like these help end your meal with more filling power. However, MCT oil packs a great fatty-tasting punch, so you don't have to make a habit of that two-teaspoon exception. Using a half teaspoon of MCT in each of those courses is also another option.

If dairy products and you play well together, that is great because lean dairy can be a boon to E meals without having to add a meat (helps your budget). One-percent cottage cheese is a great source of protein as is 0% Greek yogurt. Notice we are not encouraging a lot of "fat-free" dairy products with added fillers. Zero-percent Greek yogurt does not have any additives or other strange ingredients to make it "fat-free." It is simply yogurt made from naturally skimmed milk with the whey fluid (which contains most of the carbs) drained out. This is very easy to make at home if you love cooking from scratch. One-percent cottage cheese can be found without additives in a couple of brands like Nancy's and Friendship. However, all forms of 1% cottage cheese are on the plan if they do not contain added sugar in the ingredients. If you cannot find a 1% cottage cheese that fits your purism standards, some 2% cottage cheese brands do not contain these fillers (like Daisy brand) and can be used with E meals if you do not have stubborn weight to lose.

If dairy and you are not compatible, check out Chapter 26, "Heads Up: Allergen-Free Mamas!" (page 240), for other protein ideas. Gelatin and collagen peptides are excellent forms of superfood protein that can be used with all meal styles since they do not contain any fat and they are naturally dairy-free.

BREAD: THE PROS AND CONS

The Trim Healthy Mama approach to grain-based bread is not to put a big X over it (however, it is very easy to be gluten-free on plan if your own body finds that necessary). We simply make sure that grain-based bread flours are sprouted or a sourdough variety. The reason for this is that any grain in flour form causes a more speedy rise in blood sugar. Sprouting or souring bread flours slows this down and helps create a more balanced blood-sugar level, which is always our goal.

The exceptions to this are whole rye, whole barley, oats, or quinoa. These are more gentle even in flour form, and you can use them on the plan without worrying too much about sprouting them for blood-sugar purposes. We cannot include brown rice flour in this exception. It has a greater ability to cause blood sugar to spike. All wheat varieties should always be sprouted or soured.

Time for your second quiz. Be careful; we may trick you.

Question: What happens when you eat turkey, mayo, and cheese on wheat?
Answer:
A. You wash it down with orange juice.
B. You choose pretzels over chips as your side.
C. Your buttons get more difficult to fasten.
D. You paint your nails afterward.

If you thought the answer was A, you're the winner ... in another quiz, not ours. While fruit is a good choice and on the plan, extracting the juice from the whole fruit is a nightmare on your blood sugar. It is FATTENING, as you'll learn more about in Chapter 12, "Thirsty Mama" (page 95).

If you chose B, congratulations: You're the runner-up ... again on somebody else's quiz, not ours. While pretzels are considered fat-free and looked on fondly by the dieting world, we call them fatzels. They're white-flour blood-sugar spikers. Even if you find a whole-wheat variety, if they are not made from fermented or sprouted flour, they will quickly spike your bloodstream. This also applies to all whole-wheat-flour products including pasta, crackers, and that wheat bread in the turkey and cheese sandwich. Don't let this throw you into a pit of despair. Life is still awesome because sprouting or fermenting grains predigests much of the starch. Along with sprouted whole-grain breads, sprouted pastas are also on the plan and can work in your E meals. There are many brands of sprouted breads to choose from in stores these days. (Or be adventurous and make your own. There are some THM-friendly sprouted bread recipes easily found online, and you'll find a fabulous one in the "Breads and Pizza Crusts" chapter of the *Trim Healthy Mama Cookbook*.) You can even purchase sprouted pretzels if you just have to have them!

Answer: C is it! While a turkey and cheese on wheat is not a burger and fries, it is still a common, deceivingly innocent meal, contributing to the obesity epidemic in our culture. We've already addressed the fact that the regular wheat bread is a blood-sugar spiker. It is also the combination of the heavy fats (mayo and cheese) with the fast-spiking flour product (don't forget those pretzels on the side) that makes this meal a fat bomb ready to explode. People with super-high metabolisms are exempt from this fat explosion, but that blood-sugar high is still dangerous for their long-term health.

We can't leave option D unaddressed. We love us some painted toenails, but here's a little tip for your health journey. Most nail polish contains a laundry list of toxins. All are disturbing but the big three are formaldehyde (a known human carcinogen), dibutyl phthalate (DBP, which is linked to birth defects), and toluene, which damages the nervous and reproductive system. These are absorbed into the bloodstream. We don't want to take away pretty nails, but do seek out brands free of these obnoxious chemicals.

WHERE'S THE CORN?

Corn is a grain, so does that make it E-friendly? We have a gray answer for this one. Corn is used to fatten up animals and we don't promote it enthusiastically on plan. If eaten too frequently, corn and most corn products won't do your health and waistline any favors. The exceptions are sprouted whole-grain corn tortillas, which can be used in an E setting. A few baked blue corn chips are a nice snack with Greek yogurt and salsa or on top of an E-style chili. As you can see, we are not being corn Nazis and demanding that a kernel of corn never again cross your lips. A little bit of corn in an E-style chili really does add something incredible … little pops of sweet. We use it in moderation in some of our E recipes. We're just saying, go easy! Corn is not a gentle-burning grain, so don't make it a go-to food. Seek out organic sources of corn if GMO foods concern you but non-GMO does not take away the fattening effects of too much corn.

Popcorn—what would life be without it? Drenched with butter and sprinkled with salt and nutritional yeast, it is just about one of the most amazing Crossover snacks eva! But even when you're at Crossover stage, don't sit there every night eating that snack. Just watch what will happen to your once loose jeans: Good-bye to them! Save it for a now-and-then treat. You can eat popcorn in an E setting; just follow these guidelines:

• Keep portion size to four to five cups.
• Spray with coconut oil or olive oil spray (so you don't go over about one teaspoon of fat) and sprinkle generously with seasonings.

- Keep a three-hour distance between an E popcorn snack and an S meal if you are in weight-loss mode.
- Don't eat popcorn daily; save it for a couple times a week or only when you get strong cravings for it.
- If possible try to find organic, non-GMO popcorn seeds; but once again we leave that up to your own purism standards. Some of our ultra–Drive Thru Sue Mamas even use 100-calorie bags of microwave popcorn for a rare E snack. Hey, let's not be too hasty to judge; they're still baby-stepping their way to health.

TO SOAK OR NOT TO SOAK?

That is the question: Whether 'tis nobler to put grain in warm water overnight, or not? Poor Hamlet would have been just as stumped as many of us are on this question had he been able to connect to WiFi.

Dried grains, beans, and seeds are protected by substances called phytates that keep them dormant for storage. This is a good thing—a real good thing. God allowed us to be able to store grains without them rotting. Mankind might well have starved to death without this protective ability.

But here's where all the controversy starts. Many believe that in order for these dormant foods to unleash their full load of nutrients, they need to be soaked, sprouted, or fermented. It is true that these methods make superfoods out of foods such as grains because they:

- Add beneficial bacteria and other detoxing and healing goodies.
- Increase nutrients.
- Make protein more absorbable and lower the starch content.
- Are tolerated better by those with sensitive stomachs.

But there are some untruths involved here as well. These techniques are predominantly used not so much for the above benefits but in an anxious effort to reduce phytates (and lectins), which are not necessarily the evil villains that they are made out to be. (See more about this in Chapter 31, "Balance Is Beautiful," page 273.)

So should you feel guilty if you don't soak every bowl of oatmeal you eat as a Trim Healthy Mama?

No.

Go ahead and soak if you want all those benefits and the characteristic flavor and texture that comes from soaking and fermentation methods. But you sure don't have to if it is only the fear of phytates you are worrying about.

Soaking grains is not one of the Ten Commandments in the Bible nor is it a commandment of the Trim Healthy Mama Plan. Old-fashioned oatmeal is a budget-friendly food, an all-American staple, and has weight-loss merits due to its slow-burning energy fuel. Many Trim Healthy Mamas have lost countless pounds without bothering to soak oatmeal overnight.

Soaking does have its merits, though. Serene soaks all her grains, simply because she wants to make all her grains as digestible as she can for her family—and, let's face it, she's a sucker for extra steps. Check out her recipe for Super Prepared Purist Grains (found in the "Good Morning Grains" chapter of the *Trim Healthy Mama Cookbook*), which she soaks with rye flour or sourdough starter. Pearl mostly does not worry about soaking her oatmeal but does make sure to eat all her bread fermented or sprouted, to protect her blood-sugar health.

As part of a widely varied diet, grains and beans still have plenty of nutrition to offer you even if you never soak them. A bowl of unsoaked oatmeal will not leave you depleted of minerals. As a Trim Healthy Mama, your diet will be rich in vitamin C from lots of greens and berries, which counteracts any problems with phytate binding with minerals in your grains, beans, seeds, and nuts.

E FOODS LIST

E-FRIENDLY MEAT
- Avoid fatty meats and eat freely from all of the following lean meats:
  - Chicken breast
  - Tuna packed in water
  - Salmon (both wild-caught and most pouch or canned forms are fine; farm-raised may have more fat, so look for less than 5 grams of fat)

- All other fish (not fried)
- Venison
- Turkey breast
- Lean ground turkey or chicken (96% to 99% lean)
- Lean deli meats (natural brands are best)
- Ground meats with higher fat levels can be browned, drained, and then rinsed very well with hot water and used in E meals in up to four-ounce portions (see page 188 for further directions).

E-FRIENDLY EGG SOURCES
- Egg whites (both fresh and carton egg whites; products like Egg Beaters are also acceptable)
- Note: It is best to leave whole eggs to S settings.

E-FRIENDLY DAIRY
- 0% plain Greek yogurt (Triple Zero stevia-sweetened Greek yogurt by Oikos is also on plan)
- Low-fat or nonfat regular (not Greek) plain yogurt
- Plain low-fat or nonfat kefir
- 1% cottage cheese (2% is fine for purists who cannot find 1% that fits their standards)
- Reduced-fat ricotta cheese (keep to ¼ cup servings in E settings, as even the reduced-fat varieties have more fat than cottage cheese)
- Skim mozzarella cheese (garnish amounts only)
- Reduced-fat 2% hard cheeses (garnish amounts only)
- Laughing Cow Creamy Light Swiss cheese wedges (these are also on the "Personal Choice" list, since they are not a usual choice for purists)

E-FRIENDLY GRAINS
- Brown rice—up to ¾ cup cooked per serving
- Quinoa—up to ¾ cup cooked per serving
- Whole barley—up to ¾ cup cooked per serving
- Farro—up to ¾ cup cooked per serving
- Oatmeal—up to 1¼ cups cooked per serving

- Whole-grain bread: 2-piece servings in sprouted, artisan sourdough, or dark rye form (Note: Some sprouted breads, such as Trader Joe's, have lower carb counts, but they are still completely grain based, so they need to be kept to E meals, not S meals.)
- Sprouted tortilla—1 large tortilla
- Sprouted whole-grain flours
- Sprouted whole-grain pasta (This is best used in side dishes rather than as a main dish with spaghetti sauce, where you might be tempted to have two bowls full. Save huge bowls of pasta for Not-Naughty-Noodles.)
- Light Rye, Fiber, or Flax Seed Wasa crackers—up to 4 crackers
- Multi Grain, Hearty, Whole Grain, or Sourdough Wasa crackers—2 to 3 crackers (most Ryvita crackers will be fine for E meals, too)
- Popcorn—4 to 5 cups of popped kernels
- Baked blue corn chips (use to top chili or soup; don't overdo)

E-FRIENDLY FRUIT
- All fruits in moderate quantities, for example, 1 apple, 1 orange, 1 peach, 1 generous slice of canteloupe (very high glycemic fruits like bananas and watermelon are best not overdone; best to stick to 1 cup of watermelon or half of a large banana, or one small)
- All berries in liberal quantities
- 1 tablespoon all-fruit jelly for use with Greek yogurt or on Trim Healthy Pancakes found in the "Pancakes, Donuts, Crepes, and Waffles" chapter of the *Trim Healthy Mama Cookbook* (This type of jelly usually does contain some fruit juice concentrate but it is minimal. Please stay away from drinking fruit juice.)

E-FRIENDLY BEANS AND LEGUMES
- All beans and legumes, including lentils and split peas (stick to 1 cup densely packed cooked, but more can be eaten when liquid is involved, as in chili, or lentil or chana dal soup)

E-FRIENDLY VEGGIES
- All veggies except potatoes (save potatoes for occasional Crossover meals)
- Sweet potatoes—1 medium sweet potato
- Carrots, both raw and cooked

E-FRIENDLY OILS

- 1 teaspoon oil (exception of 2 teaspoons MCT oil on occasion, explained on page 44)

E-FRIENDLY NUTS

- Limit nuts to garnish amounts or 1 teaspoon nut butters (you can use 1 to 2 tablespoons of Pressed Peanut Flour in an E setting)

E-FRIENDLY CONDIMENTS

- Mustard
- Horseradish sauce
- Hot sauce (prepared without sugar)
- Low-fat dressings (homemade or store-bought)
- Mayo—up to 1 teaspoon or just a smear (you can mix 1 teaspoon with Greek yogurt for a nice sandwich spread)
- Soy sauce/tamari/Bragg Liquid Aminos/Coconut Aminos
- All vinegars
- All spices prepared without sugar or needless fillers
- Unsweetened cocoa powder
- Nutritional yeast
- All skimmed stock and broth prepared without sugar

E-FRIENDLY HEALTHY SPECIALTY ITEMS

- Pristine Whey Protein Powder (www.trimhealthymama.com)
- Integral Collagen (www.trimhealthymama.com)
- Just Gelatin (www.trimhealthymama.com)
- Glucomannan "Gluccie" Organic Fiber Supplement (www.trimhealthymama.com); nonorganic also available
- Plan-approved natural sweeteners: see page 103 for guidelines (www.trimhealthymama.com)
- Trim Healthy Mama Baking Blend (www.trimhealthymama.com)
- Pressed Peanut Flour (www.trimhealthymama.com)
- Not-Naughty-Noodles and Not-Naughty-Rice (www.trimhealthymama.com)

- Unsweetened nut milks, such as almond, cashew, or flaxseed (canned coconut milk is not E-friendly)
- Check out Chapter 18, "Specialty Food Stars" (page 140), in which we give descriptions and benefits of many of the above products and tell you what to look for in other brands or how to seek locally if you don't want to purchase online.

E-FRIENDLY "PERSONAL CHOICE" ITEMS

- Joseph's low-carb pita or lavash bread (these are not a significant carb source; add beans or fruit for an E meal)
- Low-carb tortillas (these are not a significant carb source; add beans or fruit in an E meal)
- Fat-free Reddi-wip—don't overdo (avoid light or fat-free Cool Whip due to the inclusion of high-fructose corn syrup)
- Laughing Cow Creamy Light Swiss cheese wedges
- Dreamfields pasta (Limit to once a week, and assess your own reaction to this pasta. Although current nutritional information displays this as a significant carb source, the resistant starch may not amount to enough glucose for an E meal. Add beans or fruit if desiring E.)
- Light Progresso soups (excluding "cream of" versions; add sprouted or soured bread on the side if desiring E)

chapter 5

....

FUEL PULLS (FP FOR SHORT)

These are the wonderful, lighter foods that round out your plate and make your S and E meals complete. A quick recap from Chapter 1: Fuel Pulls are lower in calories and, as their name suggests, they have insufficient amounts of either fats or carbs to swing a meal one way or the other—to either S or E.

We'll soon explain how Fuel Pulls make excellent snacks and desserts; but sometimes they are also used as full meals. Huh? "Isn't the whole premise of Trim Healthy Mama focused on having your main meals contain the nourishing primary fuels our bodies need to thrive?" you wisely ask. Yes, but some of us can actually benefit from some complete Fuel Pull meals thrown into the S and E juggle.

Changing up your fuels on plan helps to keep your metabolism revving, but another weight-loss trick is to also change up caloric loads in meals. S meals are usually the highest-calorie meals on the plan. Don't let that scare you: Despite being higher in calories, they are weight-loss friendly. E meals often have a somewhat lighter calorie count than S meals, so that is a nice changeup; but Fuel Pulls take the count way, way down. Smattering these meals into the plan can cause faster weight loss, so they are a benefit to some people carrying stubborn weight, such as postmenopausal pounds. Other issues, such as severely imbalanced sex and thyroid hormones, can sometimes make the best of weight-loss plans impossible. Healthy caloric loads that most of us can burn through with ease become too hard a task for women afflicted with these issues.

Including some Fuel Pull meals within the healthy environment of lots of S and E meals will allow your body to also get a benefit from these lighter calorie loads, without lowering the metabolism. When created smartly, Fuel Pulls can be ultra-filling. Even though the calorie count might be low, your tummy won't know it. But WARNING: If overdone, they will backfire on you. Take your calories down too low, too often, and your very smart body will catch on and turn down its metabolic fire. It will think you are starving it. Also, Fuel Pulls are not as nourishing as your parent S and E meals are, so they MUST NOT be your constant.

Some of us (not pregnant or nursing women) throw in a couple to a few of these Fuel Pull meals each week. For instance, our Fat-Stripping Frappa recipe (in the "Shakes, Smoothies, Frappas, and Thin Thicks" chapter of the *Trim Healthy Mama Cookbook*) is a popular Fuel Pull recipe. It is a gigantic, full quart of chocolaty, creamy yumminess despite a very low calorie count. It can be a full breakfast or even lunch if desired, or it can be used as an afternoon snack. Full Fuel Pull meals are not necessary for all people on the plan. Some people on plan only ever use FP foods to round out their plates and as snacks and desserts. We're all different and your own THM journey will not look the same as someone else's. Some with stubborn weight may want to try up to one Fuel Pull meal per day if they cannot lose on S and E meals alone. Check out Chapter 24, "Heads Up: Turtle Losers!" (page 214), to find out how much is too much when it comes to these Fuel Pull meals and how they can help you rather than harm you.

There will be many more examples of FP meals as you keep reading through the book, but here is a quick description of what a FP evening meal might be:

A generous amount of stir-fried veggies with slices of lean chicken breast tossed
 in a sweet-and-spicy Asian sauce
Not-Naughty-Noodles (optional; to really beef up the quantity on your plate)

Here's what an FP meal looks like on a seesaw:

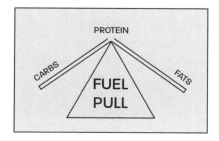

BUILD YOUR FIRST FP MEAL

This can be done in three easy steps:

1. Choose your protein. It must be lean and this is the only time we restrict you to 3 to 4 ounces of lean meat due to caloric load (or choose from Integral Collagen, Just Gelatin, or Pristine Whey Protein).
2. Add minimal fat (roughly 1 teaspoon—the same as E meals). Coconut and MCT oils are preferred due to their metabolism revving abilities, but are not mandatory.
3. Add other Fuel Pull foods to your plate: GENEROUS amounts of non-starchy veggies, moderate amounts of berries, and optional lean dairy (check out the Fuel Pull Food List on page 58).

In practical terms this might look like:

Breakfast—Large egg-white scramble or omelet loaded with veggies. Choose from non-starchies like mushrooms, grated summer squash or zucchini, onions, tomatoes, peppers, and spinach. Use coconut oil spray on a well-seasoned or nonstick skillet. Non-purists may enjoy extremely light cheeses, such as Laughing Cow Creamy Light Swiss cheese wedges, in the scramble or omelet.

Lunch—Sandwich or wrap made with one of our homemade Fuel Pull breads like Swiss Bread or Wonder Wraps (in the "Breads and Pizza Crusts" chapter in the *Trim Healthy Mama Cookbook*) or a store-bought FP option such as a Joseph's pita. Fill the sandwich with lean meats or tuna and succulent non-starchies such as tomatoes, cucumbers, lettuce, and onion. Smear with mustard, a hint of mayo combined with Greek yogurt if desired, or horseradish sauce, or spritz with extra-virgin olive oil and drizzle with vinegar.

Dinner—Citrus-Baked Tilapia with wilted greens and tomatoes. Fill up further with a Salted Caramel Fat-Stripping Frappa (found in the "Shakes, Smoothies, Frappas, and Thin Thicks" chapter in the *Trim Healthy Mama Cookbook*).

FUEL PULLS AS SNACKS

Fuel Pulls really shine as slimming snacks and desserts. Due to their limited fuel, they aren't likely to cause a tandem-fueling effect no matter the fuel of your next meal. They're like Switzerland—completely neutral and friends with everyone.

Let's say it is four thirty in the afternoon. You've rushed home from errands and are in desperate need of a snack. Your next meal needs to be ready within two hours but you haven't decided yet whether it will be an S or an E. Eating a snack of 0% Greek yogurt (FP) with some raspberries (FP) will tide you over without messing with the fuel of your next meal. To explain further, you'll soon learn in Chapter 8, "Let's Get Started!" (page 71), that you need time (roughly three hours) between meals when switching up fuels. What if you'd grabbed an E snack of an apple for a quick late-afternoon snack but then chose to eat an S meal of chicken and veggies in a cream-based sauce at six o'clock? You'd be tandem fueling—not a horrible thing, but not very weight-loss friendly. Fuel Pull snacks can help you avoid having an accidental Crossover like that.

FUEL PULLS AS DESSERTS

While we all get to enjoy cheesecakes and whipped cream as desserts on plan, the lighter Fuel Pull desserts should not be left out. You've already fueled your body with a main meal. Continuously slapping more fuel on top of that can be a weight-loss hindrance. Tummy Tucking Ice Cream, Cottage Berry Whip, Butterfly Wings Cake, and puddings—these are just a few of the light and lovely Fuel Pull dessert recipes you can choose from "Sweet Treats" in the *Trim Healthy Mama Cookbook.*

And now it's quiz time:

Question: What happens if you have a Fuel Pull dessert after an S meal?
Answer:
A. You break out in hives.
B. Your body thanks you for not overloading it with excess fuel and continues chugging on the Trim Train.

C. You do a crossword puzzle.

D. You notice your floor needs mopping.

Okay, these quizzes are getting way ridiculous. The answer is B, but you knew that!

FUEL PULL FOOD LIST

FUEL PULL FRIENDLY MEAT (SIMILAR TO E GUIDELINES EXCEPT E MEALS DO NOT LIMIT MEAT PORTION)

- Keep lean meat portions to 3 to 4 ounces; avoid fatty meats.
  - Chicken breast
  - Tuna packed in water
  - Salmon (both wild-caught and most pouch or canned forms are fine; farm-raised may have more fat, so look for less than 5 grams of fat)
  - All other fish (not fried)
  - Venison
  - Turkey breast
  - Lean ground turkey or chicken (96% to 99% lean)
  - Lean deli meats (natural brands are best)
- Ground meats with higher fat levels can be browned, drained, then rinsed well with hot water and used in FP meals in up to 4-ounce portions (see page 188 for further directions).

FUEL PULL FRIENDLY EGG SOURCES (SIMILAR TO E GUIDELINES)

- Egg whites (both carton egg whites and products like Egg Beaters are also acceptable)
- Note: It is best to leave whole eggs to S settings.

FUEL PULL FRIENDLY DAIRY (SIMILAR TO E GUIDELINES)

- 0% plain Greek yogurt (Triple Zero stevia-sweetened Greek yogurt by Oikos is also on plan)
- 1% cottage cheese (2% is fine for purists who cannot find 1% that fits their standards)
- Low-fat ricotta cheese

- Skim mozzarella cheese (garnish amounts only)
- Reduced-fat 2% hard cheeses (garnish amounts only)
- Laughing Cow Creamy Light Swiss cheese wedges (these are also on the list of Fuel Pull Friendly "Personal Choice" Items on page 60, since they are not a usual choice for purists)

FUEL PULL FRIENDLY VEGGIES (SIMILAR TO S MEALS)

- Be liberal with all non-starchy veggies in Fuel Pull meals. Non-starchy vegetables include asparagus, broccoli, cabbage, cauliflower, cucumber, eggplant, mushrooms, jicama, okra, tomatoes, yellow squash, zucchini, sugar snap peas, onions, green onions, leeks, parsley, all leafy greens, radishes, spaghetti squash, pumpkin, chestnuts, and baby Chinese corn (there are many more). Limit butternut and acorn squash to ½-cup amounts in Fuel Pull meals.
- Note: Starchy vegetables, such as potatoes, corn, sweet potatoes, turnips, and cooked carrots, should be avoided in Fuel Pull meals (small amounts of cooked carrots in stir-fry recipes should be okay).

FUEL PULL FRIENDLY FRUIT (SIMILAR TO S MEALS)

- Up to 1 cup of all kinds of berries can be used in FP meals but keep blueberries to ½ cup, as they have more fruit sugars than other berries (Note: You don't have to always use a full cup; ¼- to ½-cup amounts of berries are just fine in FP meals and don't push carb limits as high.)
- Avoid other fruits except lemons and limes.

FUEL PULL GRAINS AND BEANS (SLIGHTLY MORE LENIENT THAN S MEALS SINCE FAT IS NOT A PLAYER)

- 2 Light Rye Wasa or Ryvita crackers
- Up to ¼ cup beans or oats

FUEL PULL FRIENDLY OILS (SIMILAR TO E MEALS)

- 1 teaspoon oil (exception of 2 teaspoons MCT oil, explained on page 44)

FUEL PULL FRIENDLY NUTS (SIMILAR TO E MEALS)

- Limit nuts to garnish amounts or 1 teaspoon for nut butters.

FUEL PULL FRIENDLY CONDIMENTS (SIMILAR TO E MEALS)

- Mustard
- Horseradish sauce
- Hot sauce (prepared without sugar)
- Low-fat dressings (homemade or store-bought)
- Mayo—up to 1 teaspoon or just a smear
- Soy sauce/tamari/Bragg Liquid Aminos/Coconut Aminos
- All vinegars
- All spices prepared without sugar or needless fillers
- Unsweetened cocoa powder

FUEL PULL FRIENDLY HEALTHY SPECIALTY ITEMS (SIMILAR TO E MEALS)

- Pristine Whey Protein Powder (www.trimhealthymama.com)
- Integral Collagen (www.trimhealthymama.com)
- Just Gelatin (www.trimhealthymama.com)
- Glucomannan "Gluccie" Organic Fiber Supplement (www.trimhealthymama.com); nonorganic version also available
- Plan-approved sweeteners; see page 103 for guidelines (www.trimhealthymama.com)
- Trim Healthy Mama Baking Blend (www.trimhealthymama.com)
- Pressed Peanut Flour (www.trimhealthymama.com)
- Not-Naughty-Noodles or Not-Naughty-Rice (www.trimhealthymama.com)
- Unsweetened nut milks, such as almond, cashew, or flaxseed (canned coconut milk is not Fuel Pull friendly unless small amounts of the light variety are used)

FUEL PULL FRIENDLY "PERSONAL CHOICE" ITEMS

- Joseph's low-carb pita or lavash bread
- Low-carb tortillas
- Fat-free Reddi-wip—don't overdo (avoid lighter fat-free Cool Whip due to the inclusion of high-fructose corn syrup)
- Laughing Cow Creamy Light Swiss cheese wedges
- Light Progresso soups (excluding "cream of" versions)

CROSSOVERS (XO FOR SHORT)

With Crossovers, you can bring back the pairs of grain-based bread and butter, oatmeal and cream, beans and cheese, baked blue corn chips and guacamole—yee-ha! Crossovers merge the two fuels of fats and carbs together for healthy tandem fueling. They keep to the E guidelines of carbs and add as many fats as desired. Of course . . . they're always anchored by protein.

Crossovers are not CHEATS—please don't let them hear you calling them that. You are not going off plan when you choose a—or even have an accidental—Crossover. They are kind to your blood sugar, but for most people they are not weight-loss meals.

Here's what a Crossover breakfast may look like:

Scrambled eggs with melted cheese
2 slices of sprouted or artisan sourdough whole-grain toast with butter

Here's what a Crossover looks like on a seesaw.

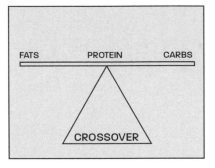

FATS   PROTEIN   CARBS

CROSSOVER

BUILD YOUR FIRST CROSSOVER MEAL

This can be done in four easy steps:

1. Choose your protein: lean or fatty meat or fish, such as chicken with skin for fatty or without skin for lean, whole eggs and egg whites, cultured dairy products (or choose from Integral Collagen, Just Gelatin, or Pristine Whey Protein).
2. Add fats as desired. Even if your protein source contains fat, other fats can be added to the meal.
3. Add your carb in E meal safe amounts: fruit, gentle whole grains, beans/legumes, or sweet potatoes.
4. Add optional Fuel Pull foods to your plate, such as non-starchy veggies, berries, and certain forms of dairy (check out the Fuel Pull Food List on page 58).

In practical terms, this might look like:

Breakfast—Your protein might be Pristine Whey Protein or Integral Collagen in an orange creamsicle smoothie that includes a full orange and your choice of superfoods such as full-fat coconut milk or coconut butter, an optional pastured egg yolk, flaxseeds or chia seeds—or even a swirl of heavy cream.

Lunch—Your protein might be a burger made with beef or venison on a split sprouted bun, stuffed with all the goodies including cheese, mayo, and avocado—yum!

Dinner—Baked chicken with skin, side salad with creamy or oil-based dressing, and an E-size portion of stir-fried brown rice.

WHO NEEDS CROSSOVERS?

There are the rare few people who will eat only Crossovers for their entire THM journey. Who is in this minority? High-metabolism folk, you know who you are—sitting there struggling to keep five pounds on rather than off. You probably get a lot of jokes from others saying they wish they had your problem, but it can actually be a serious struggle for you. The temptation for you is to give in to eating high-carb or sugary foods because you think you can or even need to. Spiking your blood sugar is not solving the problem, it is just adding another one. Keep protein-centered Crossovers in for all your meals and if you still cannot put on or maintain weight, include a tablespoon of raw honey and pure butter at every meal. Natural, sugar-free peanut butter before bed won't hurt, either!

Next on the list of those needing mostly Crossovers are growing children without weight problems. They will thrive beautifully on these meals and maintain healthy blood-sugar levels, which are important for their brain growth and function in early years, for their hormones as they near puberty, and for avoiding insulin resistance in adulthood. Reminding children to always consume nourishing amounts of protein at every meal and teaching them to keep carbohydrates in safe zones is teaching them healthy, healing habits for life.

Pregnant and nursing women, as well as maintenance Mamas, won't have to use Crossovers at every meal but will benefit from sprinkling them in with regular S and E meals. See Chapter 23, "Heads Up: Pregnant and Nursing Mamas!" (page 199), and Chapter 27, "Heads Up: Maintenance Mamas!" (page 249), respectively, for more details on how to include Crossovers.

Now for the rest of us.

CROSSOVERS DURING WEIGHT LOSS?

They're bound to happen especially when you are learning your THM ropes and you somehow merge your S's and E's. No biggie. This happens to all of us when we start. But even intentional Crossovers during weight-loss mode are okay sometimes. You won't want to include them too often, but having a Crossover every now and then can add to the metabolic fire in your body by changing things up once again. Before goal weight is reached, you could even play with one or two Crossovers a week; but this is completely up to you, and if it stalls or slows you down too much, just go back to the basics of the weight-loss part of this plan and remain true to S and E meals until you are at or closer to goal weight.

It's quiz time again:

Question: The following list contains three complete cheats and one true Crossover. Which is the XO?
Answer:
A. Burger and fries
B. Meatball sub on regular wheat bread
C. Sautéed salmon, baked sweet potato fries made with coconut or red palm oil, and Greek salad
D. Processed, sugar-sweetened cereal with whole milk

Okay that was too easy, of course you picked C. So let's ramp up the challenge with something trickier.

Question: Which one is the Crossover?
Answer:
A. 1½ cups brown rice with grilled chicken and a lemon butter sauce
B. Sweet potato with melted butter, salad with creamy dressing, and an 8-ounce sirloin steak
C. Lasagna made with whole-wheat noodles
D. Three slices whole-wheat toast with peanut butter

If you picked A, you've gone over your rice quota. Remember, even brown rice can get a little bullish on your blood sugar when not reigned in. A true Crossover would stick to the three-quarter-cup brown rice limit, keep in the chicken and sauce, but include veggies on the side if you wanted to fill up further.

If you picked C, those flour-based noodles are not going to do your blood sugar any favors. Lasagna is easily converted to a delicious S-style meal using spinach, zucchini, eggplant, or layered Wonder Wraps as the noodles. Wonderwrapful Lasagna and Lazy Lasagna are two delicious S recipes in the "Oven Dishes" chapter in the *Trim Healthy Mama*

Cookbook. If you eat an S lasagna, you can turn your meal into a Crossover, by having a garlic-buttered sprouted dinner roll or two on the side.

D? You learned in your E meal list that two slices of plan-approved, grain-based bread is a healthy maximum we want you to keep to. We understand that two pieces of bread often come in well under forty-five grams of carbs. We want to teach you not to be a "Bready." Bready Mamas don't have a limit; the toaster starts popping and keeps on going. The two-piece max is bread-sane, a simple wise habit to practice. If you do desire extra carbs in your Crossover, add a piece of fruit—and enjoy!

So there you have it, the answer is B, and it's making us hungry!

chapter 7
S HELPERS (SH FOR SHORT)

This is a quick little chapter because you already know what an S meal is. Basically all you need to know is that you add a little more carb to your meal for pleasure's sake, but don't add so much that it becomes a Crossover meal. The S Helper is worth getting to know after you make some progress in your weight-loss journey. It is an optional little blesser. We call it an S Helper as opposed to a Hamburger Helper *(giggle),* and it makes life a little more fun and freeing.

Here is an example of what an S Helper breakfast might look like.

Two or three fried eggs in butter on one piece of sprouted or artisan sourdough toast with hot sauce and optional cheese sprinkles

In practical terms, S Helper meals may look a little sumpin' like this:

Breakfast—Your protein might be a breakfast sausage with sautéed mushrooms, onions, tomatoes, and ⅓ cup cooked quinoa, all tossed together in butter or coconut oil.

Lunch—Your protein might be grilled chicken on a large leafy green salad topped with half an avocado, an olive oil–based vinaigrette, and a ¼ cup of brown rice.

Dinner—Your protein might be beef stew with one piece of buttered, sprouted bread or toast.

Here is what an S Helper looks like on a seesaw.

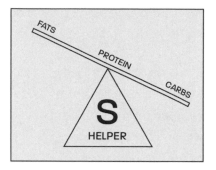

S HELPER SCIENCE

S Helper meals can still be used for weight loss but they do not work as well as your regular S meal. S Helpers allow for weight loss because they add just enough carbohydrate to your meal that your body is able to swiftly burn through it, yet still is able to burn more fuel (that is, body fat). Once you've burned the fat in your meal—you know the drill—you'll get down to the task of gnawing at your own adipose tissue.

WHO IS BENEFITED BY S HELPERS?

- Those who are happier with a little more carb tagged onto an S meal and who do not mind a slower weight-loss journey
- The rare person who loses weight too quickly on regular S and E meals. This weight loss cannot be gauged by the scale, but by whether your skin, mood, and hair are not responding well to the weight loss. In this case, you might want to slow it down a little.
- Pregnant and nursing women (see Chapter 23, "Heads Up: Pregnant and Nursing Mamas!," on page 199 for more details)
- Children with weight issues. They can incorporate pure S and E meals, some Crossovers, and also some S Helpers for a very gentle and super-nourishing weight-control approach.

- Those who suffer from severe hypoglycemia and find that regular S meals leave them a little shaky

Due to the fact that all meals on the Trim Healthy Mama Plan are solidly anchored with protein, even people who have suffered from hypoglycemia symptoms for years often experience a miraculous improvement on plan. But some people who may not be used to eating meals with lower amounts of carbs may at first find they need S Helpers to help their bodies gently adapt to the pure S meal.

Take this quiz:

Question: Which one of these people does not need S Helpers?
Answer:
A. Twenty-eight-year-old Suzanne, six months pregnant with baby number three
B. Fourteen-year-old prediabetic David, whose doctor wants him to control his rapidly climbing weight
C. Stressed-out Sasha, a THM newbie who feels a little shaky and light-headed after a long day at the office
D. Fifty-eight-year-old Lydia, who has forty stubborn postmenopausal pounds to lose.

Obviously, the answer is D. While Lydia can add some S Helpers to her diet here and there, too many S Helper meals might make her slow weight loss even slower.

S HELPER FOODS LIST

- Same list as S meals with the following additional options:
  - ⅓ to ½ cup quinoa
  - ¼ cup brown rice
  - ⅓ to ½ cup oatmeal
  - ⅓ to ½ cup beans or lentils
  - ½ piece of fruit, such as ½ apple or ½ orange
  - ½ sweet potato
  - 1 piece of whole-grain bread or toast in sprouted, dark rye, or artisan sourdough form
  - ½ sprouted wrap or tortilla

PART TWO

let's go

chapter 8

LET'S GET STARTED!

Now that you have a basic understanding of the different THM meals, you'll probably be either eager or terrified to put your new knowledge into action. Both reactions are okay. There is no right or wrong way to get started on your Trim Healthy journey. Whether you jump right in or just dip your toes in the water for a while before you slowly immerse, it will click at some point. But first, fair warning: There is a learning curve.

Not gonna lie, it takes a few weeks of practice living this out before you feel like you know the ropes. At first you'll second-guess yourself and worry about whether you're truly eating S or E or crossing over. Some days you'll wish you could throw the book at us! Hang in there. After some time this will just be like breathing in and breathing out; you really won't have to think much about it. It's like riding a bike or driving a car. It takes some focus and lots of practice at first but becomes second nature after time passes.

During the learning period you'll have lots of questions that relate to your unique THM journey. How many of each meal type should you eat? When and how will you change from S to E? Should you begin by jumping in or baby-stepping your way in slowly? How much should you eat? Must you throw out every bit of junk food from your cupboards in a frenzy? All these questions (and more) will be answered.

LEARN TO FREESTYLE

You're da boss! There is no one set way that you must change up your THM meals. We can't dictate how you should do it because that would be us shoving our own diet approach on you. Do it your way and you are going to create your own success. You'll do this by freestyling, which means you'll be changing up your own meals without a bunch of stringent rules from us. Everybody learns to freestyle differently. You don't have to switch your THM meal types in any synchronized order, such as S then E, then S. How boring!

What does your body feel like each day? Are you tired? Prepare an E meal and enjoy those energizing carbs. Are you craving comfort food, heartiness? Go with an S meal and enjoy those satisfying fats. Freestyling your meals like this gels perfectly with our Food Freedom approach. As long as you are incorporating a good mixup of each meal type each week, you are fine. You will receive all the nutrients you need.

Most of us in the Trim Healthy community like to include both meal types every day (with occasional Fuel Pull meals or Crossovers depending on individual needs). We might do an S breakfast, an E lunch, an FP or E afternoon snack, then a hearty S dinner followed by an FP dessert. Others of us are more structured and like to allot certain days for one meal style. Mondays might be E. Tuesday and Wednesday would be S. Thursday would be E, and so forth. Do what suits you best. That might take some trial and error. No biggie.

What sort of diet were you eating? Asking yourself this question can help you figure out which meal to start with. If you are coming from a standard American high-carb diet, our first meal of choice for you will be an S. You might even want to do a full day or two of these Satisfying meals to help get your blood sugar more under control and get a feel for how to build this type of meal. After that, don't hesitate to add our safely designed E meals so you can keep your metabolism revved by juggling your fuels.

If you are coming to Trim Healthy Mama from any sort of low-carb diet, your body is begging you for a different fuel; so please include E meals from the get-go.

FEELING OVERWHELMED?

A good way to start the plan without needless anxiety is to simply begin with breakfasts. Don't worry about all the other meals in your day just yet. Try some different S and E breakfasts for a few days before moving on to lunches and dinners. Enjoy a cheesy omelet or a Raspberry Cheesecake Smoothie (found in the "Shakes, Smoothies, Frappas, and Thin Thicks" chapter in the *Trim Healthy Mama Cookbook*) for S or something as simple as oatmeal, berries, and Greek yogurt. Trim Healthy Pancakes (found in the "Good

Morning Grains" chapter in the *Trim Healthy Mama Cookbook*) are another simple yet delicious E option. This "toe-dip" approach can help you gain confidence without a lot of frustration. Once you have a better grasp on breakfasts, slowly work your way to Trim Healthy lunches, then on to dinners. Pretty soon you'll be owning this thing!

CHOMPING AT THE BIT?

If you'd rather jump into the plan all at once on a Monday morning with two weeks' worth of perfectly planned menus and our food lists and seesaw pictures printed out and magneted to your fridge–that's okay, too. But don't get upset if you make mistakes along the way; we're sure you will! Just be aware that you'll probably mess up. Nobody does this perfectly in their first week and if that is going to make you feel like a big ol' failure after all the energy and hype you put into preparing, we'd rather you take it slower. Ditch the all-or-nothing, do-or-die approach. Passionate personalities are wonderful; Serene has one of those dive-in-without-looking-back approaches, while Pearl is more slow and cautious about change. No matter which type you are, forgive yourself when you mess up and keep up the mantra that this is a lifelong journey, not a race to shed fifty pounds.

MEAL SPACING BETWEEN DIFFERENT FUELS

When desiring weight loss, you need to remember to keep at least two and a half hours, three being more optimum, when switching from S to E meals or from E to S meals. This ensures that higher glycemic loads in E meals will not be digested along with the higher fats in S meals, which causes tandem fueling.

Don't get all uptight about this meal spacing. It will tend to happen quite naturally. Most meals and snacks (with the exception of desserts) are usually at least two and a half to three hours apart anyway. Eat your lunch at twelve? An afternoon snack sounds about perfect at three or three thirty. Evening meal at six or six thirty? That's a natural space that means you're right on time to eat again! We remind you of this three-hour window not only to help you avoid tandem fueling, but also because we don't want you to be grazing all day. Shoving little bites of food into your mouth every half hour or so is not a wise habit. We will cover that subject in more detail in Chapter 9, "Snacking Mama" (page 79).

One of the key principles of the Trim Healthy Mama Plan is to never let your body become famished between meals. You may not feel famished, and some of you may not even feel very hungry (especially if your metabolism has been lowered); but going longer than four hours without fueling can cause a catabolic state. This is when your body will start to break itself down (not your fat but your muscle), release cortisol, and lower metabolism. Remember to refuel the gas tank of your body every three to four hours.

This does not mean you have to dive into the kitchen at every twinge of hunger. Hunger pangs that occur less than a couple of hours after a meal (for non-nursing or pregnant women) are not true hunger pangs. They're usually only mind hunger pangs or entwined with emotional responses to life events. You are going to be "smart fed," not "feeling fed," as a Trim Healthy Mama. True hunger starts for most of us at the three- to four-hour mark (this can be sooner for pregnant or nursing women; see Chapter 23, "Heads Up: Pregnant and Nursing Mamas!" on page 199).

Allowing yourself to experience some of this true hunger is a healthy, natural state for the body and enables you to better enjoy your next meal or snack. Don't be scared of it, you won't have to be in that hungry state long and it sure won't be a constant like you've experienced with other diets. But if you are one who does not feel these normal hunger cues, practice eating at these wise three- to four-hour intervals whether you feel like it or not.

HUNGER HORMONES

There are two hormones that are in charge of your hunger and full signals: ghrelin and leptin. We can easily remember ghrelin's role because the word itself sounds like a hungry growl: It lets you know when you're hungry. That leaves leptin as the hormone that signals when you are full.

A signaling problem occurs with these two hormones when we become insulin resistant and, sadly, insulin resistance happens in varying degrees to most of us as we age. Those who have had more extreme high-carb lifestyles will often have more severe cases of insulin resistance. In this state of resistance, insulin levels are continually elevated and our cells become desensitized to the hormone. High insulin levels also create high leptin levels. You'd think that would be a good thing, right? Lots of "I'm full" signals? Sadly, no. When too much leptin is excreted we become desensitized to it as well. Picture it yelling red-faced to your brain that you are full. No response. The frequency is so high your brain can't hear it. (Only a bat can. Well, we just made up that part about the bat; but you get it.) Not until your insulin levels begin to settle will these two "hunger" and "full" hormones stabilize, at which point you'll hear their gentle nudge better than their roar.

PORTION SIZES

If we dictated every portion of your food, you'd never be able to tune in to the signals of these hunger and full hormones. If here and there we suggest serving sizes in a recipe in the companion cookbook, they are only guidelines not rules. Our ultimate goal for you is to learn to tune in and trust your own body: That is a part of the journey. Balancing these hunger and full hormones doesn't happen overnight.

In the real world this means you may very well overeat or undereat when you first start on the plan. Hey, give yourself a break. It's more than likely that you are either coming off the high-sugar roller coaster that we call "The Goliath" or some sort of extreme diet in which you were not able to make your own food decisions. You had to deny your own hunger and full signals so often that you finally got good at it. Give yourself time to learn to tune back in.

If you are coming from a high-carb lifestyle, insulin levels are going to take a while to stabilize. For some, that is a few weeks; for others a few months. In some cases it can take as long as a year to learn what being full truly feels like.

Don't worry, this doesn't mean you won't see any results during this time of healing. You'll be making strides in a better direction whether you can tell you are full or not—and we will not limit you to a half-inch slice of plan-approved cake during this time. Doing that would just be placing a Band-Aid on a wound that needs to breathe to heal. On the other hand, it is good to be mindful that if you feel like having a third piece of cake early in your journey, it is likely because you cannot hear leptin's signals telling you you've had enough. In this case you need to consciously tell yourself one generous piece is enough. That sort of mind talk is simply healthy practice—not self-starvation.

If you're coming from another rigid diet, such as a low-calorie or constant low-carb plan, your leptin levels may be too low rather than too high. That is just as big of a problem. Low leptin levels mean low energy, slow metabolism, and, in some cases, reproductive issues. Refueling your leptin levels through plenty of healthy E carb meals will help amp up the volume of this hormone to better balance.

Time will help as these bodily functions slowly come into balance again. We've had people beg us for harder portion sizes. Nope. If you are going to do this for life, you have to learn to tune in to you, not to us. We will have some portion suggestions to help you at the beginning while you are in your THM infancy, but we want you to grow and become independent. In the end, you'll be the expert on your own body and that is the way it should be.

BEWARE OF FUEL RUTS!

Don't get bogged down in dangerous fuel ruts. This is when you take one type of meal (usually S, because Mamas love their fats) and repeat it over and over and over again. Abusing S meals that way turns our wonderful THM fuel juggle into another low-carb diet, and that is NOT the Trim Healthy Mama Plan. Have a piece of fruit, for goodness sake! Sorry, getting a bit feisty here; but please, PLEASE do not think you are doing Trim Healthy Mama if basically all you are eating are S meals. They are an important but not complete part of the picture. This type of fuel rut will eventually stall your weight loss, stress your adrenals, and be a meanie to your thyroid. We get it, S meals with their rich fats are extremely appealing. We love them, too. But E meals have their own special satisfaction. Get creative with E meals; they have so much to offer. You'll find your favorites and your body will delight in the changeup.

This doesn't mean you have to eat just as many E meals per week as you do S meals. Thankfully, S meals are not completely carb-free, either. They do have those extremely gentle carbs in the form of non-starchy veggies, berries, nuts, and even some dairy, so having more of this type of meal than E meals won't be dangerous for your body. We personally tend to have more S suppers than we do E suppers, as Satisfying evening meals are such hearty, family-friendly supper fare. But there is "more" and then there is "way more." The latter is a problem.

We don't like to put hard numbers on things because freestyling is at the heart of the

Trim Healthy Mama Plan, but if you have to push us into a corner, the minimum amount of E meals we recommend per week would be five—okay, maybe four; but you'd better be having some E snacks, then! This is minimum, not necessarily optimum. You may have a physically active life and need more Energizing fuels than someone who is sitting in an office all day. Many Trim Healthy Mamas find they do extremely well including one E meal per day and often choose to make it a breakfast or lunch. Think about it: Including one E meal per day means you have two other meals that you can make S meals if you prefer. Never overdo a good thing, though.

Remember, the key to Trim Healthy Mama weight loss is juggling fuels. So if you're an E lover, sure, have a few more of those than S meals; but don't stay in E land constantly, either.

There, lecture done. Oops, hold on! Don't you dare get into a Fuel Pull rut! Fuel Pull meals play a role, but if you're having more of those than S and E meals we may have to pay you a visit and give you a Serene and Pearl intervention—which won't be pretty! Massive stop sign for Fuel Pull ruts, as that will be a surefire way to ruin your metabolism!

BEAT THE BAD DAYS

Learning anything new can be challenging at times. You may need to open up your mind to different foods, textures, and shades of sweetness. This can take some mind adjustment. You might be in the kitchen a little more until you learn a few recipes that become your quick go-to favorites. You probably won't love every new recipe, but you ARE going to fall in love with some of them. Don't let a few failures and setbacks cause you to throw in the towel. When you started to learn to walk as an infant, you fell down a lot, but there was no giving up! Take a page from your one-year-old self, brush yourself off, and get up again. You can do this!

If a cruel little voice inside your head whispers, "This is too hard," consider what Pam Graham wrote in her testimony after losing one hundred pounds with Trim Healthy Mama: "I've heard some people say this plan is too hard—the food too expensive (I disagree but understand what you are saying). I say being overweight and being unhealthy is MUCH TOO HARD! Being overweight and unhealthy is MUCH TOO EXPENSIVE! Choose your hard while you can, friends . . . choose your hard!"

SUMMARY

- Learn to freestyle by changing up your core Satisfying, Energizing, and Fuel Pull meals each week according to your own desires and challenges.

- If change feels too overwhelming, start practicing the plan with breakfast meals first.

- Don't go longer than four hours without eating. It is best to fuel your body every three to four hours.

- Make sure to leave two and a half to three hours between S and E when switching fuels so tandem fueling doesn't occur.

- Learn to tune in and trust your own body when it comes to hunger and full signals and portion sizes. Give yourself time and grace to become better at this.

- Avoid fuel ruts.

chapter 9
SNACKING MAMA

Diets that cut out snacking are Big Old Meanies. They're not only robbing you of the chance to enjoy more food, they're robbing your metabolism of fire. But there is a difference between smart snacking and mindless, silly snacking that will be detrimental to your journey. Grazing and gobbling all day is not wise snacking. Let's take a look at two women early in their journeys of THM. We don't want you to fall into their traps.

GRAZING GRACE

Grace starts her day with an S breakfast of a big ol' cheesy omelet and a nice mug of coffee with cream. Well done, Grace! An hour or so later she's cleaning up breakfast dishes, putting food away, and notices the almonds in the cupboard. Cue the dramatic music—alas, things take a downward turn for our heroine. A handful or two go in her mouth. Maybe not such a huge deal but soon after that, Grace sits down to return e-mails, and that's always more fun with another cup of creamy coffee and some Skinny Chocolate from the "Candies and Bars" chapter in the *Trim Healthy Mama Cookbook* or some store-bought stevia-sweetened chocolate. Late morning, Grace rushes out to do some errands and goes prepared with some string cheese in her purse for her toddler. Three-year-old Tommy gets to eat his string cheese in his car seat, and Mommy eats one—and another—while driving. All this occurs before lunch, but more grazing and gobbling continues throughout the day.

The sad truth is that Grace does not ever get to enjoy a proper snack. She is deprived of the memorable event itself. Her constant snatches of food every hour or so are all itsy-bitsy bites that only offer fleeting moments of pleasure and keep constant food fuel in her body. This makes it much harder for Grace's body to ever get around to using her own body fat as a fuel.

Preparing meals is another time when Grace veers off course. She wolfs down handfuls and bitefuls every time she cooks. Taste-testing dishes to check for flavor is fine, but it's very different from the several chomps and swallows of foods that Grace doesn't even realize she is eating. She's gobbling pieces of roast chicken as she cuts it up, snatching pieces of cheese that are supposed to top the family salad, wolfing down several steamed broccoli florets to see if they have enough butter and salt. As a Trim Healthy Mama, Grace does not have to count calories, but she can easily take in a few hundred calories' worth of food before she even sits down to a meal she's now sadly only halfway hungry for!

Grace never gets the chance to feel truly full or truly hungry. She shouldn't have to starve herself to make it to her next snack or meal, but that tug of true hunger is a natural, normal, and healthy feeling. It means her cells are emptying out and will soon require more fuel. Grace's body desperately needs the chance to have natural rest times from food. It is as if she constantly adds more clothes to a washing machine that is already in mid-cycle. This is only asking for digestive issues and a tougher time losing weight even if she keeps her meals on plan.

Times of eating, followed by times of not eating, are part of a natural, God-designed cycle. The scriptures in Ecclesiastes mention there is a time for everything, "a time to break down, and a time to build up." We don't build up fuel in our cells "whenever." That is a mindless approach. Just as we naturally breathe in, then breathe out, allowing our cells to empty out of fuel is equally important. This way the body gets a chance to use its own adipose tissue (fat) for fuel. This results in natural weight loss. Grace needs to give her body that chance!

"All-Day Sippers" such as Good Girl Moonshine and the Shrinker, recipes that can be found on YouTube or in the *Trim Healthy Mama Cookbook,* will help Grace with energy pickups and the hand-to-mouth satisfaction she is seeking through all-day grazing. Grace can then plan her snacks as onetime occasions between meals. They'll be more fulfilling, much more memorable, and easier on her waistline. You can do it, Grace!

THREE MEAL MANDY

Meet Mandy. She's an early riser and loves the morning stillness of a quiet house before everyone else rises. By six thirty A.M., after quiet time, she is ready for breakfast since she'll have to be out the door soon. She loves an E breakfast of Trim Healthy Pancakes (in the

"Good Morning Grains" chapter of the *Trim Healthy Mama Cookbook*) with blueberries and a little Greek yogurt, but she doesn't get a lunch break until noon, which is more than five hours after her morning meal. She packs on-plan lunches such as egg salad in a Joseph's pita with a couple of stalks of celery smeared with some peanut butter. Delish! But it will be close to six P.M. before she gets back to her slow-cooker meal of salsa chicken topped with shredded cheese and sour cream and a side salad. That's close to six hours between meals again. Cue the dramatic music once more: All is not well with this scene.

Mandy's long periods of five to six hours between meals can put her body in a catabolic state. This means her muscles break down and her metabolism slows for survival as her body wonders when the next meal is coming. Mandy may want to consider taking a container of stevia-sweetened Greek yogurt for a mid-morning snack and a Chocolate Chai-Glazed Cinnamon Muffin (found in the "Family Muffins" chapter of the *Trim Healthy Mama Cookbook*) for an afternoon snack. If she doesn't eat a mid-morning snack that might be okay—we are all different—but she absolutely needs that afternoon fuel. Making sure that afternoon snack is centered on protein is key. She can take one of our All-Day Sipper drinks with her, too (check out the videos on our website for some of those), so she stays better hydrated throughout her day. She'll notice better energy levels and will be able to focus more easily because her brain will thrive on the fuel from the snack and the hydration from the sipper. She may find her appetite slowly increasing as she includes snacks, but this is often a good sign of a perking metabolism.

HOW TO SPACE SNACKS

If you're an early riser like Mandy, you're more likely to need a snack mid-morning than those who get up later and wait a while before having breakfast. If you're eating breakfast at seven A.M., have a small snack at ten A.M. An apple with a teaspoon of peanut butter would be a great E choice; or try the recipe for Fuel Pull Peanut Junkie Butter found in "Condiments and Extras" in the *Trim Healthy Mama Cookbook*. Your mid-morning snack does not need to be huge. You'll be ready to eat again around one P.M. and, given that three hours will have passed, you can choose to have either an S or an E lunch. If you want to have an E lunch at noon, that's okay: You're still in E mode so there will be no collision of fuels and you'll have a moderate space of two hours between eating.

Remember that the THM guideline to put some fuel in your body every three to four hours is not a strict rule to make you miserable, but a wise guideline. You don't have to obsessively watch the clock, just be mindful of the time between fueling. Sometimes, life's circumstances won't allow you to stick to the three- to four-hour mark—don't sweat that. The time between snacks and meal times can sometimes be less than three to four hours if you use the same fuel for both or if your snack is a Fuel Pull. Fuel Pull snacks and desserts are wonderful bridges between meals. If your natural snack times get thrown off schedule and they land closer to your next meal, Fuel Pulls can be a perfect solution so you don't cross over accidentally if switching from S to E. But remember that Fuel Pull snacks are not freebies to be grazed on all day. Take a lesson from Grazing Grace and allow your body those wonderful digestive rest times.

Some of us don't like to eat as soon as we wake in the morning. We love to savor our coffee first for an hour or so. This means we'll eat a later breakfast and skip the mid-morning snack. That is fine, but do be sure to get a wonderful afternoon snack in. Honestly, who wouldn't want to eat a Volcano Mud Slide Muffin in the afternoon? You can find that free recipe on our website and in the "Quick, Single Serve Muffins" chapter of the companion cookbook. Even if you're a late-breakfast eater, never skip breakfast altogether. You need that protein in the morning to initiate balanced blood sugars throughout the day.

SAVOR YOUR SNACKS

If at all possible, sit down to eat your meals and snacks. Walking around eating or doing it while doing five other things barely lets your mind know you're eating. Take a deep breath, acknowledge you are actually eating. In wintertime, include a hot drink such as an herbal tea or a creamy coffee at snack time. It may help you savor the experience more. An icy on-plan drink with your snack in summer months can help you slow down more so you feel like, "I've eaten, I remember, I have relished!"

NIGHTTIME MUNCHIES

Late-night snacking can be a progress pitfall for some of us. This doesn't mean you can't have some dessert after supper, but snacking at ten P.M. unless you are pregnant or nursing isn't the wisest of nightly habits. You'll do it now and then—don't think we have a rule against it—but constant late-night snacking will get ya!

Too often it is a ravenous, fridge-searching instinct that sends you seeking only the foods classified as "no-no's" for late-night eating. Even if they are healthy and on plan, it seems to be the really rich decadent stuff that ends up being gobbled at night because when we are ultra-fatigued we lose our common sense.

Is it a simple stalk of celery with a smidge of peanut butter or a small swirl of Greek yogurt we turn to as the clock is about to strike twelve? No! It's a spoon and a jar of peanut butter or the impulsive desire for several pieces of freshly made bread and a tired Mama whose self-control went to sleep at nine o'clock! Anyone have an "Amen"? Cue the choir!

If you are truly extremely hungry in the evening, Fuel Pull snacks are your best option. Heavy S snacks right before bed offer your body too many calories when all it will be doing is sleeping. A delicious and sensible nighttime snack is our Cottage Berry Whip (you can find that free recipe on our website). Or if you are dairy-free, try some of the other lighter but still delicious treats from the *Trim Healthy Mama Cookbook,* such as Collagen Berry Whip and Tummy Tucking Ice Cream (in the "Frozen Treats" chapter) or a Choco Chip Baby Frap (in "Shakes, Smoothies, Frappas, and Thin Thicks"). These are all yummy and filling yet light in calories. Or have a Light Rye Wasa cracker or two topped with Laughing Cow Creamy Light Swiss cheese wedges and sliced cucumber. (If you are a purist or dairy-free, use the Laughin' Mama Cheese recipe in the "Condiments and Extras" chapter in the *Trim Healthy Mama Cookbook* in place of the Laughing Cow Creamy Light Swiss cheese.)

It's also important to realize that the different seasons of our lives call for different leniencies with nighttime snacking. Postmenopausal women may have a much harder time losing weight due to metabolism slowdown from lost hormones if heavy snacks are eaten later in the evening too often. If you are postmenopausal and have any nighttime snack at all, it would be better as a lighter Fuel Pull option. On the other spectrum, younger women who are either nursing through the night or pregnant will definitely need an evening snack that is rich in protein.

WHAT ABOUT DESSERT?

If you are a dessert lover, you don't have to wait a full three hours after your meal to eat it if it is the same fuel as your last meal or if it is a Fuel Pull option. But don't forget about what we keep insisting: Keep many of your desserts lighter. Heavy S desserts are a wonderful part of THM, but for some of us they are better eaten alone as an afternoon snack than constantly being tagged on to the end of a meal. We included lots of sweet Fuel Pull recipes in the *Trim Healthy Mama Cookbook* and we want you to make smart use of them. Desserts made with lots of almond flour and cream cheese can trip you up if eaten late at night after a big meal as they are so calorie dense. Some women (and plenty of men) lose weight just fine even enjoying frequent heavy S desserts after S meals, but we are all different. Get to know your body, and understand if you are one that needs to lighten up your desserts or save the richer kind for snacks between meals or even as a breakfast.

DON'T "ALL-OR-NOTHING" YOUR JOURNEY

Of course, you'll slip up sometimes. There is no avoiding eating on the run now and then; we all won't be able to space our meals and snacks perfectly every day, and most of us will eat too many heavy S desserts occasionally. But none of this means you've failed. Just keep going. Practice the art of healthy, natural meal spacing. It truly is an art and, like any skill, requires practice, time to master, and a determination to continue after failures. Learn to be more mindful of how you are snacking. Don't be so austere with your diet that you never enjoy a snack or eat enough to feel satisfied—that is the nemesis of this Food Freedom movement!

chapter 10

JUST THE NUMBERS

By now you have all the information you need to get started. But we all learn and process information differently. Maybe you're a numbers person and feel like you'll only fully "get" the plan when you have harder numbers to refer to. We'll provide those in this chapter but with a caution: Food types trump numbers!

The problem when people start trying to reduce Trim Healthy Mama to mere math formulas is that the heart of the plan can become lost in the equations. The simple "science" is that oatmeal is an E food, and peanut butter is an S food. You put them together and you have a Crossover. But if you get too number-centric, you might start counting, squeezing, and crunching numbers until you figure out that if you eat only a tiny portion size—say one-third cup of your oatmeal, peanut butter recipe—you can make that Crossover fit into Fuel Pull mode. You start calling your recipe a Fuel Pull. Cackling with glee, you post it on your Trim Healthy Mama Pinterest page. You've gone loopy; they're coming with the white straitjacket to take you away! Don't let the numbers take over the nature of food fuels, because bad things will happen!

Trim Healthy Mama should not be stripped down to algorithms. You might even be able to fit half a Snickers bar into one of the fuel categories if you work the numbers enough, but that is far from the heart of this approach. Constantly doing math in your head is not the way to do this plan healthfully nor will it keep you feeling joyful on this journey for the rest of your life—unless math somehow fills you with glee! Guess that means math professors are exempt from our current lecture.

Many of us never count a thing and do spectacularly well on plan. We've given amounts of foods in the fuel lists so you won't have to count at all. If you don't want to be bothered with the numbers, skip this chapter with our blessing and just pair foods that match each fuel in the way we have taught you so far. You can come back to this chapter in a few weeks or even months when you have a better handle on the plan and don't feel quite so overwhelmed. You may find the numbers more interesting rather than overwhelming at that point.

Having said all that, if you're still here reading you know a few numbers can be helpful at times. They're handy to have when looking at packages in grocery stores. They can also help you determine if a new product or food can fit into plan.

NUMBERS FOR S MEALS

- **Carbs—**Up to ten grams net carbs. (You don't have to count the carbs in most non-starchy veggies. Your Fuel Pull list has already outlined the higher-carb veggies that are best kept to half-cup servings.) This ten-gram limit is only there as a nice guide-line for an overall S meal. Sometimes very small amounts of non–S-friendly foods can be used in S meals, such as a few beans (up to a quarter cup), tiny pieces of fruit as garnish, or very small amounts of grains. Keep these to under ten grams of carbs and you'll be fine.
- **Fats—**There is no limit on fats, but you will want to change up amounts of fats even in your S meals rather than piling on six different types of fats in every single S meal. See Chapter 11, "Higher Learning" (page 90), for information on how to vary S meals.
- **Calories—**Trim Healthy Mama does not impose calorie limits, but, for your own sake, don't abuse calories. (That is, don't use a half cup of heavy cream in your smoothie—yikes! Two tablespoons is still going to give you a lovely creamy drink.)

NUMBERS FOR E MEALS

- **Carbs—**Up to forty-five grams net carbs. Some people with Type 2 diabetes or severe insulin resistance cannot even tolerate that amount. If you have an elevated blood-sugar reaction to certain E meals, don't quit eating them altogether but try what we call pulled-back E meals. Instead of having a full three-fourths cup of quinoa or rice, a half cup of the starch might be gentler on your blood sugar. Instead of having a full cup and a quarter of oatmeal, try three-fourths cup and have some scrambled egg whites with it. Protein will always help your blood-sugar reaction.

We have heard from many who say they are much more able to tolerate full E meals the longer they do Trim Healthy Mama. In pulled-back E meals, you will need to fill up more on the non-starchy veggies and include plenty of protein. If still hungry, you can always add a big glass of unsweetened almond or cashew milk to the end of your meal. Add a teaspoon or two of cocoa powder, sweeten it up with our natural sweeteners, and you have yummy, slimming chocolate milk in your belly. Voilà— you're chock-full now. Or try one of our many magically creamy Fuel Pull drinks in the "Shakes, Smoothies, Frappas, and Thin Thicks" chapter of the *Trim Healthy Mama Cookbook,* such as a Baby Frap to end your meal.

- **Fats**—About one teaspoon or up to five grams of fat. It is not necessary to count the fat in your lean protein but make sure it is at least 96% lean. Most salmon is fine but certain kinds of salmon are fattier, and when it comes to salmon with skin on, it may be best to pair with S meals.
- **Calories**—Counting is not necessary for E meals.

NUMBERS FOR FP MEALS

- **Carbs**—Just as with S meals, we recommend up to ten grams (but there is a tiny bit more leeway here since fats are not involved). We consider two Light Rye, Fiber, or Flax Seed Wasa crackers part of a Fuel Pull snack even though they reach eleven to twelve grams net carbs. Light Progresso soups are okay for Drive Thru Sues as FPs, even though their net carb amount goes slightly over the ten-gram limit. Those soups are low in fat and calories and their nutrition label is counting the carbs in the non-starchy veggies, which we don't usually do. (Of course, you can ignore those soups if you are a purist like Serene.)
- **Fats**—Just as with E meals, we recommend one teaspoon or up to five grams.
- **Calories**—Fuel Pulls are the only meal type in which we want calories to stay low. They are usually less than three hundred calories for a meal but that is not a hard number: Sometimes an FP meal might be somewhat higher than that, and at other times it might be quite a bit lower (as in the case of using the Fat Stripping Frappa as a meal in the "Shakes, Smoothies, Frappas, and Thin Thicks" chapter of the *Trim*

Healthy Mama Cookbook or enjoying our Minute Ramen Soup in the "Quick Single Soups" chapter of the *Trim Healthy Mama Cookbook*). This gives your body a good "calorie zigzag" shuffle. You don't have to actually count the calories in your Fuel Pull meal since the foods you will use to put the meal together are naturally low.

"PERSONAL CHOICE" (SHORTCUT OR FRANKENFOOD) NUMBERS

When using store-bought, low-carb bread items for S and FP needs, it is best to keep them at six grams or under for carbs and make sure they come in at under five grams of fat—preferably less. This means one Joseph's pita, a half to one whole large Joseph's lavash (men may want/need to use the full lavash), or two small or one medium low-carb tortilla. Let's say you make a pizza crust out of half of a Joseph's lavash and end your meal not quite filled up. Don't forget about your side salad and then fill up further with one of our many FP shakes or smoothies. No need to overdo the low-carb bread items. Light Rye Wasa or Ryvita crackers are not considered Frankenfoods, because their ingredients are simply whole-grain rye, water, and salt. One Light Rye, Fiber, or Flax Seed Wasa cracker or one Sesame Ryvita cracker can be part of an S meal, two crackers work for FP, and four are an excellent choice for an E meal. Other types of Wasa crackers like Multi Grain, Hearty, Sourdough, and Whole Grain are a little higher in carbs, so don't include those in your FP or S meals. Enjoy two to three of those in an E meal and then have a small piece of fruit on the side, if desired.

PROTEIN NUMBERS

You don't have to count the protein in every meal. Overall Trim Healthy Mama will give you ample protein. Some meals will be higher—upwards of thirty grams of protein—and some will still contain protein but may be lower than twenty grams, such as lentil soup without added chicken breast. (However, you can always add a couple scoops of Just Gelatin to your lentil soup to boost the protein content.) Most of your snacks will probably contain at least ten grams of protein, but occasionally eating an apple alone (without protein) is nothing to stress over unless you have extremely unstable blood sugar. Meals and snacks will balance out and provide you with adequate protein for the repair your body needs.

If you really want a protein number to shoot for at every meal, twenty to twenty-five grams should do it. We don't want people using that as a hard-and-fast rule, though. If you do a vigorous workout, it is a good idea to aim to get twenty to twenty-five grams of protein within a couple of hours of the workout. Pristine Whey Protein Powder can help with that, as can Integral Collagen or Just Gelatin.

CAN I CONTINUE TO COUNT CALORIES OR POINTS?

Most Mamas are tickled pink to no longer have to count calories or points. They are all too happy to let all that go. See ya, wouldn't want to be ya! But giving up tracking calories can be scary for others. They're afraid of overeating, afraid of letting go of the strictness for fear of how crazy they might go with all that freedom.

As we mentioned earlier, it truly takes time to tune in to your own hunger and full signals. We urge everyone to give no counting calories a fair try. Don't give up after a week if you gain a pound or two. Remember not to abuse calories by pouring a quarter cup of heavy cream into every cup of coffee or piling cheese on every S meal. Keep your Fuel Pull desserts and snacks handy and see how you do over a few weeks or a couple of months.

If you truly find that you do better keeping track of your calories, there is no shame in that. You can take premises from other diets that have helped you and apply them to your own long-term THM journey. We have had many Mamas come to Trim Healthy Mama after many years of counting with Weight Watchers or another plan. While so many enjoy the freedom of no longer tracking points, certain others apply their knowledge of points to their THM meals and make the combo work together for their own unique journey. Do this your way and let nobody shame you—neither yourself nor anybody else!

chapter 11
HIGHER LEARNING

As time goes on and you gain confidence in the Trim Healthy Mama lifestyle, you'll feel ready to dig deeper into the principles behind the plan. We have a couple more concepts here for you to learn when that time comes. You can happily implement the plan right now without this further knowledge, as it doesn't have to be learned straight away. In fact, if you try to grasp all of this when you first start, it might feel like learning algebra when you are only ready for basic addition. Just as we mentioned in the previous chapter concerning numbers, you can come back to this when you feel good and ready. Meet you in the next chapter if you know this is you.

THREE DIFFERENT S MEALS

All you need to know as a beginner is an S is an S and it uses the fuel of fats rather than carbs. That basic knowledge should serve you well enough as you begin to juggle your fuels and freestyle between S and E meals with occasional Fuel Pulls and Crossovers, depending on your particular needs in life. But as you journey on you'll find out that you can also vary your S meals so they are not all extremely heavy.

Most of us love heavy S meals when we first start out; but just as we can learn to juggle our fuels, we can also learn to juggle our S meals, which sometimes allows for better weight loss and sometimes serves as a way to break through stalls. Changing up your S meals between Heavy, Deep, and Light will be a boon to your long-term journey.

Heavy S—These meals contain fats that also have a few carbs, like dairy and nuts. Heavy fats are the store-bought creamy dressings, all nuts and nut butters, avocados, and all forms of dairy products, including heavy cream. Some good examples of a Heavy-S meal would be our Cheeseburger Pie recipe (find that free recipe on our website) or a dessert like stevia-sweetened cheesecake with a nut crust. Heavy-S meals are a comforting part of Trim Healthy Mama and can be enjoyed by most of us, but if overdone, they may stall weight loss.

Deep S—These meals contain only the purest fats without carbs. Your extra-virgin oils and the natural fat in meats and eggs are the fats that work their ultra-slimming magic here. Butter is also considered to be Deep S; however, coconut oil has more metabolism-revving qualities. Deep-S meals do not use some of the regular S-friendly foods that are a little bit higher in carbs, such as berries, dairy, tomatoes, onions, and nuts or seeds. They focus on leafy greens and the lowest-carb, non-starchy veggies and are liberal with superfood oils. An example of a Deep-S meal would be chicken, salmon, or beef on a huge plate of greens with some nice swirls of extra-virgin olive oil and vinegar. While most Deep S meals are dairy-free, a very small amount (one tablespoon) of Parmesan or light sheep's cheese like pecorino cheese may be okay on your salad. Another Deep S example would be two or three butter fried eggs over a bed of sautéed spinach. Deep-S meals are extremely slimming and can be used after a cheat meal to help rid the damage of excess sugars and starches.

Light S—Healthy fats of all kinds can be used in Light-S meals, but less of them. You'll still use more than you would in an E meal or Fuel Pull but you might choose to make a sandwich out of chicken breast instead of dark meat chicken with skin, very thin slices of cheese, and a moderate smear of mayo rather than thick slices of cheese and gobs of mayo. Light-S meals should be woven into the S mix for natural caloric changeup. Or you may choose to make an omelet with one egg and two egg whites and a couple tablespoons of part-skim mozzarella versus a Heavy-S omelet made with three full eggs, cream cheese, cheddar cheese, and bacon. Do you see that wonderful variation you can have within S meals themselves? Don't limit yourself to one type; enjoy all three for the joy each brings.

FUEL STACKING

Most people who lose weight steadily on the core plan of THM do not need to worry about what this term even means. Most of us with healthy metabolisms can handle fuel stacks here and there, so don't let this term wig you out. We've seen people lose more than a hundred pounds with Trim Healthy Mama and not even know what fuel stacking is. But if you are someone who struggles to lose weight (a stubborn loser), this subject may concern you. As we've pounded over and over again, the Trim Healthy Mama approach is not centered on numbers, but the general guideline is not to go over five grams of fat for Fuel Pull or E meals and not to go over ten grams of carbs for S or Fuel Pull meals. Fuel stacking occurs when different components of a meal pile up and those numbers are unknowingly surpassed.

Let's say you have an S dinner that includes a store-bought, low-carb wrap of six grams of carbs plus meat and veggies with fat. You had your dinner early, so just shy of two hours later you are hungry. You decide to have a Fuel Pull snack so as not to combine S and E fuels. You choose to have two Light Rye Wasa crackers with Laughing Cow Creamy Light Swiss cheese wedges (eleven to twelve carbs altogether). Or instead of the snack, you decide to have a Fuel Pull dessert straight after your dinner—you go for close to a full cup of Greek yogurt with one teaspoon of all-fruit jelly (about twelve carbs altogether). The meal plus snack or meal plus dessert puts you over that ten-gram carb number that is the guideline we usually aim to stay under. Actually, even if you have only a half cup of the yogurt, you're going a little over. Okay, please don't freak out! As mentioned, most of us can handle going over the numbers in this way here and there, but others of us may not be able to. This is part of the reason we suggest sticking to a half cup of Greek yogurt when it is used as a dessert, or trying our Jigglegurt recipe in the "Sweet Bowls" chapter of the *Trim Healthy Mama Cookbook*. That slashes the carbs and calories of Greek yogurt in half. We are in love with the taste and texture of that delightful treat and it is a helpful money-saver, too.

A similar fuel-stacking scenario can occur if you put two Fuel Pulls together that are already close to the top of the number limits. You can end up with a very light Crossover. Let's say you have a Fuel Pull pizza using a Joseph's pita as a crust for your main meal, then a full cup of Greek yogurt with one teaspoon of peanut butter as your dessert afterward. You were already close to Fuel Pull limits for fat and carbs with your pizza, since you used a small amount of cheese. The yogurt upped your carbs much closer to E territory, and then the teaspoon of peanut butter took you past the fat limits as well—voilà, you have a very light Crossover. Maybe not a bad thing, for many of us—but not as slimming as it could be.

HOW TO AVOID A FUEL STACK

You don't have to start counting obsessively; that's bondage. Just know that not all Fuel Pull foods are created equally. While 0% Greek yogurt and low-fat cottage cheese are considered Fuel Pulls, they have more carbs in the form of naturally occurring milk sugars than certain other Fuel Pulls. Fuel Pulls that have grains are in a similar boat, e.g., Wasa crackers. Ultra Fuel Pulls are the ones that will not cause any fuel stacking. They contain negligible carbs and fat so fuel stacking has no chance of occurring. Ultra Fuel Pull desserts and snacks are the ones you want to use in close proximity to another meal if you have weight that is hard to shed.

Which are the Ultra Fuel Pulls? Dessert and snack recipes like Choco Chip Baby Frap, Thin Thicks, Gluccie or Glycine Glory puddings, Tummy Tucking Ice Cream, or Tummy Spa Ice Cream are all Ultra Fuel Pulls. Find those in the *Trim Healthy Mama Cookbook*. Small amounts of lean meat, such as a few slices of lean deli turkey, could be "ultra" also as that is a snack that contains very little carbs or fat. If you are struggling with stubborn pounds, it simply makes sense to use more of these Ultra Fuel Pulls rather than dairy-based ones as desserts (tagged on to the end of a meal or as snacks close to another meal), especially in the evening (when your body burns less energy).

This doesn't mean you cannot use other moderately higher-carb Fuel Pull snacks and desserts in your THM plan. They are not banned for you. They are perfect as a full stand-alone snack three hours away from a meal. They often work best as afternoon snacks. Two Wasa crackers with Laughing Cow Creamy Light Swiss cheese wedges for an afternoon snack at three thirty P.M.? Sure! Add on Pearl's easy recipe for chocolate milk (found on our website). But Wasa crackers too close to another meal can be a problem. A full cup of Greek yogurt for an afternoon snack with berries as a FP snack? Sure! But don't do that right after your S meal if you have very challenging pounds to lose.

Once you get it, this is a very easy principle to apply. If you are freaking out with major informational overload right now, we must spray you with our magical memory-erase spray. There . . . *poof,* all this info has now been erased from your mind. You read it too early. Go forth and be a simple Trim Healthy Mama with our sisterly blessing. DO NOT COME BACK TO THIS CHAPTER until your newbie anxiety has lessened.

chapter 12
THIRSTY MAMA

You're going to learn how to drink yourself trim. Anything you put into your body in liquid form is absorbed much faster into your bloodstream. When it comes to weight, a drink can either be the worst offender or the best trimming tool. Finding your trim will depend upon you having the knowledge to tweak your liquid world to your healthiest favor.

If your drink contains sugar, your blood glucose levels will immediately sky rocket. This rapid sugar high is worse for your body than a regular sugar high from food, which is already bad enough. It is basically fat in a drink, and that still applies to all those "fat-free varieties," too. Most sodas are fat-free but with every gulp they pour on the pounds.

THE OBVIOUS NAUGHTY LIST

We have to tackle the baddies first. Don't worry, the goodies list is coming. We just need to nullify some options from your brain's playlist. Once these naughty guys are removed, a new world of liquid goodness will open up to you.

Soda/Pop—Do we really need to say anything else here that hasn't been said about this stuff? The hazards of soda have been preached over and over, yet soft drinks are a sixty-billion-dollar annual industry. Okay, we'll take our turn: In a nutshell, they are the death of a trim waistline. The problem is that we are told to quit soda, but willpower doesn't last long, so we have to have something equally as delicious to replace soda with. Never fear, all the bubbles you could ever want can be had the healthy way. We'll show you how in our recipes; but if you want store-bought, there are already many brands of stevia-sweetened soft drinks available. Or a more budget-friendly approach is to enjoy sparkling water mixed with natural, plan-approved sweeteners and flavored with extracts found at any grocery store.

Highly Caffeinated Energy Drinks—They usually contain high amounts of sugar combined with mega amounts of caffeine. They might seem like a quick fix, but in the long term they are energy thieves that can rob the life out of your adrenals. The sugar-free versions are usually sweetened with artificial sweeteners so are not a great choice for your body.

Coffee—Nah! Just kidding. You can drink joe on the plan, although we recommend moderation. If you're drinking coffee all day just to survive because you're not getting enough sleep, that is coffee abuse and not moderation. Coffee itself is not the problem, it is what you put in it that can make it naughty. You'll learn to drink coffee without undoing its wonderful health benefits by adding sugar and processed creamers. Most coffee-shop concoctions—think double-mocha, caramel-fudge-swirl latte—might be hip but are very cruel to your actual hips. If you want the coffee-shop experience, stick to regular brewed coffee or Americano with optional heavy cream or half-and-half. Pull out an on-plan sweetener from your purse and you have it made. (More about coffee soon.)

Sweet Tea—It might be what you grew up with, but this drink is the undoing of trim waistlines all over the globe. Tea is on the plan; sugar is not. You're going to learn to sweeten up your tea with our on-plan sweeteners and you'll love them. Check out Sweet 'n' Slender Iced Tea in the "More Drinks" chapter of the *Trim Healthy Mama Cookbook*.

THE DECEIVING NAUGHTY LIST

The following drinks aren't doing you any favors, either:

Fruit Juice—This is the greatest deceiver: Even 100% juice is 100% fattening. Never remove fruit juice from its own fiber. Eat the whole fruit in E meals, and if using in a smoothie, throw the whole thing in the blender (minus the rind and seeds).

Honey-Sweetened Tea or Coffee—While raw honey has health benefits and we'll tell you in Chapter 13, "Sweet Mama" (page 102), how it can be implemented on plan, using it in drinkable form daily is a sticky fat trap.

Diet Soda/Pop—Artificial sweeteners are not part of Trim Healthy Mama. We're not saying you have to quit your diet sodas today. Baby-step your way and if you have a diet soda or two while you're still figuring out your meals, we won't shun you! You'll do this in your own time and let your taste buds adapt to natural zero-calorie or low-calorie sweetened sodas rather than artificial ones.

Milk—It does the body good? Feeding your baby your own milk certainly does. Allowing your high-metabolism children to drink some whole, raw cow's or goat's milk does, too. Drinking it yourself, as a full-grown adult, does not (if you have weight to lose). If you are a natural, super-skinny type, have at it if you can find a source for pastured raw milk. But milk is a fat-and-carb combination, a natural Crossover in liquid form, which means it is more weight-promoting than a Crossover in solid form. We've got lots of yummy milk alternatives that will cream up your smoothie or bowl of oatmeal, or make a fantastic chocolate milk. You can easily find unsweetened almond, flax, cashew, and coconut milks at grocery stores and they are all on plan. Did you read the word *unsweetened*? "Original versions" without the word *unsweetened* means sweetened with sugar of some kind. You will smartly sweeten up your plan-approved milks at home.

Sports Drinks—These are often extremely high in sugars and artificial colors. Stay far away from those! Some vitamin waters are sweetened with stevia and erythritol—check labels. If you can find ones sweetened that way, they'll be fine.

Health Food Store Drinks—Just because your bottled drink comes from your local, organic market does not mean it is trim or health-friendly. The following drinks can put a bunch of organic weight on you.

- Natural cane juice–sweetened colas: fattening (cane juice is just another form of sugar)
- Naturally sweetened lemonades or teas: The term *naturally sweetened* printed on food and drink labels usually just means you'll become naturally fat. Sorry, but it's true. High-glycemic sweeteners such as honey, fruit juice concentrate, agave, organic raw cane sugar, maple syrup, date syrup, and brown rice syrup are just so-called healthy ways to help you gain weight, especially in liquid form.
- Organic fruit juice smoothies: hard on your blood sugar (watch out for any drinks with apple or pear juice concentrates—or any juice concentrate, for that matter, aside from lemon)
- Fresh-made juice from the juice bar featuring carrots or apples: Watch out for the myth of carrot juice. It has an effect similar to that of fruit juice on blood glucose. Many people turn to juicing as a way of fighting diseases such as cancer, but cancer

feeds on sugar so igniting the bloodstream in this way does not make sense. If you would like to add juice to your diet, do so with a base of mild green juices such as cucumber or celery and romaine lettuce with smaller concentrations of more pungent greens. You can also make Serene's Earth Milk Sip recipe. Check out the video on how to make that on our website or on YouTube, or find the written recipe in the *Trim Healthy Mama Cookbook.* It is a cleansing, blood-sugar-stabilizing way to drink greens for health.

- Coconut water: The thin liquid contained in a coconut (as opposed to the milk made from the nut) has many health benefits and is great for infants and children who have diarrhea, as it restores electrolytes. If you are drinking it frequently, it will inhibit weight loss as it contains significant sugars. A way of receiving the wonderful benefits of coconut water while preserving your trimming goals is through fermenting it, which naturally lowers the carbs. Google Coconut Water Kefir.

- Vitamin-charged waters: These products are usually sweetened with sugar or an artificial sweetener, but there are now a couple of brands like SoBe and Vitaminwater that use stevia and erythritol as natural low-calorie sweeteners. You must look at the nutrition label to make sure you are buying the right one. It should say zero calories and list only stevia or erythritol as sweeteners.

YOUR CAN-HAVES

Enough with the naughties. There are so many goodies in your drink future, you won't feel deprived. Check out our beverage section in the *Trim Healthy Mama Cookbook* for our All-Day Sipper recipes or check out some of our videos of them on our website or on YouTube. Good Girl Moonshine has become as much a household "brand" in Trim Healthy Mama Land as Coke is around a college vending machine. This drink can help you kick the soda habit and pep up your health. Good Girl Moonshine was first in the line of Sipper drinks that we created to help you stay happily hydrated on your THM journey. Also, in the beverages segment of our cookbook, check out the Shrinker, which does as its name suggests and helps to shrink your fat cells! We have a free video for that, too. The Singing Canary is another in our popular Sipper series. If you love orange juice, this can give you that fix. Turmeric, the star ingredient in this drink, is known as a cancer fighter, an adrenal healer, and an inflammation fighter and is also a skin-beautifying tonic.

Coffee and Tea the Trimming Way

These drinks have been around for centuries, so why would we be so cruel as to suddenly rip them from your life? Our stance is go ahead. Shouts and cheers! Fist pumps and high-fives all around. We join you in a resounding "Yay!"

It was all the rage in the 1980s to vilify coffee. Coffee and cigs went together. Take a sip on one and a puff of the other. Not so anymore. You can drink your coffee without the slightest bit of guilt. Latest research has exonerated coffee of its bad reputation. It is a myth that coffee leaches minerals from your body, and it is a myth that coffee is dehydrating; but you should not count it as part of your water intake.

In moderate amounts, both coffee and tea are beneficial because of their extraordinarily high antioxidant amounts and mood-lifting abilities. Black tea, oolong tea, and green tea can be consumed more liberally than coffee since they have less caffeine. These teas can aid in weight loss (especially oolong tea, which is an important ingredient in the Shrinker), can calm nerves due to their theanine content, and are antiaging tools.

Coffee elevates dopamine levels, which contribute to a feeling of happiness and can lessen the chance of getting Parkinson's disease. Numerous studies indicate that coffee consumption is associated with a sharply reduced risk of Type 2 diabetes, including an eighteen-year follow-up study on Swedish women released in the *Journal of Internal Medicine*. A 2012 study released in the *Journal of Agricultural & Food Chemistry* found that coffee is able to inhibit toxic amyloid proteins that are normally found in the pancreas of people with Type 2 diabetes. The Chinese researchers in this study found that four cups per day slashes the risk for diabetes in half! Logic says it doesn't make sense to put sugar in coffee if we want to benefit from these diabetes-fighting components.

Coffee is now also considered by many researchers to be a cancer-fighting drink. Laboratory studies show that it may have an anti-tumor effect against ovarian, colon, liver, and other cancers. A study released in the May 2011 edition of *Breast Cancer Research* showed that postmenopausal women who drink moderate to large doses of coffee are also at significantly less risk for an aggressive type of breast cancer known as "estrogen receptor (ER)–negative."

You certainly don't have to drink coffee to be a Trim Healthy Mama, but if you love the idea of coffee with a swirl of real cream in the morning you've found the right plan. When we say swirl, we don't mean a third of a cup. No, your dreams are not dashed—you can get a good creamy coffee from a couple of tablespoons of heavy cream; even one tablespoon of it makes some of us happy. Others need three tablespoons or they feel deprived, and we can't let that happen! They do just fine like that. You'll find your own heavy creamy sweet spot that your body can handle. If you are postmenopausal, you may want to err on the side of one to two versus three tablespoons. You can also use half-and-half if you prefer. If you want a super-indulgent coffee now and then with oodles of cream, have at it—but don't make that your constant.

Sometimes you will be having an E breakfast. Coffee and cream is an S beverage: Keep this in mind if you're not wanting to cross over on purpose, otherwise you'll be doing it by mistake. Not to worry: A small amount of half-and-half rather than heavy cream can still leave you in E mode. Or, we have created a way of creaming up your coffee for E or Fuel Pull needs that is delicious and health-promoting. It is called the Trimmaccino Light and it can cream up all your teas, hot chocolates, and coffees without too much fat added. Check out the "Hot Drinks" chapter of the *Trim Healthy Mama Cookbook* for lots of Trimmaccino recipes. If you happen to like your coffee black, that is fine, too, or if you enjoy a little unsweetened almond or cashew milk in your coffee . . . that works. Those are Fuel Pull options and harmonize with any meal style. But some of us think black coffee is blech!

To all our British, Kiwi, and Aussie Mamas: We were born in New Zealand and grew up Down Under in Australia before moving to the United States, so we know not to mess with your hot tea. A spot of milk in a cup of hot tea is compulsory under the Commonwealth—well, not quite; but we're not going to go against the might of the royal family. A spot of milk is not enough to do any damage; we're not talking a quarter of a cup here. You'll be fine. We raise our tea cups and pinkies to you in salute!

Fruit juice drinkers: Fruit-flavored herbal teas will be a fantastic replacement for you. Brewed, then iced and sweetened up to perfection with plan-approved sweeteners—nothing better! The same applies to peppermint tea. So refreshing! Check out our fruit-flavored slushy recipes in the "Frozen Treats" chapter of the *Trim Healthy Mama Cookbook* for more fruity goodness.

Kombucha

There is no denying the health benefits of this drink. Enjoy a half cup with your S meals and even more with your other meals. While most of the sugars in it have been eaten up in the fermenting process, a few remain, so it is best not sipped on all day.

Water

So many diet plans force water on you. We're not going to tell you to drink a certain number of ounces per body weight. You'll no longer be chugging down sugary sodas, sports drinks, and juices, so your water intake should naturally increase. You can also use any of our All-Day Sipper drinks to help you stay hydrated and to bring more flavor to your life. You won't want to fully replace water with those options. You still need some pure water, but we don't want you obsessing over ounces and cups per day or making yourself feel like a dehydrated failure if you don't meet a quota. Some plans go too far with their rigidity over water. You're left sloshing around all day, constantly having to use the bathroom! Common sense is a good approach with water.

Adult Beverages

If you like a nice glass of wine, either white or red, you can have it on plan in moderation. Be sure it is a dry wine, as sweet wines are fattening. We know it goes against all wine snobbery rules, but there are certain Trim Healthy Mamas who only like sweet wines so they add a tiny bit of pure stevia extract to their glass—please don't report them to the winery association! If you want to drink beer, stick to a low-carb or light beer. The beer belly is aptly named for a reason.

Too much alcohol can quickly go from being a health tonic to a health destroyer, so please know we are not advocating drunkenness here. If you are including too much wine, too often it can also interfere with your weight loss and that is even more true when it comes to beer. Go easy, but do enjoy from time to time if desired.

chapter 13
SWEET MAMA

You can keep your sweet tooth. Why try to deny it? Life would be awfully dull without dessert, and what woman can live without chocolate? Not us! Healthy treats are part of the Food Freedom lifestyle.

As a Trim Healthy Mama you won't be eating sugar (unless you choose to have an off-plan treat now and then). Please don't be fooled by packages of sugar labeled "organic" or "unrefined." Sugar is sugar in your bloodstream and is still as inflammatory no matter how earthy the packaging looks or what buzz words are used to advertise it. Those earthy options will just cost you more.

Thankfully this sugar-free state happens naturally on THM. We don't start with rule number 1—STOP EATING SUGAR! That's just going to make you want to reach for the nearest candy bar. Instead you'll start eating healthy sweet-treat options that can take the place of the other health-destructive ones. Little by little you'll become more successful at finding fantastic subs for the treats you crave. One day you wake up to realize, "Hey, I haven't had sugar in a month and I'm not missing it!"

Go you!

So how do you get your sweet fix as a THM? Keeping with our theme that we are all unique with different preferences and challenges, you have a few natural sweetener options to choose from. First let's look at what to avoid aside from sugar itself.

NO TO ARTIFICIAL SWEETENERS

The fake sweetener industry is a billion-dollar one, but we predict that might begin to wane. Similar to what happened with cigarettes, the more that is known about the harmful effects of artificial sweeteners, the harder it will be for these companies to keep people hooked on them.

Aspartame, sold under the brand names Equal or NutraSweet, has constantly shown dangerous side effects in independent research. It is a known neurotoxin that causes overexcitement in brain cells that lead to their death. Aspartame is now banned in many countries, yet sadly it is still the number-one sweetener of diet sodas here in the United States.

Sucralose, or what is more commonly known as Splenda, has been thrust forward as the healthier alternative but there are grave concerns that it disrupts the endocrine system. Some scientists call Splenda a "mild mutagen," depending on how much is absorbed. Some researchers have put forth that it has more in common with pesticides like DDT than table condiments like salt or sugar. It doesn't come from anything grown in the ground, so we'll nix it, thanks!

Note: If Splenda is something you are having great difficulty giving up, you can still be a Trim Healthy Mama. We'll try not to nag you too much about it as nagging never works; but we do want to encourage you to switch over to the natural sweeteners mentioned here. We understand your tastes are used to one sweetener right now and it takes time to adjust. Do your best and baby-step your way in even if you have to cut Splenda from your life more slowly than abruptly.

YES TO STEVIA

This is the main (but not only) sweetener option on the plan. Please don't call stevia an artificial sweetener—you'll hurt her feelings. Stevia is a plant with leaves that have a natural sweet taste and, incredibly, this sweetness has no calories, carbs, or fat grams; so this makes it a fantastic chief sweetener if you need to lose weight. Now before you say, "Yuck, tried that and it's nasty," give us a minute and we may change your mind. Stevia extract is the sweet powder that is extracted from the leaves, but be aware that not all powders taste the same. You know this from experience, especially if your first word was *blech* when we mentioned stevia. Don't be gun-shy about trying again once we arm you with pointers for stevia success. We're going to teach you how to use this plant so it actually tastes wonderful in your treats, but we will also have to warn you about what to watch out for. Not all stevia sweeteners are beneficial to your health or waistline.

The rise of Type 2 diabetes and obesity and the recent spotlight on the hazards of artificial sweeteners have caused stevia to become more readily available. You can probably find it in your local grocery store, whereas it would have been extremely rare just ten years ago. Due to this growing demand for stevia, cheap, low-grade extracts are flooding the market. They are often mixed with fillers that are actually harmful to your health and your waistline. This brings us to the perfect setup for a shameless sales pitch, to convince you that the Trim Healthy Mama brand is the one and only stevia you must buy, right? Nah! If you find another brand of stevia that meets our criteria and you like it, then go for it! We won't hold a grudge. (We'll try not to, at least.)

When we wrote our first self-published book, we had no idea of the response that was to come and never conceived that one day we'd have to launch our own line of natural sweeteners. We mentioned the brand of stevia we used at the time (which we had no association with) and how it was pure and tasted great. That particular company got swamped with tens of thousands of orders but, sadly, only a few months later they changed out their stevia to a lesser-grade extract. We got flooded with e-mails from women telling us their desserts suddenly tasted terrible and please would we do something about it and fix this mess!

We scouted the globe looking for the best-tasting, most pure and minimally processed stevia that our Mamas could come to rely on. We tasted hundreds of stevia extracts and most ended up right in the trash. *Ugh* was our most commonly repeated word. Serene sent her husband on a mission. He had to go to the source—across the globe to the farms where the plants are actually grown—and find something incredible for our Mamas.

We were beyond ecstatic when we tasted THE ONE. It almost felt like finding the Holy Grail. Major happy dorky dances were performed in our kitchens that day! Trim Healthy Mamas everywhere felt the same way once they got their hands on it. Their drinks and desserts tasted great again! Our stevia extract is completely organic and is made from the highest grade of stevia available—99 percent rebiana, which costs us a lot more but gives you better purity and taste. This extract and the blends we've created with it don't have that awful bitter aftertaste when used correctly. Having said all that, we do need to put a lid on the boasting for a minute to say, if your local grocery store provides you with a plan-approved stevia that floats your boat, then we're happy because we want you to succeed.

This plan needs to be doable for you and your unique situation. We do need to give you some pointers, though, on what not to buy.

The Stevia Baddies

Please read labels carefully and avoid any stevia blends that are mixed with the following:

- Sugar
- Dextrose
- Fructose
- Maltodextrin
- Agave

The Stevia Goodies

- Any stevia that is a pure extract (while not mandatory, it is best to use an organic source of unbleached, water-extracted stevia with a grade of at least 95%)
- Any stevia blend that contains only stevia extract plus either erythritol or xylitol (while not mandatory, it is best to use a non-GMO source of erythritol or xylitol)

Starting Out with Stevia

If you are used to the taste of sugar, you're going to have to allow your taste buds some time to transition over to a new sweet taste. Even when using a non-bitter stevia sweetener, some can find the taste odd at first. Hang in there. Here are a couple of tips on how to make this transition smoother.

1. Stevia Extract Powder is several hundred times sweeter than sugar per serving. Only teensy amounts are used. To measure our pure stevia extract, we use a "doonk," our pet term for the tiny one-thirty-second teaspoon used for a serving size. It takes only one doonk to sweeten up your glass of tea . . . or two if you have a real sweet tooth. Most stevia blends on grocery store shelves are twice as sweet as sugar, so don't measure cup for cup when trying to rework some of your old favorite recipes. Start with less than half. Our Super Sweet Blend is four to five times as sweet as sugar, so if a recipe calls for a cup of sugar you'll only use, at the most, one quarter cup of Super Sweet Blend. Our other blended stevia, Gentle Sweet, is approximately twice as sweet as sugar, so if you prefer that, you'll use only a half cup compared with a cup of sugar.

2. If you have a hard time with stevia-sweetened chocolate recipes at first, give them a little break and focus for a while on recipes flavored with berries, fruit, vanilla, or caramel. Try Cottage Berry Whip as one of your first THM sweet recipes to help your taste buds acclimate better. Find our video for that recipe on our website or on YouTube. Once you've been using stevia for a little while with these more adaptable flavors, chocolate recipes will taste better when you go back to them. Gentle Sweet will be the kindest option to your taste buds at first.

How Do I Know Which Type of Stevia to Get?

It's a good idea to always have some pure stevia extract in your cupboard. This pure form is the most budget-friendly way to sweeten up your drinks. There is no need to go throwing money into pound after pound of a blended stevia if you like lots of sweet drinks (such as our All-Day Sippers) when a couple or a few doonks will do the trick just fine and save you lots of money. A small pouch of pure extract can last you months, even using it daily.

But we gotta be honest, it is harder to get great baking results using a pure stevia extract alone. This is where a blended stevia option can really shine. Adding a little bit of pure stevia to either xylitol or erythritol, two natural sugar alcohols (or a combination of both of those in the case of our Gentle Sweet) can allow for baking success.

Xylitol tastes the most like sugar. It is extremely gentle on your blood sugar so it is plan-friendly but with a caution: It does have a few calories (which can add up if you throw xylitol into all your treats) and when used in excess it can cause some tummy issues (gas and diarrhea). Using xylitol alone can also be another money burner because it is not quite as sweet as sugar so you have to use a bunch to get a good sweet taste. Adding pure stevia to xylitol as we have done with Gentle Sweet, makes most of its issues go away. You'll be able to use less of it, which solves the calorie problem, the money problem, and, for most, the gas and bloating problem.

Xylitol has another issue if you have a dog in your house. Dogs cannot eat xylitol. It can make them very sick and in some cases can be fatal. Please keep treats made with xylitol away from your dogs. Dogs have vastly different digestive systems than humans.

There are other foods they are not supposed to eat, such as chocolate—so keep those chocolate cupcakes you make with Gentle Sweet well out of reach of your canine family members.

If you don't want to take any chances with your dog and xylitol, look for a stevia/erythritol blend; it won't pose the same doggy health issues. Trim Healthy Mama's Super Sweet Blend contains no xylitol and no calories and is extremely budget-friendly. It is best to use small amounts of it or else it will be too potent, so try just a couple teaspoons in your shakes or smoothies or single-serve muffins and just three to four tablespoons in a big batch of muffins. If you can't get the right sweetness with it, purchase erythritol (which measures cup for cup like sugar) and mix one and a half pounds with your bag of Super Sweet Blend. It will then be only about twice the sweetness of sugar, more forgiving a taste if you put too much in your treats and easier to work with for your tastes. You should be able to find stevia/erythritol blends locally at most grocery stores, too. Again we must caution that you avoid needless fillers like maltodextrin and, although not mandatory, we do want to encourage you to seek non-GMO sources and to use brands that do not contain "natural flavors," which is sometimes but not always code for monosodium glutamate (MSG). There is no good reason to put "natural flavors" in stevia, which is already naturally sweet. But that will be a personal choice for you so don't feel condemned either way.

You can find more details about how to use Trim Healthy Mama sweeteners at www.trimhealthymama.com.

HONEY: YES OR NO?

Teeming with enzymes and minerals, raw honey has some undeniable healing abilities. Nothing shines like raw honey as a holistic allergy medicine, since it actually counters pollen allergens. Its antibacterial and antifungal properties make it an incredible wound healer. It promotes the growth of good bacteria in the intestine, and here's a biggie: It helps counter high homocysteine levels to help maintain a healthy heart. These are compelling reasons to keep a little raw honey around to ingest regularly.

Little is the key word here.

While honey is a known biblical sweetener, Proverbs 25:27 wisely says, "It is not good to eat too much honey." The problem in our culture is that when honey is used, it is usually in the "too much" rather than the "little" category. Many whole-foodsy sort of recipes that are supposed to be so natural and good for you call for anywhere from a half to a full cup of honey, which is then paired with grain-based flours! This combination of high carbs upon high carbs is cruel to cells that are already too stuffed with blood sugar from our modern diet. All the health benefits of honey can be quickly overshadowed by its ability to raise blood sugar—especially when paired with other starches or fruits, as it so often is. Putting it bluntly, honey can very easily make you fat!

But honey does not need to be ditched altogether. If you can find a good source for local raw honey, including one teaspoon per day as a holistic health supplement is fabulous. To figure where honey fits in your own THM journey, look at the season of life you are in with a good dose of honesty. Are you currently in the weight-loss part of your journey? Do you have blood-sugar issues such as insulin resistance, prediabetes, or full-blown diabetes? In these cases it doesn't make sense for you to be chiefly sweetening with honey on a day-to-day basis. It should only be used in the small medicinal doses we just mentioned. The exception to this would be for those who don't have a sweet tooth and who rarely have desserts or sweet drinks. If you'd prefer to just have the rare honey-sweetened treat, rather than frequently using stevia, that is a viable choice and it should not set you off track too much. But the majority of us THM's love our daily sweet drinks and treats. Sipping on a honey-sweetened drink all day will not work in your trimming favor.

Are you at or close to goal weight? You may want to include a little more raw honey here and there. Don't be afraid to put one tablespoon in your smoothies or shakes some-times. But even though we are both at goal weight, we have not simply traded out stevia for honey. Most of our sweetness still comes from stevia but we enjoy more honey than we did in the earlier stages of our THM journey. If you are exercising a lot, running around burning up energy, and feel like you can handle (or even benefit from) the glucose/fruc-tose energy gift of honey, do so but always in moderation.

Children can enjoy regular honey-sweetened treats if they don't have weight issues, since their cells are not nearly as insulin-resistant as ours. But remember, even children shouldn't overdo glycemic-impact sweeteners. Our children enjoy both honey- and stevia-sweetened treats. They often use a little of both in their oatmeal, in their drinks, and in some baked sweet treats they enjoy making. In our homes we call that "honey 'n' doonk." These two sweeteners harmonize fabulously together. Stevia extract is actually a much more affordable sweetener than honey, since it is so potent—so combining them this way helps out our budgets.

CAUTION

Beware of store-bought, pasteurized honey. It has a much higher glycemic index compared with raw honey—almost as high as that of sugar. Some people believe that buying "natural" honey from the grocery store is a less processed approach than using a stevia extract. Testing has shown that more than three quarters of the honey on grocery shelves is ultra-filtered. This is a high-tech procedure in which honey is heated, watered down, and then forced at high pressure through extremely small filters to remove all traces of pollen. We are not saying this process of ultra-filtering itself is necessarily horrible. We're just evening the playing field. The processing of stevia has come under some harsh scrutiny from some online bloggers. But most grocery store honey these days is far from minimally processed. One word of warning, the American Academy of Pediatrics says that infants younger than 12 months should avoid all sources of honey (raw or unpasteurized).

What if you have a super-high metabolism and actually need to put on weight? In this instance it does not make sense to use stevia over honey. Try a little raw honey with every meal, always make sure to center these meals with protein, and don't forget to load the buttah on, too, for a good Crossover effect!

Coconut Sugar: Yes or No?

While coconut sugar does not spike your blood glucose nearly as much as regular sugar, it does have a glycemic index (GI) in the mid-thirties, which means its ability to raise blood sugar is about the same as that of raw honey. It contains both carbs and calories, so if weight loss is desired, it is best not to use coconut sugar as a chief sweetener. Like honey, though, it is another sweetener that can be used with our blessing when you are close to or at goal weight, for children, or for those who only like rare sweet treats and prefer to use it over stevia sparingly.

Agave Syrup: Yes or No?

While this is promoted as a low-glycemic sweetener and safer than sugar, we don't recommend it due to its extremely high fructose component. Due to processing (even at low temperatures) it has an unnaturally high concentration of 90 percent fructose to 10 percent glucose. Nowhere in nature does this occur naturally. The only other food that is similar is high-fructose corn syrup, which most people know is extremely unhealthy.

Other Viable Sweeteners on Plan

Chicory root and monk fruit extract are two other natural sweeteners that do not have an impact on blood sugar. If you have allergies to any of the above-mentioned sweeteners, you can use these on the plan, but be careful to read labels when purchasing. Make sure they are not blended with any items on the list we mentioned above in the Stevia Baddies section on page 105. Chicory root (otherwise known as inulin) can also cause some stomach bloating for certain people.

TACKLING THE MYTHS

We can't end this chapter without addressing some of the myths and concerns about stevia that continue to propagate. Please don't simply take our own word for it: We encourage everyone to do their own research when considering adding any new food or supplement. There are hundreds of studies and much research available on this subject. We were compelled to get to the bottom of it all for our own peace of mind.

Stevia has been called a fake sweetener—ouch, that stings—and of late it's been given a hard time by some food-blogging sites. Stevia extract powder is not "created" in a laboratory like artificial sweeteners. It's every bit as natural as honey, maple syrup, or sugar itself. Recently it's been called overly processed, bleached, and responsible for insulin spikes (despite the fact that it does not raise blood sugar). Stevia is sometimes blamed for triggering "sweet taste addictions" that will never go away and that cause people to overeat. What else? Oh yes, it's been labeled an unbiblical sweetener. But here's what hurts the most: Stevia has been blamed for infertility and miscarriage. All joking aside now, some of these are pretty serious accusations. Let's tackle them.

Processed and Unnatural?

Much of this finger-pointing at stevia comes from it being lumped in with the pink and purple packets of artificial sweeteners at your grocery store. Stevia is not sugar, which is perceived to be "natural," so what else could stevia be but an artificial sweetener—a fake! This notion could not be more wrong. You may have heard the speculation that artificial sweeteners keep you fat by raising insulin levels—and there may be some truth in that—but don't lump stevia into that category. A study published in the August 2010 issue of *Appetite* comparing sugar, aspartame, and stevia revealed that stevia reduced both blood sugar and insulin levels as compared with the other two sweeteners. This same study revealed that the group who were preloaded with stevia before meals did not overeat at subsequent meals.

Stevia plants are grown to maturity, then the leaves are dried naturally. The sweetest parts of the leaf are extracted via water (which simply means they are soaked for periods of time). This water extract is then filtered with the use of food-grade alcohol (in the case of THM's stevia, every ingredient used—even this alcohol— is certified organic). Those of you who have ever made a vanilla extract in your kitchen will know that this part of the process is exactly the same one used when extracting vanilla flavor from the vanilla bean.

But how does the leaf start out as green and the powder end up as white? Serene's husband led a team for a second visit over to the farms where our stevia is grown and processed to find out more about this. Stevia extract is often unfairly bashed due to the presumption that it is bleached. While it is true that some stevia products are bleached at the end of processing, organic stevia farmers do not typically bleach the extract (THM's stevia is never bleached). Since not all parts of the stevia plant are sweet and some are even bitter, extraction needs to occur for this sweetness to be isolated. The sweet taste of stevia comes from the glycosides inside the leaf. Glycosides are naturally a whitish color, and they can be anything from a creamy hue to a stark white depending on the strain of plant.

Once the green part of the leaf (chlorophyll) is separated during the extraction process, the glycosides remain. But even though they've been separated from the other non-sweet parts of the plant, these glycosides are not chemically altered from their original state. The end result after they are dried is a white, fluffy powder. This powder is then usually granulated, making it easier to spoon out or pour through shaker holes. THM's Pure Stevia Extract Powder is a little different from most other extracts in that it is not granulated. We chose to leave out this extra step because in our opinion it changes the flavor of the stevia—making it slightly more bitter (according to our taste buds)—and we also wanted as few processing steps as possible from leaf to powder. True, it's harder to shake out; but that is why we "doonk."

So yes, stevia undergoes some processes to get to the white-powder state. This does not mean it has been debauched into something not recognized by the human body. If you prefer to grow stevia leaves in your garden, dry them, soak them, and then follow further steps until you can pulverize the redried leaves into a green powder—go right ahead. This homemade stevia option is certainly fine for some of our ultra-purists who prefer the whole-leaf option rather than the extracted glycosides; but there will be more bitterness in this powder. We used to think that while the green powder didn't taste as good, surely it was the only type that contained all the health benefits of stevia. Our thinking was that the white glycosides did not pose actual harm but they probably didn't contain many health goodies, either—sorta neutral health ground. We were wrong. A study published in volume 64, issue 7, of *Nutrition and Cancer* in 2012 showed that the extracted sweet part of stevia kills up to 71 percent of human breast cancer cells after seventy-two hours of treatment in vitro. Researchers also found that this stevia compound acts as an antioxidant for healthy cells and helps protect them from damage. It does the exact opposite to the breast cancer cells and floods them with toxic-free radicals. This halts DNA replication and disrupts the cancer cells' mitochondria, causing the cancer cells to die. The extract itself has also shown significant anti-inflammatory, immune-boosting, and blood sugar–stabilizing effects.

The Scary Stuff

Does stevia cause infertility and miscarriage? These are fair questions and they continue to arise as stevia gets more time in the spotlight. No use putting our heads in the sand and ignoring these questions just because we love having a natural sweetener that is calorie-free and doesn't raise blood sugar. If it's dangerous, let's logically find out. We could not encourage something that is damaging to fertility and health.

The whole controversy over stevia and fertility started when it was rumored that women in two indigenous tribes of South America chewed on the herb as a contraceptive (or drank the tea—there are different claims). There is no data showing that this did in fact work for these women and many researchers point out that if stevia did have contraceptive properties, then the native population of Brazil and Paraguay would certainly be affected, which is simply not the case. Many researchers have been quick to make the argument that it is likely that if the contraceptive effect of stevia were real, scientists would have long ago discovered that fact and isolated the compounds responsible.

It was this rumor that grew into folklore that triggered many hundreds of studies attempting to see if there is any real connection between stevia and fertility issues. In the 1960s a study was published in which rats were given extremely high doses of liquid stevia (in place of water), which caused a downward trend in their fertility. If you hear someone say, "Stevia causes infertility," this is the study that entrenched that claim in some people's minds.

Hundreds of subsequent studies with better methodology and larger numbers of test subjects have not shown that stevia poses a risk to fertility, especially in the dosages of normal consumption. A recent study done at the Primate Research Center of Chulalongkorn University in Bangkok, Thailand, once again studied the effects of extremely high doses of stevia on rodents but again revealed opposing results to the initial controversial 1968 study. The researchers not only looked at the rodents ingesting the high doses but on two subsequent generations. They found that health, mating, and fertility were not affected at all, in any of the generations, even with a dosage of 2,500 mg/kg. The recommended daily dose for humans is 2 mg/kg. Another study published in the *Journal of Endocrinology and Reproduction* (volume 12, 2008) concluded that *Stevia rebaudiana* had no adverse effects on the fertility of adult female mice.

We're talking rodents in those studies, so what about human fertility? Professor Joseph Kruc, the Purdue University biochemist who headed up the initial stevia study on rats in 1968, summed up the likelihood of stevia affecting human fertility. He admitted that the reason the rats in the study experienced fertility issues was because of the overdose of the stevia they were given. For the same effect to be had in humans, a 120-pound human would have to consume upward of seven pounds of stevia a day. Also, these rats were fed extremely high doses of dried green stevia from the entire plant, not just the leaves. It's not unusual for stems and roots to contain higher amounts of toxic components that leaves do not (elderberry is a great example of this).

In fact, the use of stevia and its positive influence on blood sugar (which can also be researched in hundreds of studies) has been touted to improve fertility in women with PCOS. Once insulin levels decrease when sugars and starches are lowered in the diet, cycles normalize and fertility has a much better chance of returning. We receive hundreds of testimonies from women who could not conceive before THM and now that they have regulated their blood sugars they are pregnant!

Miscarriage is a heartbreaking topic. We have both suffered miscarriages and we would never wish that painful loss on any family. We have each had two miscarriages but we had them before we ever began using stevia. We never blamed our diets, which were high in honey and maple syrup at the time probably because those two are such common sweeteners.

When dealing with the trauma of miscarriage sometimes we're just desperate to have a reason—grief is blinding, feelings of loss are overwhelming, and confusion is high. It's human to grasp at anything different in our lives that may or may not have been a cause. Some women can have many full-term pregnancies and then suddenly their body will not carry a pregnancy—"WHY????!!!!" we scream. While there is no scientific evidence to put any blame on stevia for miscarriage, there are anecdotal reports of women who begin stevia use and then relate their miscarriage to that. The tribal folklore and the early rat studies that are often stated as factual keep the suspicions about stevia twirling around in women's minds.

Sadly, the bottom line is that miscarriage is extremely common. An article entitled "Miscarriage Statistics" adapted from the book *Hope Is Like the Sun* states, "Sources vary, but many estimate that approximately 1 in 4 pregnancies end in miscarriage; and some estimates are as high as 1 in 3. If you include loss that occurs before a positive pregnancy test, some estimate that 40 percent of all conceptions result in loss." Before stevia is blamed, one should look at all the known causes.

Solid evidence does back up many reasons for miscarriage, though, but in the end, only God knows.

Real Blame

One thing is for sure, while solid evidence that stevia causes infertility or miscarriage is not to be found (even though multiple studies have attempted to do so), there are many reputable studies pointing to high blood sugar and insulin resistance as certain reasons for both miscarriage and infertility. We would never want to go around saying "Sugar caused my miscarriage!" or "Too much honey caused my friend's or sister's miscarriage," but it is good to know the facts. We have talked to several doctors about the concern over stevia and miscarriage, and their belief meshes with ours. If there is blame to place, let's place it solidly where it is founded—on a high-sugar and high-starch modern lifestyle, which causes disastrous metabolic and hormonal changes to the human body.

The American Diabetes Association says that high glucose levels can increase a woman's chance of miscarriage anywhere from 30 to 60 percent. These are not maybes or rumors—these are hard numbers. According to Dr. Christine Lee in a 2013 article entitled "Diabetes and Your Fertility," high blood sugar also creates an increased risk of having a baby with birth defects. She says, "During the first few weeks of pregnancy, when a baby's vital organs are just beginning to form, high blood glucose can cause damage to the embryonic cells."

There are too many studies to cite supporting the connection between miscarriage and high blood sugar and insulin issues, but here are a few of interest: A 1998 study published in *Cell Biochem Function* found that plasma levels of glucose (blood sugar) were significantly higher in habitual miscarriage than in controls. A 2006 study in *Akush Ginekol (Sofiia)*, published in Bulgaria, showed that high Hb A1-c levels (average levels of blood sugar) in the first trimester of pregnancy had a primary role in the occurrence of early miscarriages. Women who are insulin resistant are four to five times more likely to have a miscarriage.

Choose Peace

Sorry we had to go all hyper-study on you—hope your eyes are not glazing over—but we felt we had to clearly lay out some of this evidence to help clear stevia's name. Having said all this, pregnancy should not be a time for stress and worry. Everyone on plan should feel comfortable with the particular sweetener they choose to use. To use stevia or not will be your own decision to make. But a word of caution: Keep the amounts of any glycemic-impact sweeteners small, especially if you have any form of gestational diabetes. In light of all the evidence concerning high blood sugar and risk of miscarriage, infertility, and higher birth defects, we do advise that you not go overboard with honey or other natural higher-glycemic sweeteners for your own and your baby's health's sake.

chapter 14
FAMILY FRIENDLY

The Trim Healthy Mama way of eating is nutritionally sound for the entire family. Even if other family members are not on the weight-loss part of this plan, you don't have to make completely separate meals. In fact, they can enjoy on-plan meals without even knowing they are on plan at all. This plan is simply regular whole foods, kept in safe blood-sugar boundaries. You may have toddlers, grade school children, teenagers, and full-grown adults all eating around the Trim Healthy Table and all getting their individual needs met.

HOW DOES IT WORK?

There are times, of course, when it is natural to have your own quick "alone Mama" meal. In our homes, lunchtime is usually a free-for-all. Our children are homeschooled and the older ones love to make their own sandwiches or fry up some eggs with toast. This leaves us with endless options. You could make up a quick fillet of salmon and put it on a salad or use leftover chicken in a Wonder Wrap found in the "Breads and Pizza Crusts" chapter in the companion cookbook, or in a store-bought low-carb wrap if you're more like Drive Thru Sue. Have a quick two-minute soup: Just Like Campbell's Tomato Soup is a Trim Healthy Mama favorite (you can find that free recipe on our website). Have it with a grilled cheese made with Swiss Bread if you want—yum! (Check out the Swiss Bread recipe in the "Breads and Pizza Crusts" chapter in the *Trim Healthy Mama Cookbook,* or if you are more of a Drive Thru Sue, use a Joseph's pita to make a grilled cheese.)

Breakfast can be an occasion for gathering around the table or a separate mad rush. A big pot of oatmeal can either go E for you or Crossover for your children, depending on what you pour on top of it: Butter or cream on oatmeal would be a Crossover, and unsweetened almond milk or 0% Greek yogurt would keep it in E mode. Eggs can be S for you or Crossover for them, depending on whether you add a side of veggies or bacon, or your children put theirs on whole-wheat toast. Smoothies? Maybe the whole family is going to love a chocolate berry smoothie—S or FP for you. Add some honey to the blender for extra glucose if your children need a bit more fat on their bones. A wisely sweetened smoothie using our on-plan sweeteners is healthy for all family members, so the honey is an option, not a necessity. Trim Healthy Pancakes found in the "Pancakes, Donuts, Crepes, and Waffles" chapter in the *Trim Healthy Mama Cookbook* are perfect full-family fare. Our children LOVE them slathered with butter and topped with honey. You can keep your pancakes in E mode with 0% Greek yogurt, or if you are a Drive Thru Sue, a squirt or two of fat-free Reddi-wip can keep you happy. Close your eyes if you are a purist—you didn't just read that. We also have a Fuel Pull, dairy-free easy yogurt recipe that will be great on your pancakes. Check out NoGurt in the "Sweet Bowls" chapter of the *Trim Healthy Mama Cookbook*.

The evening meal is the perfect time to get the family together. It is simple to harmonize your fuel choice with the needs of the whole family. Say you choose S, everyone at the table can eat that same yummy protein source. Maybe it is chicken with crispy skin or meat loaf. Make a huge salad with S goodies topping it and your meal will be complete. If you'd like an additional side, roast, steam, or sauté your favorite non-starchy veggies with butter or coconut oil and spices. Your children can enjoy the veggies and salad because they'll be tossed in those decadent fats that children are naturally drawn to, but they can cross this meal over with choices like brown rice, mashed potatoes, or even something as simple as whole-grain bread and butter or a glass of raw, whole milk. The core of your plates is the same, it is only the edges that are a bit different. This is not two meals, this is just one with the ability to choose which sides suit each person.

Let's say you make a big pot of lentil soup for a budget-friendly, E-fueled night and you add some optional chopped chicken breast to the soup for extra protein. You can enjoy a large bowl of the soup, topped with Greek yogurt and maybe a very small amount of part-skim mozzarella (purists can enjoy one tablespoon of raw Pecorino Romano cheese, which has a robust flavor with little fat and calories). You might enjoy a piece of plan-approved toast for dunking. Children can really go to town with grated cheddar and sour cream on their soup for a Crossover effect.

OFF TO WORK

Brown-bag lunches are easy on plan whether you are packing them for yourself or for your family. Your favorite sandwich stuffings, such as egg, chicken, or tuna salad, or deli meat, can easily be placed on S-, E-, or FP-friendly breads or wraps. Or take a salad, a kefir smoothie, or a portion of a leftover soup or casserole. Sides can be little zippy bags of cubed cheese and nuts or Skinny Chocolate (there are many creative versions of our Skinny Chocolate, on Pinterest) jerky, on-plan muffins, mini meat loaves, quiche, fruit, veggie crudité with on-plan dips, boiled eggs, Greek yogurt swirls with frozen berries, or on-plan cookies. Check out Chapter 22, "Heads Up: Working Mamas!" (page 194), for more ideas.

chapter 15
EATING OUT

As a Trim Healthy Mama you won't have to agonize over slim pickings at restaurants. It is very easy to eat out on plan. A steak house date with Hubby? Yes, ma'am! A chicken-topped Caesar salad for lunch at a café? Absolutely! Bacon, eggs, and mushrooms or a cheesy omelet at a pancake or waffle house for breakfast? You bet! Here's how to eat THM at your favorite restaurant.

STEAK HOUSE

Choosing a delicious on-plan meal here is so easy simply because steak house menus are centered around protein sources. S meals are the easiest. Choose from unbreaded chicken, beef, salmon, or other fish such as trout. Order a non-starchy veggie or two for your side instead of the usual potato, mac and cheese, or rice. What's your pleasure— asparagus, broccoli, sautéed mixed veggies, mushrooms? All those veggies are staples at most of these restaurants and can be tossed with butter if you ask your waiter. Your meal will often come with a house salad. Remember to choose a dressing that is not sweet. Oil-and-vinegar, Ranch, or Caesar are usually the safest options. You can be very liberal with oil and vinegar but don't go crazy with Ranch or blue cheese. Although on plan, they're far from superfoods and can turn into caloric abuse if you overdo. But we also want you to enjoy yourself, so don't obsess over the dressing—just be mindful.

Here are some tips to help you out:

- Nix the bread. It is always best to ask your waiter not to bring any bread to your table. If you are dining with someone who would prefer to have bread, simply ask your waiter not to bring your portion. If you forget to do that, know this: The wafting aroma of fresh yeast bread can bring down the strongest of us. It's too hard to resist, except possibly if you're Serene (I couldn't resist writing that from me, Pearl, because bread has undone my best intentions at restaurants while Serene annoyingly remains as strong as a statue.) It is best to ask your waiter to remove the bread and mention that you haven't touched it so he or she can eat it on break. We've made many friends of waiters doing just that.

- Don't eat the croutons on your salad—okay, we'll try not to spy if you just eat one or two. But liberal amounts of croutons can take a perfectly good S meal and ruin its slimming capabilities. Or bring a zippy of Blendtons, found in the "Condiments and Extras" chapter of the *Trim Healthy Mama Cookbook.*

- For special occasions you can sip on a glass of dry wine while you wait for your meal. Other great drink ideas are mineral or soda water with lemon or unsweetened tea (which you can sweeten up yourself with a little trusty stevia that you carry in your purse).

- E meals can be a little more challenging but are not impossible. Sweet potatoes make great E sides with a whitefish or grilled chicken breast. Use the lightest dressing on your salad and hold the cheese. Baked sweet potatoes with butter make fantastic Crossovers with either steak or salmon.

FAST FOOD

Although you'll never see Serene eating fast food, many of us can still enjoy it (had to get another dig at Serene there—Pearl). Many burger joints offer low-carb burgers on their menus. They'll cook up any juicy burger of your choice, whether beef, turkey, or chicken; pile it with your favorite burger fixins; then wrap it in lettuce. Who needs those buns?

Blech to buns when the real flavor of the burger is only enhanced wrapped this way. Okay, so if you don't agree with "Blech to buns" and do miss a bread casing, be not dismayed. Take along a couple of homemade Swiss Bread slices (found in the "Breads and Pizza Crusts" chapter in the companion cookbook) or store-bought Joseph's pitas in a little plastic bag. Throw away those devitalized, health-destroying buns and put your burger and fixins between your blood sugar–friendly bread options. Smart!

No fast-food joint, including McDonald's and Burger King, will think you strange if you ask for your burger without a bun (order it that way and they'll put it in a little box and give you a fork to eat it with), but the following restaurants have low-carb burgers on their actual menus:

Carl's Jr.
Five Guys
Hardee's
In-N-Out Burger
Jimmy John's
Red Robin

Fast-food restaurants usually offer a variety of great protein-topped salads, too. Avoid toppings like craisins or fruit if you intend to use a fatty dressing. Dressings such as Italian, Ranch, blue cheese, or Caesar will be better options than French or honey mustard, as any sweet dressings contain sugar.

Sandwich and sub places don't have to throw you right off plan, either. It might not be a perfect approach but you can order a six-inch whole-wheat sub with lean fillings such as turkey, mustard, a smear of low-fat mayo, and lots of veggies. No, the bread won't be sprouted or sourdough, most likely; but you're doing your best and hopefully this won't be your daily fare. Most popular sub shops such as Subway won't bat an eyelash if you ask them to take out the center of the bread filling so you don't have to have as many of those less-than-stellar wheat carbs. They do it all the time for more health-conscious folks. Panera Bread has a hidden power menu with lots of on-plan S and E options. You can look up the menu online or ask to see it at the restaurant.

MEXICAN

The biggest temptations you'll face at a Mexican restaurant are the chips they place directly in front of you as soon as you sit down. Steer clear of Mexican restaurants if you can't resist those, or ask for cucumber slices and guacamole instead to scratch that dip-and-crunch itch. If you can wait for your food without chowing down on chips, Mexican food works fabulously with a Trim Healthy approach.

The best item to order at a Mexican restaurant is fajitas. Who needs refried beans, rice, and white flour tortillas when you can have seasoned grilled meat with caramelized onions, peppers, and tomatoes? Tell the waiter you won't need the tortillas, rice, or beans. You can top with sour cream, salsa, guacamole, and pico de gallo. Who would miss the bland starches? Not us! Taco salad is another great option—nix the fried corn tortilla shell.

Those who are at Crossover stage can add beans to their meal, but the white rice that is usually served at Mexican restaurants is best avoided.

CHINESE AND JAPANESE

If you follow our tips and avoid the foods that will fatten you up in a jiffy at Chinese restaurants, you can find wonderful dishes of tasty meats and vegetables to fill you all the way up. S meals are once again the easiest.

- Avoid anything that is battered.
- Avoid all sweet sauces.
- Avoid the white rice that only looks brown due to the soy sauce.

What are you left with? Lots of fantastic non-breaded meats and veggies. Try pepper chicken, beef and broccoli, mushroom chicken, and garlic string green beans, just to name a few. Once again we need to throw in the caution not to get too crazy and visit Chinese restaurants too often. Although you will be avoiding the real nasties for your health, most Chinese sauces still do contain a bit of cornstarch used for thickening. But you'll survive this every now and then and if it is a dish you absolutely love, get creative and try to make it at home using glucomannan instead of cornstarch. Try meats and veggies tossed with sauces made from broth; plan-approved sweetener; soy sauce, Bragg Amino Acids, or

Coconut Aminos; chile flakes; and vinegar. Thicken up with glucomannan (aka "Gluccie," available on our website) and you'll have wonderful sweet and spicy flavor. Check out our Orange Chicken recipe in the "Family Skillet Meals" chapter in the *Trim Healthy Mama Cookbook*—amazing!

Japanese hibachi grills are easily THM friendly (if you avoid the rice). Ask for extra veggies and then pick your protein—salmon, steak, or chicken (or shrimp if you eat it). A broth-based soup to start your meal won't be a problem, either.

INDIAN OR THAI

Coconut- or cream-based sauces from these cuisines are perfect for S options. Chicken masala or butter chicken are dishes that won't mess with your weight too much if eaten on occasion. If you eat them too often, these cream-based Indian dishes can bring on calorie abuse from their richness. We're talking oodles and oodles of cream in those sauces, which is fine on occasion but problematic if eaten too often. Add lots of veggies and you won't miss the rice.

Thai curries and soups can be another wonderful option. Avoid the real sweet sauces and starchy noodles and focus on coconut-based red or green curries with lots of health-promoting veggies and chicken or fish.

PIZZA JOINTS

How could one possibly eat at a pizza joint and stay on plan, you wonder? It can be done. Many pizza restaurants have started offering pizza in a bowl for people concerned about their blood-sugar levels. Basically that is just pizza toppings without the crust—super yummy. Go real high on the veggies and meats to get your protein in. If your local pizza buffet does not do that—yep, some of us Trim Healthy Mamas have been known to just eat the toppings, over a green salad, and throw away the crusts—that's not exactly wasteful because white pizza crusts cause health decline, so you're not gaining anything but weight by eating them. Another option is chicken wings. Many pizza places offer those as an option. Just make sure they are not breaded or covered in sweet sauce. Buffalo-style hot sauces are your safest bet, and have a side salad to balance your meat-heavy meal.

chapter 16

TO CHEAT OR TREAT?

Time to deal with the subject of off-plan eating, otherwise known as cheating. Oh boy, this is a painful subject for some of us. The idea of cheating can be either terrifying or liberating depending on our past relationship with certain trigger foods. If you were terribly addicted to sugar and abused your body with junk foods in the past, you're probably so relieved to finally be free from those strongholds with Trim Healthy Mama that one cheat meal doesn't seem worth it. You worry it may send you into a downward tailspin you won't be able to bounce back from. For others, choosing to have off-plan foods every now and then is mentally freeing. Tell us never to cheat and you take away the joyous approach that this is a lifestyle, not a rigorous diet.

No matter how you view off-plan foods, the most helpful thing to know is that as a Trim Healthy Mama you can treat yourself with on-plan goodies all the way to goal weight and then beyond without guilt. The temptation to cheat on sugar or processed, refined starches has far less of a hold when you are not deprived in your everyday life.

Eating some meals off plan is bound to happen at some point. The main problem with cheating is often not the cheat itself, but the shame that derails us. Most of us can handle an off-plan meal occasionally without it affecting our progress to goal weight or our overall health. But for some of us the self-loathing that ensues after cheating can throw us right off track.

PEARL CHATS: *Serene is leaving the bulk of this chapter to me since she has no real desire to cheat ever—in fact, I have never seen her eat an off-plan food. The temptation for such foods simply isn't there and there is no pretending; she is perfectly happy never eating any of that stuff that the rest of us are sometimes tempted with. (Secretly I sometimes think she is an alien dressed up in human skin, since I truly think this is not normal. But what am I saying . . . of course Serene is not normal!)*

SERENE CHATS: *Hey, Pearl, I gave this chapter over to you but that doesn't mean you can use it to bash me. I'm actually only partly alien, not fully like you are leading our readers to believe. Kidding aside, why would I want to cheat if it involves poisoning my body and adding to the aging process? Spiking my blood sugar—I don't get how that's fun. That is not being kind to myself, that is being cruel to myself. Just the way I look at it.*

Pearl has some great advice on how to navigate your way out of cheat disasters, but I do want to add a caution here. Although Pearlie is able to go off plan here and there and survive it just fine, don't let her own liberty to cheat overtake your THM journey. Throw in too many cheat meals and our plan will no longer have the ability to work. I know that Pearl enjoys popcorn at the movies with her husband once a month or so and occasionally eats a donut, but she doesn't do this sort of thing several times a week. Following Trim Healthy Mama part-time, interlaced with a bunch of destructive cheats, is not an approach for success. It is fine to start out that way for the first couple of weeks while you wet your feet; but after you've matured in your journey, you need to do the whole plan, not halfway, nor three quarters of the way.

We are part of a very large extended family. There is always an occasion or party to attend. If we decided to cheat at every birthday, celebration, or family movie night we'd be cutting loose almost as often as staying on plan. I'm not saying you shouldn't have a piece of Aunt Marge's pecan pie at Thanksgiving. Go for it; I don't give Pearlie the evil eye when she eats our sister-in-law's famous cheesecake (made with sugar) at Christmastime. But choosing to eat a traditional family recipe is much different from cheating willy-nilly without good reason.

PEARL CHATS: *Serene's points are valid. (Pretty good for an alien.)*

Now let's find out how to overcome the pitfalls of cheating. Here's Pearl's advice:

GETTING BACK ON TRACK IS AS EASY AS 1, 2, 3

Some of us are going to go off plan at Christmas and Thanksgiving, on our anniversary, and possibly on that cruise we've saved for years to take. My hand is raised. If you choose to stick to luscious S foods on these occasions (which are the easiest celebration foods), I am thrilled for you and fiercely proud of you. You're determining what your body and mind need—you're staying the course and I imagine you don't even feel a little bit deprived with all your S goodies. The rest of us need a way out of the thorns that try to keep us from returning to the green pastures of THM. Here are three easy steps:

1. SHOVE THE SHAME! Maybe in other years you fudged whatever stringent diet you were doing, ate off plan for Thanksgiving or Christmas, and never got back on due to self-loathing. That AIN'T going to happen as a Trim Healthy Mama! Eating off-plan treats to celebrate family and life blessings is a mere blip on the radar of your THM journey.

Refuse to listen to shame when it whispers, "What's the use. You've messed up, might as well drive through and get that shake and biggie fries you know you want." Shame is a liar! You are only three hours away from your next slimming meal. That is grace. God has it for us. He knows we mess up, yet there is no limit to his forgiveness and though we fail he takes us wholly back when we turn back to him.

We also need to offer grace to ourselves. Grace and kindness are more powerful than any boot-camp or purge approach when you fail despite your own best intentions. We love that passage in Romans 2:4 that tells us it is God's kindness that leads us to repentance. Let's learn to be more like our heavenly Father and not sabotage our journeys with self-scolding and punishment because we simply can't forgive our own mess-ups.

Sure, you ate three pieces of Aunt Marge's pecan pie when you told yourself to stop at just a sliver. You got a bit of a belly ache from it and went to bed with some sugar cravings stirred up. This is not the end of it all. You don't have to eat Pop-Tarts the next morning to punish yourself. You can happily jump back on plan because your everyday eating is not a path of deprivation. Your norm is now delicious and satisfying and makes you feel great.

2. DON'T PURGE! Stay out of the vicious cycle that I call "Binge then Purge." Yes, you need to come back to the THM green pastures, but you don't need to eat nasty, dry rabbit-food meals to get yourself back on track. I hear this question a lot: "Help, I ate terribly . . . should I do all Fuel Pulls for a few days?"

"No!"

Deep-S meals like fried eggs in generous amounts of butter are the best ones for getting back on track and getting all those excess sugars out of your cells. Or get some of that leftover meat, put it on a huge plate of salad, and use heaps of extra-virgin olive oil in your dressing. Eating too few calories and denying yourself fats to try to combat your splurge will only make your cravings worse. Remember that fats satisfy. Sure, you can still have your usual amounts of Fuel Pull snacks or enjoy a Fat Stripping Frappa (found in the "Shakes, Smoothies, Frappas, and Thin Thicks" chapter in the companion cookbook) as a meal now and then, but don't overdo these low-calorie items when you are trying to bounce back from a cheat fest. I think that a couple of Deep-S meals in a row are the best way to do a THM reset (from my own experience).

3. ENOUGH IS ENOUGH! Don't let one or two cheat meals turn into a whole season of cheating. The freedom THM offers is one thing, but seriously harming your body is another. Don't give yourself license to spike your blood sugar with off-plan foods from Thanksgiving all the way until January 1. You'll wake up on the first day of the New Year feeling desperate and more apt to make extreme food choices, which will only create another vicious cycle.

No, life will not always be perfect; you may travel for the holidays and not have access to your own kitchen. Do your best and baby-step your way back. Eat on plan when you can, but if you have to continue with less-than-perfect THM meals for a few days, that does not have to derail you forever. Say the word *blip* with me: This is temporary. But if constant cheating goes on for another week or two weeks . . . then I'll need to send Serene to shake you up and give you one of her Sergeant Serene lectures. Now you're only harming this incredible body God gave to you to look after.

What if the holidays pass but you still have sugar-laden pumpkin pie in your house and cookies galore? They are doing you in: You feel derailed, you can't fight 'em. Take action: They go in the trash or they go to a shelter, they do not stay in your house! You don't want to waste? It is a greater waste of health to continue to eat them, and ill health is much more expensive than throwing away a box or two or cookies. You have plenty of incredible THM treats to replace them with. Don't allow your body to be the garbage can when you have one already.

You are never too far gone to deserve another chance. We're all going to mess up, that's a given. Practicing your comeback will be what gets you all the way to goal and beyond.

chapter 17

AFFORDABLE SUPERFOODS

Just because you can't afford a bunch of specialty foods doesn't mean you can't thrive on plan. Most of the wonderful foods you'll be eating on a daily basis can be found at any grocery store and can fit within the tightest of budgets. Check out Chapter 21, "Heads Up: Budgeting Mamas!" (page 185), for more tips on how to do the plan super-inexpensively.

It's time to take a closer look at the health benefits of some of your everyday budget-friendly foods that are actually superfoods! We want you to know the reasons behind our ardent enthusiasm that they be front and center on plan so that you make sure to include them.

EGGS, EGGS, GLORIOUS EGGS

You don't have to eat meat at every meal. Eggs are a cheap source of protein. The bright orange yolks from chickens running free are undoubtedly the healthiest, but regular ol' eggs still grow healthy children and trim down adults that need trimming. We'd all eat free-range eggs in a perfect world but even battery-raised eggs contain health-promoting nutrients. Both of us raise chickens for eggs, but we fall short some weeks so off to our Aldi budget chain we go to buy dozens of regular old eggs. They are still rich in EPA and DHA (responsible for nervous system health and mental health) and sulfur-containing proteins crucial for cell membrane integrity. Eggs are the highest source of leucine, which stands above all branched amino acids for muscle building.

The Cholesterol Myth

Do not be too concerned about the cholesterol scare. Sugar and trans fats are the worst offenders, not eggs. God provided choline, found in the egg, as the perfect built-in cholesterol aid. It helps to raise HDL cholesterol, or what is known as good cholesterol. This is needed for proper hormone production. It is actually dangerous for total cholesterol levels to be too low. This increases the risk of heart attack, since adequate cholesterol ensures adequate hormones and without adequate hormones the immune system breaks down. Most people find their lipid profile improves after following the Trim Healthy Mama Plan despite eating more eggs. You'll likely see your triglyceride levels come down. This is a good indication that your cholesterol particles are becoming bigger and fluffier and not as dangerous as the small, dense cholesterol particles indicated by high triglycerides. High triglycerides are caused by a high-carb lifestyle and the high blood-sugar and insulin levels that come with it. More and more knowledgeable doctors are looking to other cholesterol markers rather than just overall cholesterol.

SALMON

All forms of meat are on plan, but wild fish have incredible cardiovascular health benefits and salmon is the king of them all. Salmon is rich in omega-3 fatty acids and therefore is highly anti-inflammatory. It is our highest food source of dimethylaminoethanol, or DMAE. This firms and lifts our skin and brings tone to our appearance. DMAE is essential fat for brain health and has been shown to be very effective in combating conditions like Attention Deficit Disorder and lack of concentration.

A piece of wild salmon either sautéed, poached, baked, or fried, served over a bed of buttery sautéed greens, or diced yellow squash or zucchini is a perfect quick and (if bought as frozen fillets) inexpensive lunch. Most budget grocery stores will have a pack of four frozen wild salmon fillets for under five bucks. That's just a little over a dollar for a superfood protein source. Frozen fillets are quick to thaw since they usually come wrapped in their own protective package. Just drop them into room temp water, and in an hour or so they should be ready to cook.

If you've given salmon a fair try and still can't acquire a taste for it, all other clean, wild fish are great options. What? Did we just hear a "blech"? Some distant voices saying they don't like fish at all? At least give our Super Salmon Patties a try. You can find that free recipe on our website as well as in the "Extra Skillet Stuff" chapter of the *Trim Healthy Mama Cookbook*. They are an inexpensive and easy evening meal that gets raves from the whole family. Or try our Salmon Mousse (found in the chapter on "Crackers, Chips, and Dips" in the *Trim Healthy Mama Cookbook*) with plan-approved crackers or slices of cucumber—delish! And the lemon juice really takes away any fishiness. If you can't stomach fish in any form, there are plenty of other protein options for you on plan; but consider taking a good cod liver, fish, or krill oil supplement so you don't miss out on the benefits.

BERRIES

These are nature's candy, but more than just being sweet and exotic, they pack powerful health punches. The bright color of berries gives away their health secret: They are brimming with phytochemicals, those nutrients that protect our cells from disease and damage. The wonderful thing about berries is that due to the fact that they are not prone to causing a spike in blood sugar, they can be used in both S and E meals—*woot!*

Frozen berries can be enjoyed on plan all year long and are the budget-friendly way to enjoy berries. Throw them into smoothies, thaw and mix into yogurt, stir into your oatmeal, whiz them into Cottage Berry Whip, or bake into muffins and pies. In summer, you'll find sales for fresh berries or, if you're lucky like us and live in the woods, you can pick them wild. Just pop them into your mouth or throw them onto your salad.

Just one handful of blueberries per day significantly decreases inflammation in the brain. Strawberries have more vitamin C than oranges. Cranberries significantly boost your immune system. Blackberries owe their deep purple color to anthocyanin, which is believed to be effective in fighting cell mutation and cancer. Red raspberries contain high amounts of ellagic acid, which has been shown in clinical studies to cause death to cancer cells. They are also high in quercetin, which protects the heart, and they contain ketones (which are thought to aid in weight loss). Our children love to eat frozen berries right out of the bag and we don't mind a bit!

LEAFY GREENS

We keep insisting that you include non-starchy veggies and, of these, your greens in leafy form are most important. They won't cost you an arm or a leg. We love purchasing the large containers of organic field greens from our local budget store for just two bucks fifty. Already washed and cut, they make for super-quick meals. If all you can afford is nonorganic lettuce, we believe it is still much better to eat it than to not eat lettuce at all.

We don't nag you to include more leafy greens just because they are Fuel Pulls and can go with any meal. You NEED their vital health benefits. A large plate of leafy greens decadently tossed with superfood oils and topped with hearty protein such as eggs, salmon, tuna, chicken, or steak is a superfood meal.

Most people don't realize it but meat contains all the necessary amino acids for life, all the essential fats, and twelve of the thirteen vitamins. The one vitamin missing from meat is vitamin C, which is integral for your immune and adrenal health. Greens are extremely high in vitamin C. Problem fixed. Here's a little poem for you to remember:

> *Add some greens when you eat meat*
> *They will make your meal complete!*

OKRA

Get ready for our rant on one of the healthiest foods on earth—and we love it even more because you can buy a nice-size frozen bag of it at your grocery store for under two bucks! While we want you to eat oodles of all kinds of non-starchy veggies, after much research we've realized okra deserves its own special time in the spotlight and, sorry, but we couldn't reduce its benefits to one or two paragraphs. We want everyone clued in on this humble, inexpensive food that slashes high blood sugar and the ravages of Type 2 diabetes, helps melt super-stubborn pounds, and heals your gut.

Now before you go all "yuckety yuck" and "grossity gross" on us because you are one of those people who hates okra and thinks it tastes like slime, give us some faith. We won't make you eat something you hate because you'll feel guilty if you don't. That's not the Trim Healthy Mama way. We want you to love your food and we are determined to get you loving okra. Due to certain members of our own family who started out as okra haters, we have had to get very creative with disguises. You okra haters can now reap the full benefits of this amazing vegetable by making some of our bluffing recipes that work on our pickiest slime-detecting children. Okra in brownies? You are the only person who will know this classified information. No need to tell your family members. Just smile as you watch them happily devour the goodness. Check out Cry-No-More Brownies in the "Brownies and Cookies" chapter of the *Trim Healthy Mama Cookbook*. Or try the Choco Secret Big Boy smoothie in the "Shakes, Smoothies, Frappas, and Thin Thicks" chapter. You'd never know it contains slimming, healing okra.

Why are we so gung-ho about okra? It has beneficial insulin-like properties that allow your body to reduce the amount of insulin it has to secrete itself. Remember that overexcretion of insulin causes fat storage and that dratted insulin resistance. Okra also contains a unique kind of fermentable fiber that helps your body regulate high blood-sugar levels. This medicinal food boasts one of the highest levels of phytonutrients and antioxidants such as beta-carotene, xanthin, and lutein. It contains dense nutrition yet miraculously comes with very meager calories.

A Hero to Support All Seasons

In Chapter 23, "Heads Up: Pregnant and Nursing Mamas!" (page 199), we encourage all our pregnant Mamas to become frequent okra eaters because of its abundance in folate, which not only helps prevent birth defects like spina bifida but also promotes the growth of strong bones. The rich vitamin C in okra helps with optimal fetal development and keeps a pregnant Mama's immune system firing strong during this special time when her body is often maxed out by a new full-time responsibility. But okra is universally talented and its merits reach way beyond pregnancy to benefit all seasons of life. This folate-rich non-starchy veggie can also keep a full-grown Mama's bones strong and prevent osteoporosis. Including okra is a no-brainer if you are a postmenopausal woman at risk for bone loss and it makes sense as a bone-loss preventative for the rest of us as we age. Its high vitamin C levels are a great counterattack to the stress and chaos we all face in our lives, especially with adrenal fatigue becoming such an epidemic. Our adrenal glands require vitamic C to function and we all need more highly bolstered immune systems to help fight off the ravages of disease.

Research in Brazil uncovered okra's uncanny ability to kill human breast cancer cells, prostate cancer cells, and some melanoma cells in a study published in 2012 in a British journal called *Biology Letters.* The researchers expounded on how a lectin found within the okra pod seems to induce apoptosis, or cell death, in cancer cells. This miracle buried in okra helped slow the growth of breast cancer cells by a dramatic 63 percent and killed up to 72 percent of human breast cancer cells in an in-vitro setting.

By supporting the production of red blood cells, okra fights anemia. Its extra-special kind of fiber lowers serum cholesterol levels and helps battle heart disease and arteriosclerosis. Its high antioxidant levels protect the immune system and prevent cell mutation, making this special little "gumbo" veggie a robust anticancer weapon in more than just one way.

Please Don't Call It Slime

Okra's famous mucilage (we won't call it slime from here on out, as we cannot hurt a superhero's feelings) coats your intestines with a moisturizing, healing layer that soothes an irritable bowel, soothes ulcers, prevents colon cancer, may help with food sensitivities, and relieves constipation. As a prebiotic it provides a perfect environment for good bacteria to multiply and form a strong healthy inner ecology.

We've nicknamed our okra recipes "Tummy Spa" recipes because that is exactly what they are. They nourish and pamper the bowels and intestines like healing beauty creams would do for the skin. Any recipe made with okra is a "spa" for the colon. Check out our Tummy Spa Ice Cream recipe made with okra in the "Frozen Treats" chapter in the *Trim Healthy Mama Cookbook.*

Weight-Loss Friend

This mucilage, the very thing that freaks some people out, is a phenomenal aid to weight loss. It satiates the appetite and helps curb overeating. But this ability to help curb overeating is not the only reason that okra is touted as a friend to those trying to lose weight. It helps protect the body against lectins that may bind to insulin receptors and destroy the lining of the gut. In Chapter 31, "Balance Is Beautiful" (page 273), we'll discuss the mistaken notion that all lectins are a bunch of baddies. Lectins, otherwise known as glycoproteins, are found in most foods and are important for the proper messaging and signaling in our bodies. They also break down the membranes of hurtful invaders such as cancer cells and dangerous viruses and bacteria.

But some people with hormonal conditions such as PCOS can be overly sensitive to lectins. They may be more affected by certain lectins that bind to insulin receptors in fat cells and send them the same message that insulin gives, which is to make more fat. Due to a lack of feedback control from other hormonal and biological pathways associated with regular insulin messaging, these lectin signals don't know how to shut off. The humble okra pod comes to the rescue once again. This mucilaginous wonder-fiber has the ability to bind to lectins in a way that renders them harmless. Lectins become good guys again instead of troublemakers.

But I'm Pretty Sure I Still Hate Okra

Okay . . . you're sold on the fact that you need to feature okra in your diet, but how? What if the very thought of chewing it up in your mouth is making you want to hurl? Then you'll want to make plenty of our "okra in disguise" recipes in the companion cookbook. Believe us when we say Secret Silk Pie and ice cream are beyond delicious when made with this secret agent.

Rohnda Monroy is a Trim Healthy Mama who has been such a trouper helping with our cookbook project. As soon as we finish a recipe, we pass it to her. She makes it, offers us any feedback, and takes the beautiful photographs you see in the companion cookbook. She was very skeptical about okra at first but has come to love it in so many of the recipes. She was overcome with joy when she made our okra-filled Choco Secret Big Boy Smoothie (in the "Shakes, Smoothies, Frappas, and Thin Thicks" chapter of the *Trim Healthy Mama Cookbook*) and tried it on her son Jonah, who has autism. Jonah is extremely wary of any new food and has issues with any strange tastes or textures but he slurped up the whole thing with a huge smile!

CULTURED DAIRY PRODUCTS AND VEGETABLES

By enjoying our basic meals, you will lower and balance your blood-sugar levels, but with the addition of fermented foods, you can actually heal the havoc of overgrown yeast that years of sugar consumption may have caused. Cultured foods contain beneficial bacteria and provide a natural antibiotic and anticarcinogenic effect to the body. They contain abundant amounts of living enzymes, so we think of them as raw foods on steroids! A salad is great and contains enough living enzymes to help you digest that meal efficiently, but the addition of a little lacto-fermented sauerkraut or a few sips of kefir have more living enzymes than even a salad can offer. These lacto-fermented foods make sure you will not only preserve but replenish the enzyme count in your body. Serene's two most popular cultured recipes, Artisan Sourdough Bread and Double Fermented Kefir, which she has tweaked to make even easier for you, are featured in our companion cookbook.

Many of our purist Mamas may already be making lacto-fermented kimchi and sauerkraut. Cabbage is a very inexpensive veggie, so sauerkraut will offer you wonderful health benefits but won't break your budget. But hey, some of us are never going to get around to that. Regular pickles, if unsweetened, can be enjoyed on plan, but they should not be confused with the lacto-fermented superfoods we are talking about here. They are usually prepared in a canning process in which they are exposed to high heat, which means there will be no living enzymes. True living sauerkraut must be refrigerated. Bubbies brand, which contains these healing living enzymes, can be purchased in some grocery stores.

Greek yogurt has twice the amount of protein of regular yogurt, has far fewer carbs, and is wonderfully healthy for your inner digestive ecology. Yogurt and kefir made from raw milk are optimum, but even if made from pasteurized milk, they are beneficial. They basically rise from the dead and start living again after culturing.

Don't buy sweetened yogurt (unless you find a brand sweetened with on-plan sweeteners); you can easily sweeten up your Greek yogurt at home with a doonk of stevia or a teaspoon or two of Gentle Sweet or all-fruit jelly. We consider plain 0% Greek yogurt a Fuel Pull food. You can have a full cup of it if it is the main protein component of your meal, but if it is used as a tag-on such as a dessert, it's best to stick to a half cup. Or try our Jigglegurt recipe in the "Sweet Bowls" chapter of the *Trim Healthy Mama Cookbook*. It slashes the carbs of yogurt in half and is a sheer delight to eat. It is a budgeting Mama's friend, as it stretches two cups of yogurt into four cups. Our purist Mamas will want to make their own Greek yogurt. There are hundreds of recipes available on the Internet that explain how to make yogurt and then strain it. Regular nonfat yogurt should be considered an E since it still contains the whey water.

GOLDEN FLAXSEEDS

We debated putting this info about flaxseeds into the next chapter along with the other specialty ingredients, but nope, flaxseeds are very budget-friendly and thankfully flaxseed flour can now be found at almost any grocery store (often next to chia seeds, which also pack a powerful health punch and are in some of our recipes). A full pound of ground golden flax should cost you less than five bucks and will probably last you a good length of time. We like to think we have a little something to do with ground flax meal becoming so readily available. We encouraged it for baking in our previous book and our Mamas create a high demand. You can use brown flaxseeds if that is all you can find, but we think baked goods are much prettier with golden flax and we find it has a milder taste.

Flaxseeds carry one of the biggest nutrient payloads on the planet so they truly fit the budget super-star title. To obtain these nutrients from flax, it has to be ground. Your body cannot absorb them in its whole seed form. Ground golden flax is one of the flours mixed into our Baking Blend, found on our website, but it can be used as frugal stand-alone baking flour, too. Check out our Frosted Cinnamon Muffin (found on our website) or Chocolate Chai-Glazed Cinnamon Muffins (in the "Family Muffins" chapter in the *Trim Healthy Mama Cookbook*) if you want to try inexpensive flax flour for baking. Toss ground flax in your salad, sprinkle a teaspoonful in your oatmeal or in a smoothie, and get started baking yummy treats with it.

Flax is not a grain, but its vitamin and mineral profile is more similar to that of a grain than of a seed. Like grains, flax is high in most of the B vitamins, and for you that means better mood and ENERGY! It is rich in omega-3 fatty acids, which fight inflammation in your body.

Flax is full of fiber and disease-fighting lignans. It is this fiber in flax that is responsible for its ability to help lower harmful cholesterol. The lignans are known for their ability to balance female hormone issues, decrease premenstrual symptoms, and possibly help prevent breast and colon cancer.

Some people are fearful of flax because they have read that it has estrogen-like qualities. Studies show that it is these very qualities that offer protection against cancers of the reproductive organs. The estrogen-like lignans in flax attach to hormone receptors and help to block more harmful estrogens in the body while allowing less aggressive estrogens to flourish. A healthier estrogen ratio is thus supported.

APPLE CIDER VINEGAR

Raw apple cider vinegar, or ACV for short, is one of the key throat-tingling players in our refreshing Good Girl Moonshine (watch our YouTube video on how to make this drink or look up the recipe in the *Trim Healthy Mama Cookbook*). That wild drink has made many an ACV convert—or maybe we should say addict. But there are many other ways that we enjoy ACV, so it is a regular necessity in our grocery carts. A little drizzle in homemade salad dressing, soups, chilis, meat loaves, and stews gives the perfect tang to round out the flavors and satisfy the taste buds.

ACV is the quickest, cheapest, and easiest of all superfoods to add a no-fuss health boost to your meals. The gourmet flare with which it brightens up the palate is only one reason to include raw ACV. It is a lively and robust health-promoter and can definitely boost the healthiness of your own Trim Healthy Mama journey.

For ultimate taste and health promotion, your ACV needs to be raw and contain the "mother," which is a cloudy spiderweb-like growth that usually sits at the bottom of the bottle or, when the bottle is jostled, floats in the vinegar. ACV with the mother is raw, so it contains many more vitamins and minerals than regular vinegar. Most grocery store chains stock this form of ACV now. Even the famous Heinz brand has a raw version at an affordable cost.

Raw ACV contains a number of beneficial acids, such as acetic and malic acid, that are revolutionary to waning health. It is a potent liquid filled with vitamins A, E, C, and B_6, thiamin, riboflavin, niacin, pantothenic acid, as well as other goodies like beta-carotene, lycopene, mineral salts, amino acids, and pectin. It is also rich in minerals such as phosphorus, potassium, sodium, calcium, iron, and magnesium.

Here are just some of the perks Apple Cider Vinegar can offer you:

- It is abundant in potassium, which is imperative for growth and building muscles, the transmission of nerve impulses, heart activity, and preventing brittle teeth and hair loss.
- It encourages weight loss by breaking down fats to be used instead of being stored in your adipose tissue.
- It slows the digestion of starch and lowers the rise in glucose levels that occurs after mealtimes because of its potency in acetic acid.
- It is antiviral, antifungal, and antibacterial due to its high levels of malic acid (we frequently hear testimonies from our Good Girl Moonshine drinkers who have had warts disappear that they could previously not get rid of).
- It is super-alkalinizing.
- It helps to lower bad cholesterol and regulate blood pressure.
- It is a powerful detox tool and improves bowel function.
- It is a digestive aid and a simple but effective remedy for heartburn.
- It clarifies the skin.
- It shows strength in new research at killing cancer cells or slowing their growth.

chapter 18
SPECIALTY FOOD STARS

Let's get this out in the open in case you are worried. You don't NEED to purchase any specialty foods from us to make this plan work. The vast majority of your meals will be made with regular foods from any grocery store. You will see some of our recipes in the companion cookbook calling for items like whey protein, collagen, and glucomannan (Gluccie). Yes, they are awesome superfoods; but hey, if you can't afford them or can't access them, don't stress it. Keep it simple! You can take the meals you are eating right now and apply the THM principles to them rather than trying those particular recipes at first. Don't fear, we have oodles of easy recipes that use everyday foods, too.

We shudder at the thought of diets that make their own brand of products mandatory. We never thought we'd end up carrying products, but demand happened. Sometimes we just have to shake our heads and laugh at the direction our lives have taken. This accidental Food Freedom movement threw us neck-deep into the food business—not something we ever conceived we'd be doing. But other companies do not have our Mamas' needs in mind. They often change product formulas on a whim and we have no control over that. We promoted other brands and, over and over again, this problem arose. Our readers begged us for products they could come to rely on, so we started the Trim Healthy Mama food line.

But the truth is, you can find success on a very tight budget and never buy even one of our food items. Or, you can save your pennies and order our fun items only when you are ready. You can make Trim Healthy Mama work within your budget no matter how tight. We understand what it feels like to struggle financially, so don't feel any pressure from us to fill your cupboards with specialty foods. For years we struggled to make ends meet and our husbands had to work two jobs to keep our families barely afloat. We shopped at saver stores like Aldi (and still do). If we could make it work, anyone can. Our ultimate desire is for you to flourish and succeed without having to break the bank to do it! But if you do have a little leeway in your budget, boy oh boy, do we have some goodies for you!

GELATIN

By now you know Trim Healthy Mama is based upon protein grounding all your meals. If you've only thought of gelatin as something that makes a red or yellow wiggly dessert— that's all about to change. Gelatin is a pure protein, rich in glycine and proline, two amino acids with incredible healing abilities. Just one tablespoon of gelatin gives you ten grams of this nourishing protein, and it is the perfect substitute for anyone allergic or sensitive to other forms of protein supplementation. Although gelatin is not technically a complete protein, it is a "muscle-sparing" protein; so when you consume it as a main protein source in your meals, your body will not break down its own muscle tissue. Also, since Trim Healthy Mama is rich in other forms of protein, changing up with gelatinous forms is a healthful balance.

The time-tested folklore remedy of home-simmered chicken soup to rescue a weary soul from nearly every ailment imaginable rests on this one treasured ingredient: gelatin. As the pot simmers away, releasing the nutrients from bones, the liquid transforms into a collagen-rich flavorful stock that is phenomenally good for your body. The benefits of gelatin-rich stock are not just folklore; gelatin is an imperative part of the diet not only for the health benefits it brings but also for the balance it maintains.

Bones, Glorious Bones

If homemade stock made from clean meat bones is regular fare at your home, then supplementing gelatin may not be as crucial to you as it is to others. All of us get busy, however, and sometimes even the most ardent scratch cook cannot find the time to make stock when life gets crazy. That's just the time when your body needs the benefits of gelatin the most, since gelatin supports your immune system! If you're not the type who wants to boil down bones too often, daily supplementation with gelatin is a very smart move. It is easy and practical to get the benefits of gelatin daily in a powdered form without having to always rely on bone stock. (But we hope you'll still try your hand at making stock by trying the stock recipes in our cookbook, Purist Bone Stock and the supereasy Bone Stock for Drive Thru Sues found in the "Condiments and Extras" chapter in the *Trim Healthy Mama Cookbook* or search for some online. There are heaps of stock recipes on Pinterest.)

The gelatin available in most grocery stores is usually derived from pork and is not considered a clean source. It may look a little more budget-friendly coming in such a tiny box, but ounce for ounce it is not. However, you can still use it on the plan. Gelatin derived from the bones of cows fed a clean diet primarily of grass is the optimum nutritional source. You can add this clean gelatin to your soups, chilis, smoothies, puddings, or even your morning coffee. Watch your skin, hair, gut, mood, immune system, and so many other bodily functions improve.

There are two forms of powdered gelatin we recommend: hydrolized collagen (which dissolves in all liquid whether hot or cold and will not thicken anything) and basic gelatin (traditional gelling type of gelatin which needs to "bloom" before dissolving in cold liquid). This type of gelatin will thicken cold liquids. You can order Integral Collagen and Just Gelatin from our website. They are 100% pure, pork-free, and processed with integrity from grass-fed cows. If you want to look for these items locally or elsewhere online be sure to seek out grass-fed beef-bone sources of both collagen and gelatin.

What's the difference between these two sources of gelatin? They are fundamentally the same thing but they shine in different ways. They both offer incredible healing capabilities and both contain significant amounts of glycine and proline, which are the two amino acids greatly responsible for their health benefits. As a pure protein both are the perfect substitute for anyone allergic or sensitive to other forms of protein supplementation.

Let's learn a little about their unique abilities.

Just Gelatin

This is the old-fashioned type of gelatin that sets up when cold and helps make delicious treats like the Lemon Pucker Gummies or Skinny Chocolate Truffles found in the "Candies and Bars" chapter of the *Trim Healthy Mama Cookbook.* This kind of gelatin takes longer to digest, which benefits your digestive system and is known as the gut healer. It is hydrophilic in nature, which means it attracts water and forms a soothing layer inside the mucosal lining of the digestive tract. If you have any gut problems, such as irritable bowel syndrome, or if you suffer from food sensitivities, including Just Gelatin in your diet can be an incredible help.

As well as soothing the intestines and bowel, Just Gelatin aids in more efficient digestion and breakdown of nutrients. It is the most budget-friendly of the two supplements, so this is the one we add to our big pots of family soups, chilis, and stews to amp up the nourishment and balance their amino acid profiles. As long as it stays hot, it won't thicken your liquids, so don't imagine that you'll be eating a jellylike soup or chili.

Integral Collagen

This type of gelatin is in the form of collagen peptides. This simply means gelatin's amino acids are broken down into smaller chains called peptides. This is accomplished by a natural enzyme found in pineapples, so there's no need to worry about the processing as it is accomplished very naturally. These collagen peptides are quickly absorbed into your bloodstream and are more efficiently utilized by your body for therapeutic uses. Collagen shines as a wonderful healer of joint pain and arthritis. It improves hair and nail growth and skin elasticity. It is known for its wrinkle-smoothing abilities.

The other factor that makes the peptides more desirable at times is that they do not set when chilled. Since they dissolve in liquid, they are perfect to swirl into Greek yogurt or pour into your hot tea for a nutritional overhaul. Integral Collagen is the more potent "let's-get-serious" approach to collagen supplementation.

Both supplements, including good old-fashioned homemade stock (which we hope you will make), are packed full of the amino acids glycine and proline and harness the following abilities:

- Support the immune system
- Release fat-burning glucagon
- Soothe anxiety
- Aid sleep and ease insomnia
- Improve digestion
- Help heal a compromised (leaky) gut
- Detoxify the liver
- Decrease allergies and food intolerances
- Increase production of human growth hormone
- Boost the metabolism
- Satiate and dampen cravings

- Beautify and strengthen skin, hair, and nails
- Remineralize teeth
- Fight arthritis
- Strengthen bones and joints
- Reduce cellulite by improving connective tissue
- Help prevent heart disease
- Reverse atherosclerosis deposits
- Battle against prostate cancer

There are more, but we don't want to write a fat encyclopedia this time around.

Whey Protein

Whey protein's health and weight-loss merits are extensive, but, putting those aside for a second, we love it best of all because it creams up our smoothies and shakes like nothing else can! Whey protein positively influences hormones and body signals to flush fat, decrease appetite, boost mood, rev the metabolism, and raise the thermogenic temperature. Whey's microfractions work synergistically to support muscle growth and recovery, tissue healing, immune function, and digestive health.

There is a lot of conflicting information about what to buy or what not to buy when it comes to a whey protein supplement. We spent a couple of years studying hard, trying to get to the bottom of it. Not every whey protein supplement provides these health benefits. Many are cheap concentrates that are either harshly processed or, even if prepared with integrity, retain fat, lactose, and cholesterol. In powdered form, cholesterol is extremely vulnerable to oxidation and it becomes injurious to our health. Some whey concentrate products try to separate themselves from the pack with extremely high price tags. They come with many misleading slogans. Some even try to claim that their whey is raw. The bottom line is that it is illegal and impossible to retail a whey supplement from raw dairy.

After a year or two of study in this subject and headache after headache due to promoting other brands that subsequently changed their formula, we settled on sourcing a cross-flow micro-filtered type of whey for ourselves and our Trim Healthy Mama community. This form of whey protein isolate is the most biologically preserved and beneficial form that successfully and healthfully removes any denatured particles. Cross-flow micro-filtered (or CFM) whey protein isolate is the most undenatured form of whey available.

Its native protein structures remain intact to a large degree by a cold-processed isolation method using ceramic micro-filters. During this micro-filtration process, undesired particles such as lactose, cholesterol, and even any denatured fractions are successfully removed. After filtration the whey is spray-dried using low temperatures. CFM whey isolate is the protein with the highest biological value of all proteins. It retains high percentages of immunoglobulins and minerals and is higher in calcium than other whey protein supplements.

CFM whey is rich in alpha-lactalbumin. This wonderful protein fraction, which is also found in abundance in immune-protecting mother's milk, has the highest bio-availability and has the greatest efficiency of any other protein fraction. Alpha-lactalbumin is nature's chief source of an essential and often missing amino acid called tryptophan. Tryptophan is needed for the manufacture of our brain chemical serotonin. Proper serotonin levels help keep our appetites in check, regulate our sleep patterns, and improve our mood—especially under stress. It is in this power-packed alpha-lactalbumin that we find the treasure cysteine. This is the amino acid that is the direct precursor to glutathione. It is glutathione that is our body's most effective immune-builder and antioxidant.

Trim Healthy Mama's Pristine Whey Protein Powder is authentic CFM whey with nothing else added. No flavors, colors, or sweeteners are added. It is not enriched with artificial vitamins and minerals, or diluted by being mixed with cheaper forms of whey so that we can make an extra buck. You can purchase this from our website; but if you want to buy locally or elsewhere online, search for a whey protein with a CFM-certified stamp, then you know you are getting the real deal. Since it does not contain lactose, this form of whey can be used by most dairy-sensitive Mamas. Don't buy whey that is sweetened with any artificial sweeteners (sucralose is common), and similar to our warning with stevia sweeteners, look out for baddies like maltodextrin in the ingredient list. Your whey should have only one gram or less of carbs per serving. Avoid concentrate forms of whey or cheap-grade isolates. If you cannot afford a CFM whey isolate, the next best version of whey will be a micro-filtered whey isolate. Beware of ion-exchange whey protein, which is processed using electrical charge. This involves using the acidic chemicals hydrochloric acid and sodium hydroxide. Whey's pH levels are drastically changed and as a result most of the important native whey protein fractions like alpha-lactalbumin, glycomacro-peptides, immunoglobulins, and lactoferrin are destroyed. Beta-lactoglobulin, which can cause allergies in some, can survive the pH change and become the most abundant native protein structure in ion-exchanged whey.

Glucomannan (aka "Gluccie") Powder and Noodles

We have nicknamed this incredible food "Gluccie." Why? It is our kitchen buddy, and every buddy needs a nickname. Did you notice we said "food?" This powder might have a funny name but it is simply a root that has been used in Asian cultures for centuries that goes by the name of konjac. In this powdered form, konjac root is an incredible calorie-free, carb-free, and fat-free thickener that allows us to eat yummy puddings, ice cream, and thick smoothies and "frappas." Usually savory sauces and gravies are in the fattening category since they are thickened with cornstarch or flour—but Gluccie turns all that upside down and makes these foods slimming! It is a fantastic weight-loss tool. Studies show that it enhances the weight-loss effect of all diets but amazingly, even if used in the absence of a calorie-restricted diet, glucomannan stands alone as a weight-loss tool.

This konjac root also transforms into zero-calorie noodles—think pad thai—yum! We get to indulge in all these goodies and experience a host of health benefits at the same time. It is nature's second most alkalizing food and a wonderful balance to meat and dairy, which leave a more acidic ash in the body after digestion. It is a grain-free, gluten-free product that is a great find for those with celiac disease and wheat intolerance.

Gluccie is a wonder food for those with diabetes—a source of fiber that absorbs several times its weight in water and forms a gel in the stomach, creating a feeling of fullness. This is a boon for those with diabetes or prediabetic conditions as it slashes the rise of blood sugar in half and allows for a slower, more safe release of carbohydrates. It helps keep fasting blood glucose levels stable. A study conducted on diabetic patients who were given glucomannan for ninety days showed a drop in their fasting glucose levels by an average of 29 percent. If you have high blood-sugar readings in the morning, try some Gluccie pudding as an evening snack and you may notice a remarkable improvement the next morning. Check out our "Trim Healthy Mama Puddings Part 1 and 2" videos on YouTube or enjoy the many new Gluccie puddings, creamy drinks, and sauces we make in the *Trim Healthy Mama Cookbook.*

Gluccie can be a great dinner helper. We both have large families and try to stretch our meals as far as they can go. Gluccie helps us accomplish this in dishes like spaghetti sauce and chili. Once you have made up your regular sauce or chili, simply put one and a half cups of boiling water in a blender and add three quarters to one teaspoon of Gluccie. Blend until it is thickened. Add that to your sauce and you create a greater volume of food! This also helps to blunt the blood-sugar rise from the meal and cuts calories per serving. This is a wonderful trick to help lower the glycemic load of your family meals.

Gluccie is the most powerful fiber you will come across yet it does not have a fiber-ish mouth feel. For this reason it is an incredible cholesterol regulator and colon cleanser. You'll want to drink lots of water when you eat anything made with Gluccie to help it broom out your colon. Those with sensitive stomachs will want to start gently with it. If a gassy problem is quite severe at first, pull back and use smaller amounts at a slower pace. Little by little your body should become more accustomed to it. Although it is very cleansing, Gluccie is known to soothe conditions such as diverticulitus.

On plan we use this powder as a food always mixed with a liquid, such as in the Fat-Stripping Frappa in the "Shakes, Smoothies, Frappas, and Thin Thicks" chapter in the *Trim Healthy Mama Cookbook*. There have been some concerns that when people use it as a supplement in capsule form there can be a choking hazard. The way we use Gluccie on plan negates this concern; however, you will want to store this dry powder in a high cupboard away from small children. Always consult with your own doctor, but there is no evidence to show that you need to be afraid of consuming glucomannan while pregnant or nursing. Konjac root is a traditional food used daily in Japan and China. This is not a drug or an herb but an everyday food. If pregnant, use common sense by not replacing other important and needed healthy higher-caloric foods and snacks with glucomannan puddings or noodles all the time.

You can find both organic and nonorganic forms of Gluccie on our website, so it can fit within your particular budget. Our organic Gluccie is unbleached and very potent—this form is the one we use in all our recipes. A little goes a long way, so the one-pound bag should last you several months, making it a budget-friendly food over time. If you have a less potent grade of glucomannan you may have to use more powder than what we call for in our recipes. It is difficult to find glucomannan powder in stores other than in supplement form (capsules), and those do not work well for our recipes. If you want to purchase online, look for a high-viscosity grade of glucomannan. Glucomannan powder ranges in viscosity anywhere from 15,000 to 36,000 IU. Your best thickening results will come from higher grades.

We also offer Not-Naughty-Noodles and Not-Naughty-Rice on our website. These are fabulous noodle replacements that are made with pure glucomannan without any of the common fillers such as potato starch or tofu. Imagine chowing down on a big bowl of noodles that actually make you slim rather than fatten you up! Watch the free video on our website in which we show you how to make Hot Pot Soup using these noodles. This recipe is so easy, quick, and tasty and is similar to a big bowl of ramen noodles without all the junk that goes into them. Not-Naughty-Noodles have a chewier texture than most starchy noodles, but once you are accustomed to that, you'll fall in love!

More and more grocery stores are starting to carry glucomannan-based noodles. Look for the words *konjac root* in the ingredient list. They are white, almost transparent noodles packed in water and they will usually be in a refrigerated section. Sadly, these brands too often contain needless fillers such as potato starch. The carbs are still low enough that they can work on plan, though, so go ahead and give them a try so you don't have to miss out completely if you don't want to order online. Another problem (for some people) with most store-bought glucomannan noodles is that they have a fishy smell when you open them. This smell will go away when you rinse them, but it can be off-putting at first. This smell comes from the water they are packed in, not from the noodles themselves. We have loved using konjac noodles for several years and just got used to the smell, but we were so excited to be able to source our own brand of Not-Naughty-Noodles that don't have that odor. This has made many a smell-sensitive Trim Healthy Mama very happy and able to embrace these slimming noodles where the smell had previously put them off.

Final note on Gluccie powder or noodles: Consult your doctor before using it if you take medication. Taking your medication at the same time as a meal that contains glucomannan may cause your medication to work more slowly. This is due to a longer digestion time, part of the reason Gluccie makes you full and allows the body to absorb more nutrients from your food. Best to take meds away from glucomannan or keep in mind the delay.

COCONUT

Coconut is not only lip-smackin' good for the taste buds, it is beyond good for just about everything else. From nourishing babies by superpowering breast milk (explained more in Chapter 23, "Heads Up: Pregnant and Nursing Mamas!" on page 199) to nipping in waistlines by revving the thyroid, coconut is a jack-of-all-trades.

Medicine You'll Enjoy

Munching on Toasted Coconut Chips, which we call Crispy Addictions (in the "Crackers, Chips, and Dips" chapter in the *Trim Healthy Mama Cookbook*) or savoring the velvety smoothness of a Skinny Chocolate Truffle is a yummy way of swallowing this medicine. The middle-chain fatty acids abundant in coconut oil are antibacterial, antiviral, antiprotozoal, antiparasitical, and antimicrobial. Coconut in all forms battles against flu viruses, so it is the first thing we reach for when the cold and flu season starts lurking around our homes. Coconut meat is incredibly cleansing with nine grams of detoxing fiber per one cup. That is three to four times as much as most fruits and vegetables. The middle-chain triglycerides kill body pathogens and the fiber helps to broom the nasties out of your body.

Trimming Coconut Oil

Coconut oil is a true trimming oil. It raises the thermogenic temperature of your body and this ignites your fat-burning potential. But losing weight can mean less padding and sometimes that can result in you feeling colder. Try this experiment if you're cold. Eat one tablespoon of extra-virgin coconut oil before an S meal for a few days or make sure to eat some Skinny Chocolate (found in the companion cookbook or on Pinterest) after an S meal. Notice how you start to feel warmer after eating coconut oil. Even the addition of one teaspoon helps us tolerate the cold better. Coconut oil is an excellent energy source, fuels a tired brain, and beautifies your skin from the inside out.

Are you confused between regular coconut oil and 100 percent MCT oil? MCT oil will be described next, as it deserves its own write-up. It is extracted from coconut oil and is purely the shorter middle chains, namely capric and caprylic acids. These are the quickest to absorb and are used therapeutically for weight loss and brain repair but also have many other therapeutic purposes. Coconut oil is rich in lauric acid, which is a slightly longer middle-chain fatty acid and is extremely effective at enhancing and defending the immune system. Both these oils provide different benefits even though some of them might overlap. We would never suggest substituting MCT oil for coconut oil as that is like substituting green supplements for fresh salads. In a perfect world, you would use both; but life ain't perfect and if budget is your issue, then choose virgin coconut oil as your mainstay, given that it carries the full spectrum of immune-supporting fatty acids. It is also more budget-friendly. If you have a serious condition that needs more concentrated treatment (such as early-onset dementia), then MCT oil will double up your arsenal attack.

You can find extra-virgin coconut oil in many grocery stores these days or online. Thankfully, as more is being learned about this incredible food, competition between brands is driving prices down. Even budget stores like Aldi carry this oil inexpensively now. That calls for a fist pump from our budgeting Mamas.

Hate the Taste of Coconuts?

If you hate the taste of coconuts, use the expeller-pressed versions of coconut oil that have no residual tropical taste or smell but still contain the helpful middle-chain triglycerides. Another perk in cooking with coconut oil is that it is extremely stable and will not transform into insidious trans fats. We use the neutral-tasting coconut oil for cooking when we don't want our zucchini fries tasting like they were drowned in Hawaiian suntan lotion.

Red Palm Oil: The Sacred Food of the Pharaohs

While on the subject of tropical oils we can't leave out coconut oil's ruby-red cousin, red palm oil. This deeply pigmented oil was prized by the pharaohs of ancient Egypt as a sacred food. In Southeast Asia and Africa it is as widely used as olive oil is in the Mediterranean. It carries many of the same benefits as coconut oil as it is also abundant in middle-chain triglycerides. Its rich ruby hue is due to it being nature's richest source of tocotrienols, tocopherols, and carotenoids. This makes it a super antioxidant, proven to reverse heart disease and fight cancer. It has a deep earthy taste, so you won't want to pour it all over your salad. But it makes delicious fried eggs and is one of the safest oils to fry foods with and retains much of its "superness" even after frying at high temperatures.

MCT OIL

MCT stands for middle-chain (or medium-chain) triglycerides. These are the healthful fatty acids found in tropical oils. Virgin coconut oil is roughly 65 percent MCTs but the pharmaceutical-grade MCT oil we're talking about here is 100 percent medium-chain triglycerides. It is carefully extracted from coconut and palm oils.

We wish we had time to tell you just how AMAZING MCT oil is for your health, but we'd have to write a whole chapter on the subject. But before we get to its health benefits, there's something else we love most about it and the reason we use it in many of our All-Day Sipper drinks. It does not clump into tiny balls when mixed with cold liquid like coconut oil does, and it does not give a coconutty taste to your coffee. Remember, we don't want you to replace coconut oil with MCT oil; you can use coconut oil in your sipper drinks, you just have to mix it with a little hot water to dissolve first. But do try to save your pennies so you can give MCT oil a chance at some point on your THM journey. Some websites have given MCT oil a bad name since it is extracted from coconut oil and is not in its original form. We do not advocate that you leave coconut oil behind in the dust, but in our minds there is nothing wrong with using ingenuity to isolate the most healthful compounds in foods and then use them to our benefit. Many beneficial supplements are extracted in this manner.

We have squeezed just some of its benefits into a little list but this does not do it justice. What follows is a very inadequate list just to introduce you to a very talented and capable dietary friend.

- MCTs burn three times more calories for six hours after a meal than other fats do.
- These fatty acids get metabolized more like a carbohydrate but without involving insulin. It provides INSTANT yet SUSTAINED ENERGY—*woot!*
- MCT oil converts into energy faster than glucose itself . . . but with no sugar rush and subsequent lull.
- It helps counteract the decreased energy production that results from aging.
- It lowers blood glucose and insulin levels and is an aid to diabetics or those in the category of having a tendency for prediabetes (which includes most of us over age thirty-five).
- It helps suppress appetite.
- It is the LOWEST-CALORIE oil.
- It helps decrease body fat while at the same time increasing lean muscle mass. A study released in March 2008 in the *American Journal of Clinical Nutrition,* volume 87, followed forty-nine overweight men and women (between the ages of nineteen and fifty). The participants who consumed a middle-chain triglyceride oil as part of their sixteen-week weight-loss program lost more weight and fat mass than the group that consumed olive oil. It is very difficult for MCTs to be stored as fat because of the way they accelerate the metabolism and are so quickly and efficiently converted into fuel for immediate use by organs and muscles. After our mid-thirties, we lose muscle

mass every year and replace it with adipose (fat) tissue. MCT and resistance exercise can powerfully reverse this sign of aging.

- It acts as a powerful antioxidant and reduces tissue requirements for vitamin E.
- It helps optimize the production of thyroid hormones.
- It helps prevent atherosclerosis (a high risk for stroke) as MCTs have an anticoagulation effect.
- It has a positive effect on autoimmune reactions.
- The lifespan of experimental animals is longer when their diet is richer in MCTs.
- It is used for malabsorption in neonates (newborn babies) and for those recovering from serious burns, major surgeries, and serious infections.
- MCT oil fights against brain deterioration. The middle-chain fatty acids produce ketones to provide fuel for your brain without having to stick to an extreme and dangerous ketogenic diet. These ketones repair, renew, and revive the brain. Some recent research on MCT oil shows its incredible ability to reverse Alzheimer's and other types of dementia. Dr. Mary Newport, a neonatalist and author of the book *Alzheimer's Disease: What If There Was a Cure*, treated her husband (who was diagnosed with Alzheimer's) with 20 grams of MCT oil per day. He quickly began recovering his memory and cognitive function.
- MCT oil is used to treat seizures in children because of its ability to increase ketone production.

Note: Start slowly with MCT oil, as adding too much too quickly can cause diarrhea for some people. Enjoy it in your Trimmies, in the Shrinker, in the Singing Canary, and in many of your S shakes and smoothies. Use it as a salad dressing. Change up between MCT oil and extra-virgin olive oil on your salad to receive the benefits both provide.

MCT is now available at www.trimhealthymama.com or find it online elsewhere.

SPICE MUSKETEERS

We now need to make room on this superfood stage for the Three Musketeers that hail from the land of Phenomenal Spicedom. Each one of them wields a powerful sword against the woes of sickness and disease in the body. You'll notice that these are the three spices we use in our most popular All-Day Sipper drinks. When all three are welcomed in the diet they are an unstoppable force you will want to have on your side. With no further ado, we introduce to you Terrific Turmeric, Scintillating Cinnamon, and Genius Ginger.

Terrific Turmeric

Daily consumption of turmeric is directly associated with increased healthy fat loss and decreased insulin issues. Curcumin, a plant-based polyphenol found in turmeric, regulates the body's metabolism. This golden treasure spice is rich in antioxidants and its anti-inflammatory mechanisms fight actively against obesity. In a Columbia University study of turmeric, researchers discovered that mice that were fed turmeric had reduced incidence of diabetes and were not susceptible to weight gain. Under turmeric administration, the decline in body weight was shown to be literal fat rather than muscle or water weight. The fat cells shrunk! This is the real deal.

Turmeric karate-chops cancer and delivers a blow strong enough to induce apoptosis. This is a process that triggers the self-destruction and elimination of cancerous cells. Turmeric is one of the best protectors against radiation-induced tumors. This simple spice is an effective preventative against tumor cells such as T-cell leukemia, colon carcinomas, and breast carcinomas. It is known to reduce the risk of childhood leukemia; and look out, prostate cancer—turmeric is your deadly foe. Turmeric can even scavenge the hydroxyl radical, which is considered to be the most reactive of all oxidants. With fewer of our cells becoming damaged by free radicals, cancer and other degenerative diseases can be thwarted.

Terrific Turmeric also supports the adrenal glands by assisting in the production of its hormonal cascade. For this very reason, along with many others, our adrenal-building Singing Canary (one of our All-Day Sipper drinks) stars turmeric as its main spice. Check out the recipe in the *Trim Healthy Mama Cookbook*. Amazingly, turmeric brings a calming and relaxing effect while simultaneously providing mental alertness. Low liver function is often associated with low adrenal function, and turmeric is a liver rebuilder and detoxifier. Turmeric helps produce bile, and bile is the vehicle that flushes toxicity from your body.

You can gain access to turmeric's power by drinking the Singing Canary or Singing Canary Shot, which is a fun, faster way to get in the goodies of that drink. Add turmeric to your olive oil to preserve the oil's integrity and also to boost your salad with super spice wonders. Sprinkle it in your egg salad or on your roasted or sautéed meats or veggies;

or make the nourishing, calming nightcap Turmeric Toddy Trimmy (found in the "Hot Drinks" chapter of the *Trim Healthy Mama Cookbook*).

You can use any old turmeric found at your grocery store, since some turmeric is better than no turmeric; but a nonirradiated turmeric will be your best choice. Organic sources of turmeric have not been irradiated.

Scintillating Cinnamon

Cinnamon is famous for regulating blood sugar. It battles high blood sugar by slowing the rate at which the stomach empties after meals. Not only does it stimulate insulin receptors, but it inhibits the enzyme that inactivates them and successfully increases the body's ability to use glucose. It only takes a scant half teaspoon to reduce blood-sugar levels, so throw it in your smoothies and sprinkle it on your pancakes and Greek yogurt. For that matter, go and make yourself our fat-blitzing All-Day Sipper, the Shrinker, and reap the benefits of this fragrant spice. Watch us make that drink on a video on our website or check out the recipe in the companion cookbook. Oh, while we're on the subject of fragrance, let us say that even just getting a whiff of cinnamon's aroma heightens brain activity and cognitive processing. Let's quickly hit some more of cinnamon's dazzling highlights.

- It reduces LDL cholesterol: Good news!
- It contains effective infection-fighting compounds that fight against dangerous pathogens: Cheers!
- Cinnamon is highly anti-inflammatory and reduces cytokines (message signalers that promote inflammation in the body) linked to arthritic pain. It also reduces chronic inflammation linked to neurological disorders: standing ovation!
- Cinnamon reduces the proliferation of cancer cells: Oh yeah!
- It is an effective remedy for menstrual pain and infertility. This is because cinnamon contains a natural chemical called cinnamaldehyde, which, studies show, increases the hormone progesterone in women: round of applause!
- It is also a natural food preservative. Cinnamon is such a powerful antioxidant that it prevents oxidation more effectively than the chemical food preservatives butylated hydroxyanisole (BHA) and butylated hydroxytoluene (BHT) and it surpasses many other spices for preserving. Wow! Let's sip some SHRINKER.

Genius Ginger

Ginger is the star spice in our Good Girl Moonshine drink. One of the major effects we notice from sipping Good Girl Moonshine all day is that it battles the snacking monster. When we began to dig into the merits of ginger it was no surprise for us to learn that it dulls an overzealous appetite. This delicious spice of pungent heat fires up the thermogenic temperature of the body and kindles the metabolism.

Another benefit we noticed from swiggin' our moonshine was a less gassy tummy. Ginger is a potent digestive aid and fires up the digestive juices. It improves the absorption and assimilation of essential nutrients in the body. Most folks know of ginger's talent in reducing nausea, and our Good Girl Moonshine, spiked as it is with this super spice, is a pregnant Mama's BFF when the morning sickness hits.

Ginger clears the micro-circulatory channels of the body, including the easily clogged sinuses. It clears throat and nose congestion and is a wonderful stimulant to the immune system. Ginger is up at the top of the list with the most potent anti-inflammatory supplements on God's green earth and can help relieve common aches and pains and even help with more serious arthritic conditions. It is also considered to be an aphrodisiac, which is a boon for all our Foxy Mamas!

OOLONG TEA

This is the tea that stars in our drink that went viral, the Shrinker. As the name of this drink suggests, it shrinks your fat cells. Just one cup of oolong tea can help burn off an extra sixty-seven calories. Yeah! As yummy as this drink is, you don't have to limit oolong only to that drink concoction. Sip it as a pure tea without the added ingredients of the Shrinker, hot or iced, sweetened with just a doonk or two of stevia—delicious!

Oolong has health benefits far beyond just weight loss. In ancient Chinese books, oolong is regarded as an elixir that contributes to prolonged life. It is known as having the richest and most complex flavor among all the varieties of tea. The following is an embarrassingly modest list of just a few of oolong's wonders.

It helps prevents obesity and is powerfully active in burning fat. Research shows that the polyphenols that are highest in oolong tea help activate thermogenesis, which increases fat oxidation in your body. Caffeine content is significantly lower in oolong tea than in coffee but it robustly boosts vitality and energy. It is oolong's abundant polyphenols that help with this elevated feeling. In 2003, scientists from the University of Tokushima in Japan found that oolong tea can double the amount of fat excreted by the body. They reported that people who drank two cups of oolong tea burned more than 157 percent more fat than those who drank the same amount of green tea!

Oolong lowers blood-sugar levels and can be an effective treatment for diabetics. A Taiwanese study in 2003 found that oolong tea controls blood-glucose levels very effectively. The thorough study showed that plasma glucose and fructosamine levels dropped significantly for oolong tea drinkers. Oolong contains antioxidants that powerfully destroy free radicals. Research conducted in 2004 by Dr. Kenichi Yanagimoto of the University of California showed that only fifteen days of oolong tea drinking enabled an incredible 50 percent reduction in free radicals. Another study conducted by the Academy of Traditional Chinese Medicine of Fujian Province, China, concluded that stress levels reduced significantly with four servings of oolong each day for a week. We could cite study after study, but we won't risk causing your eyes to roll back in your head. Our encouragement for you would be to buy this tea and allow it to help revitalize your life. When it comes to oolong, you do want to seek out a USDA-certified-organic source, as some oolong tea (with bogus organic labels) has been shown to have too-high levels of lead. You can find authentic organic oolong tea on our website www.trimhealthymama.com or seek out another quality brand online or at your favorite health food store.

NUTRITIONAL YEAST

We love this stuff for its health benefits, but we gotta be honest and admit—mostly it's because of its wonderful, cheesy, nutty flavor. You'll notice we include it in our recipes for so many savory dishes. Around our homes, fried eggs are not fried eggs without nutritional yeast, and our children cannot eat their Crossover popcorn without it! We use it in soups, savory baked goods, stews, stir-fries—too many ways to list.

While nutritional yeast is not a mandatory ingredient on the plan, it will enhance flavors and supply your body with all sorts of health goodies. It contains eighteen amino acids and is a complete protein. It is also a very good source of vitamins and minerals and a plentiful source of B complex vitamins, which help in managing stress levels. Its greatest boast is that it supplies a good source of the mineral chromium to the body. Another name for this mineral is GTF (glucose tolerance factor). This substance is highly effective for those with high blood-sugar levels, such as diabetics and those with insulin resistance and prediabetic conditions (such as hypoglycemia and hyperglycemia). Chromium is also used to help lower cravings for carbs and sugary foods.

Don't be scared of the word *yeast* here. There are good yeasts and bad yeasts. Nutritional yeast is one of the good yeasts and has no connection with harmful bodily yeasts like candida albicans. It does not promote harmful yeast growth in the body and is naturally gluten-free. You can find nutritional yeast in some grocery stores in their "healthy food" aisles, at most health food stores, and online.

HIGH-MINERAL SALT

Salt is not a no-no on plan. Instead we say a big yes-yes to natural salt full of minerals and health benefits for your body. The no-salt approach to dieting is tasteless boredom: No wonder so many people want to ditch their diets. You will notice the addition of mineral salt in most of our recipes, even those that are sweet desserts! We find a little salt rounds out high sweet notes and brings a warmer "honeysuckleish" sweet flavor.

High-mineral salt comes from mineral deposits deep under the ground or from the sea. It will be either light pink in color (from the ground) or light gray in color (from the sea) and will have a heavier, almost moister feel to it than regular, refined table salt. These colors hint at the minerals within the salt that are, sadly, greatly reduced in refined salts. Not all sea salt is high in minerals; much of the sea salt in grocery stores has been refined and is not as rich in minerals. High-mineral salt alkalizes the body, maintains electrolyte balance, and helps fight adrenal fatigue—part of the reason our adrenal-building Singing Canary drink calls for two to three generous pinches of this amazing stuff. It helps to combat elevated blood sugar, relieve muscle cramps, combat osteoporosis, and, yes, even manage cases of hypertension. It is true that regular, devitalized table salt is not great for your body, so let's use the real stuff our bodies crave for good reason.

The no-salt approach is old-school "the-world-is-flat" thinking. Latest research says it is actually a low-salt diet that does damage. Let's take a look at the facts about salt through a round-world lens.

- A recent 2011 study published in the *Lancet* on the effects of a low-salt diet made headlines, disclosing that a low-salt diet increases mortality for patients with congestive heart failure.
- Another study, conducted at Harvard University and published in 2010, linked low-salt diets to an increase in insulin resistance.
- An Australian study published in *Diabetes Care* in 2011 followed 638 patients with Type 2 diabetes for an average of ten years. Researchers found that lowered salt consumption was associated with all increases of mortality. A similar study was carried out on those with Type 1 diabetes and came to the same conclusions.
- Yet another study, published in the *American Journal of Hypertension* in 2011, showed eating less salt will not prevent heart attacks, strokes, or early death. On the contrary it revealed that low-sodium diets increase the likelihood of premature deaths.
- Salt-restrictive diets may actually raise cholesterol and triglycerides (fat in the blood).
- Some studies show that a low-salt diet will reduce blood pressure slightly. However, this effect is minimal and is counteracted by compensatory mechanisms that release too high amounts of hormones and chemical mediators into the bloodstream that try to counterbalance the low-salt diet. The released chemical mediators include insulin, epinephrine, norepinephrine, renin, and aldosterone. In excess, these are damaging to the vascular system.
- A deficiency in sodium causes other minerals to become bio-unavailable, so your body cannot absorb them.

You can purchase high-mineral sea salt from www.trimhealthymama.com or find another mineral-rich, natural salt (such as Celtic or Himalayan salt) that you like in your local shopping area.

SUNFLOWER LECITHIN

What is lecithin? A weird manmade substance? Nope. It is a group of phospholipids found in certain foods and in your body. Your brain is approximately 30 percent lecithin. When you supplement with lecithin, you nourish your brain. This God-designed substance improves memory, helps combat learning disabilities, and promotes longer attention spans.

It has been shown in many studies to relieve age-associated memory impairment, dementia, and early symptoms of Alzheimer's disease. Research also shows promising results with lecithin supplementation being able to prevent further deterioration of mental function in Alzheimer's patients.

Within your body, lecithin is richly concentrated in the myelin sheaths that form a protective coating around your nerves. Eating a diet high in lecithin-rich foods, such as runny egg yolks (cooking to opaque destroys much of the lecithin), and supplementing with lecithin are wonderful nerve calmatives and healers.

The two main forms of lecithin available today are from sunflowers (obtained from the seeds) or from soy. We encourage a sunflower-based supplement for more frequent use over soy. We prefer to use a dry lecithin powder over a liquid in our recipes. You can find it at our website or elsewhere online or in some health food stores. It is an incredible emulsifier of foods, which helps make our smoothies, mousses, chocolates, sauces, and drinks so much more wonderfully creamy and delightful. It helps our Healing Trimmy coffees stay creamy and white ("Hot Drinks" chapter in the *Trim Healthy Mama Cookbook*) and our Thin Thick shakes be the creamiest Fuel Pull drinks you could dream of ("Shakes, Smoothies, Frappas, and Thin Thicks" chapter in the *Trim Healthy Mama Cookbook*). It sure is not a mandatory ingredient on plan, but it is a delightful one that we have fallen in love with.

What's in lecithin that makes it so effective to boost health? Lecithin is rich in choline, which is needed throughout the entire body as an integral ingredient in the phospholipid portion of each and every cell membrane. Phosphatidylcholine is a component of lecithin that is an integral neurotransmitter and fortifies your brain and nerve cells. Phosphatidylcholine is also a potent antioxidant that paralyzes the movement of free radicals throughout our bodies. This makes lecithin a powerful antiaging supplement as it fights against oxidative damage to cells (which causes premature and natural aging as well as cancer).

Acetylcholine deficiencies are a cause of insomnia, so dosing up on sunflower lecithin may help your sheep count go down and your numbers of deep slumbering hours go up. This is due to the choline in lecithin being a direct precursor to acetylcholine.

Lecithin is also a natural fat-emulsifier and can help reverse as well as prevent nonalcoholic fatty liver disease, which is associated with insulin resistance, Type 2 diabetes, cardiovascular disease, and liver cancer. It also helps to break down harmful types of cholesterol. This emulsifying power makes it a friend of nursing women who are prone to breast infections. Lecithin has a unique ability to be able to decrease the stickiness of breast milk so it is less likely to clog and to help heal already clogged breast ducts. It is also known as a general breast-health promoter and breast-cancer fighter.

Do you have creaky joints? Lecithin is an important part of the production of synovial fluid, which is like WD-40 to our joints. It stops the creaks and the squeaks of joint rustiness. It is also considered to be beneficial in decreasing pain and increasing mobility for those suffering with rheumatoid arthritis.

menus, eating tips, and what to expect

Get Ready to Find Your Groove

Each of us brings a unique metabolism, set of tastes, different resources, budget, and existing mindset about food to the table. All of these factors will dramatically affect your eating choices and give you a unique experience with the Trim Healthy Mama Plan, and a totally different THM style to the next woman—and let's not forget we have men doing the plan, too. We want to give you an idea of what you can expect as you start out and help you troubleshoot and avoid the pitfalls no matter what "type" you are.

Trim Healthy Mama breaks the diet mold in that it does not give you set menus, set portion sizes, set grocery lists, and the same set foods to eat over and over again. Don't let this throw you. There's a reason all these "set" diet standards are not included in the book. Even portion sizes will vary according to the dietary needs of individual women. Mamas who are nursing and pregnant will need more food than postmenopausal women, whose caloric needs drop during that season of life. It doesn't make sense to tell women in vastly different stages of life with greatly varying metabolisms to ALL eat only half-cup portions. It also doesn't make sense to tell husbands to eat only tiny helpings. There wouldn't be so many happy Trim Healthy Husbands everywhere if their portion sizes were restricted to typical diet-size amounts.

While at first it might seem easier to mindlessly follow a menu than it is to learn and practice new principles, the goal here is to retrain your brain to think of foods in a whole new way. We think preset menus are frankly rather boring; but, yeah, we get that you want to have a visual idea of what to eat as you get started.

We've provided sample menus here for different "types of people" on plan. We want to be very clear that they are only ideas . . . examples. If you don't like some of the meals we mention—by all means create your own meals and ditch ours. We'd actually prefer if you came up with your own. Our ultimate desire for you is not to do our plan but to do yours! A preset stringent menu can never do what truly learning and living the plan can do. Following someone else's idea of what you should eat every day of the week makes it far more likely that you'll get bored or be dissatisfied at the end of a couple of months and walk away from THM as "just another diet."

With all that said, we understand everyone is different and some of us need more structure than others. The menus included in the next few chapters can give you a good visual on what eating on-plan might look like for you. They include some recipes from the *Trim Healthy Mama Cookbook*. We want you to have success on plan and we've made sure these recipes are going to help you achieve that. But if your budget does not allow you to purchase that book right now, there are many enthusiastic Trim Healthy Mama bloggers who frequently post up their free menus, including lots of yummy recipes to inspire others. And don't forget about Pinterest THM menus and recipes—although we can't vouch for the accuracy of all of the THM recipes posted on people's Pinterest pages.

The following blogs are written by seasoned Trim Healthy Mamas who know their way around the plan. They have many example menus you may find helpful:

www.sherigraham.com
www.workingathomeschool.com
www.darciesdishes.blogspot.com

If you want more menu ideas, check out www.trimhealthymama.com. New idea menus are loaded up monthly in our menu section. But we hope you'll get to the point where you are not following someone else's menu but coming up with your own. To help you customize your own menus, we had some very "techie" people design a unique menu builder for our website. You can use it to pull recipes from the organized archives of Trim Healthy Mama recipes there or input your own. This is a great tool to help you organize menus that actually appeal to you and your own set of unique challenges and preferences. It will also generate a grocery shopping list for you. As sisters, we certainly would not want to write each other's weekly menu. We enjoy different foods and have different approaches. Dictating preset weekly menus to people is not our idea of Food

Freedom and we are not in partnership with any online menu sites who charge for using any part of our Trim Healthy Brand

It's also important to mention that not all of us are planners. While it is a good idea to have some meal ideas in mind when grocery shopping, you sure don't have to have a weekly menu all printed out to have success on plan. Don't think of yourself as an outcast if you are not the meal-planning type and get no pleasure from seeing a crisp weekly menu coming out of your printer. Neither of us bothers with set, strict menus for each week. We enjoy winging it! We keep certain meal ideas in mind and then fly by the seats of our pants for the rest our week, which always brings us unforeseen twists and turns. You don't have to turn into Mrs. Uber Organized to be a Trim Healthy Mama; but a little planning (especially in the beginning of your journey) can help you achieve your goals.

Note: You will notice there is usually only one E meal per day in the following sample menus. We hope you enjoy plenty of E snacks, too. Don't forget your fruit for snacks (with protein preferably). Wasa or Ryvita crackers also make great snacks with 1% cottage cheese or Laughing Cow Creamy Light Swiss cheese wedges and tomato (we have dairy-free recipes for those sorts of cheeses in the *Trim Healthy Mama Cookbook*). If you don't want to eat protein with your fruit, a drink containing some gelatin or collagen will give ample protein for your E snack. We listed some snack and dessert ideas at the bottom of each menu but they are just a start: There are vast amounts of snacks and desserts to be enjoyed as a Trim Healthy Mama.

Jump first to the "Heads Up" chapter you relate to most if you want, but reading through them all at some stage will help you on your journey. You can learn something from each chapter.

chapter 19

HEADS UP: DRIVE THRU SUES!

If you relate to Drive Thru Sue, who is described in Chapter 1, you're probably coming from a diet of sodas and refined starches and perhaps your cooking has primarily involved boxed mac and cheese and putting frozen pizzas and lasagnas in the oven. When and if you cook, it is not so much for the love of it—just get 'er done and eat!

Don't worry, we're not going to chain you to the stove. Yes, you will find yourself in the kitchen a bit more; but you sure don't have to attempt complicated meals. Easy slow-cooker recipes for dinner and quick (less-than-five-minute) recipes for breakfast and lunch will not be a huge burden on your time and kitchen skill levels. The Muffin in a Mug (MIM) recipes can become your BFF for busy mornings or a speedy afternoon snack. Check out a free frosted version of that muffin on our website or peruse the many Trim Healthy Mama MIMs on Pinterest that lots of creative women in the community have come up with. Maybe you will nuke your muffin in the microwave instead of baking it in the oven—hey, you are making huge strides coming off processed, blood-sugar-spiking, and devitalized foods, so hooray for you! This is only going to get easier—not harder—as you slowly find your THM feet.

DO WHAT WORKS FOR YOU

If you want to use some shortcut/Frankenfood items—or what we refer to as "Personal Choice" Items—in our food lists to help you stay on plan, no problem. Wrap some rotisserie chicken in a low-carb tortilla with a little mayo, hot sauce, cheese, and lettuce for an S meal. Rotisserie chicken can be a Drive Thru Sue's lifesaver. If it is not tasty enough for you, pull off some chicken pieces, add your favorite seasoning (Creole is great), and sauté those chicken pieces in a skillet with just a couple teaspoons of butter. Enjoy with a salad. This takes rotisserie chicken from boring to blazin'!

You can make turkey and cheese sandwiches with a Joseph's pita, and you can even use Dreamfields pasta once a week or once every couple of weeks if that helps you not feel so deprived (each person needs to assess her or his own blood-sugar reaction to this product). What could be easier than browning some meat, adding it to a jar of sugar-free pasta sauce, and then pouring it over plan-friendly pasta? You've got this! Purchase precooked steak and chicken strips. You can roll them in a low-carb wrap, throw them on a bed of precut and prewashed leafy greens from a bag, or toss them with Not-Naughty-Noodles, veggies, sesame oil, and soy sauce in the frying pan—yum. This way of eating needn't be complicated.

While the shortcut bread items can help your entrance into the plan be smoother, we need to add a caution that we don't want you to overdo them. Center your meals around simple whole foods as often as you can, and try not to rely on store-bought low-carb bread options for every single meal every day of the week. We know you are eating far better now than you were before, so no beating up on yourself for baby-step choices—and don't let anyone else beat you up, either!

INITIAL SWIFT WEIGHT LOSS

If you're giving up sodas and fries, you may find that you drop quite a bit of weight in the first couple of weeks. By "quite a bit" we mean five pounds or more. Don't be alarmed if you see close to a ten-pound drop! Some of this is water weight. Your body flushes it out with the excess glucose from your cells. Weight loss will settle down after the initial period to a more usual average of one pound per week (possibly two pounds per week if you have a lot to lose and don't have metabolic issues). Of course, that average may not come off every week; some weeks the scale won't budge, and other weeks you might see two or three pounds melt off. Or you might decide not to watch the scale and instead to go by how your clothes fit—that's perfectly fine, too. While many Drive Thru Sues do experience fast early weight loss, don't feel like a failure if that does not happen to you or if your averages don't quite make it to a pound per week. We are all different and your body will do its own thing. Enjoy the journey rather than comparing yourself to others.

DETOX

You may experience a week or even a few weeks of "detox" response from pulling the sugar rug out from under you. This can feel like flu symptoms—headaches and fatigue. Troupe through this phase knowing it will pass. Your body needs to shed toxins and learn to adjust to the new fuels of fats and moderate glucose rather than the constantly high glucose it has been used to. Sugar does provide a sense of energy to the body, but it is a false high and a crash inevitably follows the high. Start out with a couple of full-S days if you want to, but then make sure to add some good E meals so you don't completely pull away the stable energy good carbohydrates provide. You'll come out feeling better than ever and the constant craving for sugar pick-me-ups should soon fall away.

GOOD-BYE SODA

You can do it! If you've been a soda addict, try a couple of our All-Day Sipper drinks. Good Girl Moonshine and the Shrinker have helped thousands of women kick the soda habit, and the health and weight-loss benefits of these drinks can be a huge help on your journey. If at first you aren't partial to the tastes of these drinks, try tweaking them to your liking. Add extracts, try less or more sweetener, or use sparkling water in place of regular water to give you that fizz. Or try some stevia-sweetened colas that are now readily available at so many grocery stores—some brands even contain a little caffeine, if that is part of the pick-me-up you love about soda.

GIVE YOUR TASTE BUDS TIME

It may take you a few weeks to get used to the natural sweetener options we suggest in place of sugar. At first your taste buds may rebel. Give them some time. They'll change. Make sure you read Chapter 13, "Sweet Mama" (page 102), for tips on how to use our sweeteners as you start out. Our Gentle Sweet stevia blend may be the best option for you to start the plan with if you initially dislike the taste of stevia, because this blend tastes the most like sugar and is very forgiving if you use too much.

Day 1

BREAKFAST—S

Frosted Cinnamon Muffin ("Quick Single Muffins" chapter in the *Trim Healthy Mama Cookbook* or on our website) / Greek yogurt or ½ Triple Zero Greek yogurt with berries / coffee and cream

LUNCH—S

Joseph's pita stuffed with turkey breast, lettuce, mayo, and cheese / Choco Chip Baby Frap or a Thin Thick ("Shakes, Smoothies, Frappas, and Thin Thicks" chapter in the *Trim Healthy Mama Cookbook*)

DINNER—S

Cajun Cream Chicken ("Crockpot Meals" chapter in the *Trim Healthy Mama Cookbook*) / Cauli Rice or Troodles ("Sides" chapter in the *Trim Healthy Mama Cookbook*)

Day 2

BREAKFAST—E

Triple Zero Greek yogurt / bowl of oatmeal with a little unsweetened almond milk / ½ orange / coffee and a little half-and-half to stay in E mode

LUNCH—S

Large salad topped with store-bought, precooked steak strips, creamy dressing, and grated cheese

DINNER—S

Egg Roll in a Bowl, using bagged coleslaw for ease ("Family Skillet Meals" chapter in the *Trim Healthy Mama Cookbook*)

Day 3

BREAKFAST—S

Fried egg, cheese, and sausage patty breakfast wrap made with frozen, precooked sausage patty heated in the microwave and rolled into a store-bought low-carb wrap

LUNCH—E

Light Progresso soup / 2 Wasa crackers with Laughing Cow Creamy Light Swiss cheese wedges

DINNER—S

Rotisserie chicken / buttered steamed broccoli / side salad with watered-down store-bought creamy dressing

Day 4

BREAKFAST—E

Chocolate Waffles with Strawberries ("Pancakes, Donuts, Crepes, and Waffles" chapter in the *Trim Healthy Mama Cookbook*)

LUNCH- S

Leftover rotisserie chicken, lettuce, and mayo in a store-bought low-carb wrap

SUPPER—E

Wicked White Chili ("Crockpot Meals" chapter in the *Trim Healthy Mama Cookbook*)

Day 5

BREAKFAST—S

Eggs any way with sausage or bacon

LUNCH—E

Store-bought sprouted bread sandwich with lean deli meat, lettuce, tomato, mustard, and a thin smear of mayo / a small piece of fruit with some low-fat cottage cheese or a Choco Chip Baby Frap ("Shakes, Smoothies, Frappas, and Thin Thicks" chapter in the *Trim Healthy Mama Cookbook*)

DINNER—S

Cheeseburger Pie ("Oven Dishes" chapter in the *Trim Healthy Mama Cookbook* or found on our website) / large side salad / canned green beans with a little extra butter and high-mineral salt

Day 6

BREAKFAST—FP

Strawberry Big Boy Smoothie ("Shakes, Smoothies, Frappas, and Thin Thicks" chapter in the *Trim Healthy Mama Cookbook)*

LUNCH—E

Waldorf Cottage Cheese Salad—using garnish amount of store-bought spicy nuts, finely chopped ("Quick Single Salads" chapter in the *Trim Healthy Mama Cookbook*)

DINNER—S

Ridiculous Meatballs and Spaghetti ("Crockpot Meals" chapter in the *Trim Healthy Mama Cookbook*)

Day 7

BREAKFAST—S

Brainy Blueberry Muffin ("Quick Single Muffins" chapter in the *Trim Healthy Mama Cookbook*) / ½ Triple Zero Greek yogurt or ½ cup regular Greek yogurt sweetened with Gentle Sweet

LUNCH—S

Just Like Campbell's Tomato Soup ("Quick Single Soups" chapter in the *Trim Healthy Mama Cookbook* or found on our website) / grilled cheese made with ½ Joseph's pita or with Swiss Bread ("Breads and Pizza Crusts" chapter in the *Trim Healthy Mama Cookbook*)

DINNER—E

Cowboy Grub ("Family Skillet Meals" in the *Trim Healthy Mama Cookbook*) / Choco Chip Baby Frap ("Shakes, Smoothies, Frappas, and Thin Thicks" chapter of the *Trim Healthy Mama Cookbook*)

Snack Ideas for the Week

Triple Zero Greek yogurt / peanut butter–stuffed celery / Babybel cheese with store-bought roasted or crispy nuts / part-skim cheese stick with an apple / Wasa or Ryvita crackers with Laughing Cow Creamy Light Swiss cheese wedges and cucumber / butter lettuce leaves wrapped around deli meat, cheese, and mayo / hard-boiled eggs and celery sticks / stevia-sweetened store-bought chocolate or a couple squares of 85% cacao chocolate / plan-approved store-bought ice cream like Enlightened brand (or any brand that uses stevia and erythritol as chief sweeteners / any single-serve muffin ("Quick Single Muffins" chapter in the *Trim Healthy Mama Cookbook*) / any single-serve cake ("Quick Single Serve Cakes" chapter in the *Trim Healthy Mama Cookbook*) / Joseph's crackers with sliced cheese or Drive Thru Sue Cheesy Crackers or Thinnies ("Crackers, Chips, and Dips" chapter in the *Trim Healthy Mama Cookbook*) / any shake or creamy drink from the "Shakes, Smoothies, Frappas, and Thin Thicks" chapter in the *Trim Healthy Mama Cookbook*) / Skinny Chocolate ("Candies and Bars" chapter in the *Trim Healthy Mama Cookbook*)

chapter 20
HEADS UP: PURISTS!

The crunchy type! We know you well. One of us is a staunch disciple of all those sprouting, culturing, sourdough-catching, chicken-plucking, kombucha-mushroom-growing ways. It won't take you long to guess who when you watch one of our YouTube videos or hang out on our website.

SERENE CHATS: *Waving hi!—can't leave you wondering. It's me! I haven't yet been able to convert Pearl from her microwave-using ways. Still working on it, though. Like me, you can ignore some of her suggestions for packaged Frankenfoods, which she terms prettily as "shortcuts." I've never eaten a Joseph's low-carb pita or had a Dreamfields noodle in all the years of my THM journey, and I haven't missed them, either. We purists can be happy for all of our Drive Thru Sue friends finding their way to health while we merrily cook from scratch and go about our purist ways. If Pearl and I can call a truce, there's hope for all the disagreements in the world!*

PURIST PARADISE

Grass-fed meats, pastured eggs, wild-caught deep-sea fish, and raw homemade kefir and cheeses will anchor the THM plan for our Purist Mamas. You're sure to be sipping a small glass of your homemade kombucha and garnishing your plate with a portion of sauerkraut fermented in your home crock. Your grains and beans are soaked, your sourdough starter is bubbling, your garden veggies are home-preserved, your hens are laying golden eggs, and your goat's udder is full and ready for milking. Right? Ha ha ha! This is a purist fantasy. In reality not all who are instilled with an "all-natural" mindset get to experience this puristy perfection.

Dreams are fun, but sometimes purists bear this mindset as a burden of idealism that their circumstances and finances halt or at the very least hinder. They are left anxious and longing for the greener pastures afforded by getting a raise, moving to the country, or receiving a Deepfreeze for Christmas with a full grass-fed cow tucked nicely inside. If you are not living on your hobby farm or blessed with the finances to shop solely at the organic market, take a deep breath and let's reassess together.

BE A PROACTIVE PURIST

If the full purist fantasy can't be had in your season, there are some things you can control. You can have fun learning to be savvy and find your way around high-priced retailers. Many times there are Amish farms in surrounding smaller towns that sell very reasonably priced raw milk that you can turn into kefir. Google any orchards or berry farms that, even if not certified organic, use no or very minimal crop spray and are within a couple of hours of your city. There you can pick bushels and buckets of berries or fruit for a very low cost. Freeze, dehydrate, culture, or preserve your bounty for a fun and inexpensive way of stocking your natural kitchen. Find a few like-minded friends who want to go thirds in a grass-fed cow to cut down on the price.

Even if you can't find a source of raw milk, you can still make homemade kefir and bring regular pasteurized milk back to life and teeming with enzymes by using the double-fermenting method. We share that method in the "More Drinks" chapter of the *Trim Healthy Mama Cookbook.* For more info you can check out our website, where we have a hands-on, practical video showing you step by step how to do it—or you can search it on-line. Don't worry if you don't have the bucks to fork over for organic store-bought milk. Usually these brands are sterilized at an ultra-high temperature (UHT), at very denaturing degrees from 280 F to 302 F.

Regular old milk is heated at much lower temperatures in one of two types of pasteuri-zation. It can be "low-temperature, long-time pasteurized," which is called "vat" pasteuri-zation, during which milk is heated to 145 degrees F for at least thirty minutes and then instantly chilled. The more common "high-temperature, short-time," or "flash," pasteuri-zation method is when milk is heated to roughly 160 degrees F for at least fifteen sec-onds. These methods leave the milk with more nutrients and a much better taste. More than 80 percent of all organic milk brands are UHT and are an expensive and unhealthy scam. Most of the milk from these brands is not from grass-fed cows anyway, and you pay double the price for a burned and deranged liquid that bears an organic stamp designed to make all its miserableness go away.

Many fellow purists are overtaken by multiplying kombucha mushrooms and kefir grains. They would love to give them away for free so they don't have to have fifteen cultures on their countertops. Start putting feelers out on who the mad scientist purist is in your area and then you'll have too many yourself. You'll be giving mushrooms and kefir grains away to another fledgling purist.

Once you fork over an initial investment for bulk organic grain from an online co-op (do your homework, because some are way cheaper than others) and look online for a secondhand grain mill, your own artisan sourdough bread is just pennies a loaf. Serene has perfected her artisan sourdough recipe over the years so it is now streamlined and easy enough for anyone to make. It appears in the "Breads and Pizza Crusts" chapter of the *Trim Healthy Mama Cookbook,* but there are also plenty of authentic sourdough recipes online.

Carve out an afternoon to spend online or check out a book from your local library on the wild edibles in your area. You may be surprised at the bounty you have at your fingertips. Here in our Tennessee backyard we gather and eat in-season wild persimmons, blackberries, autumn olives, passion fruit, purslane, plantain, dandelion greens, sumac, a yummy mushroom called chicken of the woods, and black walnuts. We do not have deep botanical expertise on wild edibles, so we are probably tramping right past many trea-sures. But we look forward to the different seasons when nature's gifts drop for free from our surrounding trees or pop up their pretty foliage in the ditches on our roadside. Their nutrition benefits could defy any packaged superfood from the most elite organic market and slapped with a price tag of thirty dollars. Oh, and while we are talking wild, the king of wild is wild game! Hunt down or hound a hunter and get that freezer full of ground venison and that dehydrator full of jerky.

It looks like you will be happily busy with all these relatively inexpensive purist projects, so no need to sweat all those other ideals right now. You've got your hands full proactively doing the positive things you can do today. Our advice is to be a "can-do" joyful soul, not a "can't-do" anxious worrywart.

THE PEACEFUL PURIST

Rest in the fact that you are taking healthy doable steps in your purist journey. Obsessing about the depleted soils, the toxins in most foods, and the cell-phone towers stretching their radiation tentacles into the atmosphere brings your health down. If you belong to e-mail lists from "everything-is-out-to-kill-ya" health gurus and they bring excess tension into your life, then delete your name from their file. You can find anything wrong with anything if you search the Internet and blogosphere for it.

Sensational blog posts evilizing even healthy foods are all the rage these days. It is good to research, but it is not good to obsess.

Straining over the gnat of a little soy lecithin in your favorite dark chocolate but swallowing the camel of burdensome mental torment called worry is an injurious choice. Go ahead and do away with plastics in favor of glass if you feel strongly about it, but don't—please don't—fall into a purist neurosis that can be as unhealthy as drinking a daily shot of 100 percent liquid BPA. We believe in being wise and educated, but anxiety over things that we can't ever change or at least can't change now needs to be eradicated. We both spent too many years with that mindset and it did nothing for our health but compromise it. Abolish purism stress. It KILLS.

Our Creator did not create this generation in the time of the *Little House on the Prairie*. He created us for now with all our modern techno iClouds and frustrating laws hindering the easy access to raw milk. The Bible says, "Above all, beloved, I wish you to prosper and be in good health." He has plans and purposes for you to fulfill in the here and now in 2015 and beyond. God is ultimately in control and numbers our days. We are never in control, even though we sometimes think we are.

PURIST GO-TOS

Your eyes will glaze over when they spot the quick microwave muffins in the companion cookbook, but you'll love to bring a full batch of steamy and fragrant Chocolate Chai-Glazed Cinnamon Muffins out of your oven (see the "Family Muffins" chapter in the *Trim Healthy Mama Cookbook*). Slather them with raw pastured butter or virgin coconut oil. You will make a Skinny Chocolate icing that will set hard when the muffins are cooled. If you love soup, you can get your stockpot simmering with your own chicken, beef, and wild venison bones and throw in veggie tops and skins from your own garden. This gelatin-rich stock can be the nurturing base to many of our soup and stew recipes.

Kefir superfood smoothies are as easy as it gets and fill you up with all the nutritious goodies you love. You can throw in your pastured, golden yolks from free-range hens and even some wild edibles if you've found some backyard treasures. For speedy S lunches on the go, you won't be buying store-bought low-carb wraps but making Wonder Wraps (see "Breads and Pizza Crusts" in the *Trim Healthy Mama Cookbook*) stuffed with avocado, fresh garden greens, and leftover free-range chicken. They are the yummiest things ever; we're getting hungry just writing about them.

If you don't have your own jersey cow or a source of raw pastured cream, you don't have to mar your morning coffee with ultra-pasteurized store-bought cream if that messes with your brain. You will drink the guilt-free Healing Trimmy, which is simply coffee blended with a little pastured butter or MCT oil and grass-fed collagen—and you can add some healthful, brain-protecting sunflower lecithin to keep your coffee a creamy color.

PURIST PITFALLS

Your love for all your raw pastured cream, butter, cheeses, egg yolks, and home-reared marbled steaks makes S meals the most appetizing for you. You know by now that fuel ruts of any kind are metabolism-slowing dead ends that say sayonara to your weight loss. Your challenge will be to not get bogged down in an S rut. You will need to learn to balance your weekly meals with lighter E fare and in these meals just use a tad of the super-food fats that you usually use liberally in S recipes. Sourdough ancient-grain bread is a true superfood and so is the humble lentil and simple sweet potato. Learn to relish your nourishing E meals that supply their own unique source of sustenance and invigorate your metabolism.

The common purist myth that low-fat anything is finagled, denatured, and unhealthy loses any ground when we look at nature. It is not rocket science and doesn't take civilized machinery to separate an egg yolk from a white. It takes only a little jiggle between the egg shells, and shazam, there you have it. Cream is designed by our Creator to rise naturally to the top. From there we can skim the precious treasure and churn it into butter or ladle it over fresh berries. What is to be done with all that leftover low-fat milk? Shall we chuck it out now because it is deprived of its fat? We'd be crazy! For centuries, low-fat cultured kefir, yogurt, and cheeses were crafted from this skimmed milk and nourished thriving civilizations. The term "low-fat" does not always mean it is a modern warped food.

Another myth that is taught and believed by many purists is that protein should never be eaten without sufficient fats, as these macronutrients are always paired in nature. That is not the case. The truth is that there are just as many lean fish as fatty, and lean game as greasy duck. Many whitefish are completely fat-free! In one of the famous meals in the Bible, Jesus fed five thousand people with dried fish and loaves. We would call it a yummy E meal.

Interestingly, tilapia was one of the three main types of fish caught in biblical times from the Sea of Galilee. In ancient times they were called "musht," but they are now nostalgically coined "Saint Peter's fish." These species of fish are very lean and have been the target of small-scale artisanal fisheries in the area for thousands of years.

Who could say that a poached, lean river trout atop a bed of steamed quinoa and sautéed tomatoes, drizzled with lemon juice, sea salt, and just a hint of olive oil was health-destroying? Low-fat all the time is dangerous and unbalanced. High-fat all the time is equally unhealthy and unbalanced. Enjoy your S fat-fueled meals, even use them to cross over sometimes; but rev your metabolic furnace with the energetic electricity of pure E meals.

Okay, go milk that cow, decorate your balcony with lots of potted curly parsley, and ask for a year's subscription to "How to Become More Puristy." We get you because one of us got the bug real bad and the other has to live next door to her.

Note: For puristy concerns regarding THM-approved sweeteners, visit Chapter 13, "Sweet Mama" (page 102).

Day 1

BREAKFAST—E

Super Prepared Purist Grains with blueberries ("Good Morning Grains" chapter in the *Trim Healthy Mama Cookbook*)

LUNCH—S

Superfood-Loaded Salad ("Quick Single Salads" chapter in the *Trim Healthy Mama Cookbook*) with pastured hard-boiled eggs or leftover free-range chicken meat

DINNER—S

Rich and Tender Stew using wild venison or grass-fed meat ("Crockpot Meals" chapter in the *Trim Healthy Mama Cookbook*) / Golden Flat Bread ("Breads and Pizza Crusts" chapter in the *Trim Healthy Mama Cookbook*) drizzled with extra-virgin olive oil and fresh herbs

Day 2

BREAKFAST—S

Three fried eggs in pastured butter or extra-virgin coconut oil and garnished with raw sheep's cheese (Pecorino Romano is a good variety) / Healing Trimmy ("Hot Drinks" chapter in the *Trim Healthy Mama Cookbook*)

LUNCH—E

Sweetie on Steroids ("Quick Single Skillet Meals" chapter in the *Trim Healthy Mama Cookbook*) / Beauty Milk ("More Drinks" chapter in the *Trim Healthy Mama Cookbook*)

DINNER—S

Popeye's Power Soup ("Family Soups" chapter in the *Trim Healthy Mama Cookbook*) / Swiss Bread or Golden Flat Bread with pastured butter ("Breads and Pizza Crusts" chapter in the *Trim Healthy Mama Cookbook*) / side salad with superfood oils

Day 3

BREAKFAST—E

Two slices of Artisan Sourdough or sprouted toast ("Breads and Pizza Crusts" chapter in the *Trim Healthy Mama Cookbook*) with an egg-white and veggie scramble / Healing Trimmy Light ("Hot Drinks" chapter in the *Trim Healthy Mama Cookbook*)

LUNCH—S

BBBB Thin Thick ("Shakes, Smoothies, Frappas, and Thin Thicks" chapter in the *Trim Healthy Mama Cookbook*) / 1 or 2 Chocolate Chai-Glazed Cinnamon Muffins ("Family Muffins" chapter in the *Trim Healthy Mama Cookbook*)

DINNER—S

Grass-fed pot roast / side salad with superfood oils / roasted Brussels sprouts with high-mineral salt, nutritional yeast, and extra-virgin coconut oil

Day 4

BREAKFAST—S

raw whole milk, Double Fermented Kefir superfood smoothie ("More Drinks" chapter in the *Trim Healthy Mama Cookbook*)

LUNCH—FP

Soothe Your Soul Soup ("Quick Single Soups" chapter in the *Trim Healthy Mama Cookbook*) / Swiss Bread as a dunker ("Breads and Pizza Crusts" chapter in the *Trim Healthy Mama Cookbook*)

DINNER—S

Pastured, whole baked chicken / green beans with melted ghee or pastured butter / green side salad with extra-virgin olive oil and apple cider vinegar

Day 5

BREAKFAST—E

Super Prepared Purist Grains with blueberries ("Good Morning Grains" chapter in the *Trim Healthy Mama Cookbook*)

LUNCH—FP

Chocolate Fat-Stripping Frappa made with organic cacao ("Shakes, Smoothies, Frappas, and Thin Thicks" chapter in the *Trim Healthy Mama Cookbook*)

DINNER—S

Pink Salmon Chowder ("Family Soups" chapter in the *Trim Healthy Mama Cookbook*) / side salad with liberal superfood oils

Day 6

BREAKFAST—S

Venison or pasture-raised sausage with fried eggs / Healing Trimmy ("Hot Drinks" chapter in the *Trim Healthy Mama Cookbook*)

LUNCH—E

Stewed tomatoes and onions sautéed with precooked, organic chicken breast with favorite zesty spices over 2 slices Artisan Sourdough or sprouted toast ("Breads and Pizza Crusts" chapter in the *Trim Healthy Mama Cookbook*) / hot tea with added collagen

DINNER—S

Super Salmon Patties made with ⅓ cup soaked quinoa instead of oats (recipe found free on our website or in the "Extra Skillet Stuff" chapter in the *Trim Healthy Mama Cookbook*) / roasted non-starchy veggies with ghee or coconut oil / green salad with superfood virgin oils

Day 7

BREAKFAST—FP

Breakfast-size Collagen Berry Whip ("Sweet Bowls" chapter in the *Trim Healthy Mama Cookbook*) / herbal tea

LUNCH—E

Sweet Potato Bar using pasture-raised chicken breasts ("Oven Baked or Roasted Meats" chapter in the *Trim Healthy Mama Cookbook*) / Beauty Milk ("More Drinks" chapter in the *Trim Healthy Mama Cookbook*)

DINNER—S

Mulligan Soup with wild ground venison or grass-fed beef ("Family Soups" chapter in the *Trim Healthy Mama Cookbook*) / Garlic Swiss Bread toasted with raw pastured butter ("Breads and Pizza Crusts" chapter in the *Trim Healthy Mama Cookbook*)

Snack Ideas for the Week

Double Fermented Kefir ("More Drinks" chapter in the *Trim Healthy Mama Cookbook*) with berries / raw cheese and soaked then dehydrated crispy nuts / grass-fed beef jerky (sugar-free) / organic crudités with hummus / Skinny Chocolate, Milk Chocolate Chunk Skinny Truffles, or Chocolate Superfood Chews ("Candies and Bars" chapter in the *Trim Healthy Mama Cookbook*) / Avo Cream Pudding and Chia Pud ("Sweet Bowls" chapter in the *Trim Healthy Mama Cookbook*) / Collagen Berry Whip and Tummy Spa Ice Cream ("Frozen Treats" chapter in the *Trim Healthy Mama Cookbook*) / Kale Chips and Purist Cheesy Crackers ("Crackers, Chips, and Dips" chapter in the *Trim Healthy Mama Cookbook*) / Purist Primer ("Quick Single Soups" chapter in the *Trim Healthy Mama Cookbook*) / Beauty Milk ("More Drinks" chapter in the *Trim Healthy Mama Cookbook*) / BBBB Thin Thick or any other Thin Thick ("Shakes, Smoothies, Frappas, and Thin Thicks" chapter in the *Trim Healthy Mama Cookbook*) / Chocolate Chai–Glazed Cinnamon Muffins ("Family Muffins" chapter in the *Trim Healthy Mama Cookbook*)

chapter 21

HEADS UP: BUDGETING MAMAS!

Perhaps this very book you are reading is borrowed from the library because purchasing it would eat into precious grocery money. We get it! Eight years ago, when we started writing the first edition of *Trim Healthy Mama* (which took a little more than five years to write), we were both bound by extremely tight budgets. Those were tough times, with our husbands sometimes out of work or then blessedly finding work but working two jobs just to try to catch up yet never quite making it. This plan was designed during those hard financial times. If we could do it then, you can do it now!

FOCUS ON YOUR CAN HAVES

These days, our grocery budgets are much more flexible and it's obvious from our recipes that we sometimes enjoy fun specialty items. But we didn't always have that liberty and you don't have to have any specialty items to see success. You can use everyday foods from any grocery store. You don't have to belong to a food co-op or shop at fancy-shmancy health markets or even buy the products from our own THM company. Simple, inexpensive foods can be your staples. Incorporated in the Trim Healthy Mama way, these ordinary foods can accomplish miracles.

Look at what you can buy rather than what you can't. Foods like old-fashioned oats, eggs, cans of tuna, cabbage, lettuce, brown rice, cottage cheese, the cheapest cuts of bone-in chicken, ground turkey or beef on sale, beans, and butter all are affordable. These inexpensive foods don't have to be bland or boring, either. We don't mean you'll have to boil up a sloppy plop of cabbage or have to eat plain tuna out of the can. But when cabbage is roasted with butter and seasonings it becomes a delicacy, and when it is finely chopped into angel hair noodles and tossed with ground turkey and taco seasoning—oh wow! When that tuna is drizzled with balsalmic vinegar and olive oil, mixed with cottage cheese, and stuffed into tomatoes—yummo! Even extra-virgin olive oil is affordable at discount chains.

Frozen cauliflower florets are very inexpensive. When creatively prepared, they can replace rice and potatoes in many S recipes such as potato salad, cheesy potato casseroles, mashed potatoes, and loaded potato soup. If purchasing Greek yogurt is too much of a stretch for you, you'll want to try our Jigglegurt recipe (found in the "Sweet Bowls" chapter of the *Trim Healthy Mama Cookbook*). It literally doubles your Greek yogurt so you can buy less of it. Yes, you will need some gelatin to make that recipe happen, but a little goes a long way. It takes only two teaspoons of gelatin to transform two cups of Greek yogurt into four cups.

Perhaps you cannot afford our Trim Healthy Mama Baking Blend to make breads, muffins, and cakes with. No worries, you can find ground flax meal at any grocery store and make muffins and breads with that. Oat fiber (not to be confused with oat bran) is another very inexpensive on-plan baking flour. Mix it with flax meal to lighten the calorie load and to give a less dense texture to your baked goods. You can find that on our website or look for it at discount online health food stores. Coconut flour is another on-plan flour easily found at many grocery stores, like Walmart or Target. Prices are coming down on that, too, as demand increases and competition between companies creates better bargains.

You'll notice we do use a lot of coconut oil on plan. Thankfully, extra-virgin coconut oil is not as expensive as it used to be when we both started on plan and is so much easier to find. But if it is still a stretch for you, refined coconut oil is cheaper than extra-virgin. It does not have all the medicinal qualities, but it will not become a trans fat when you cook with it, and it still retains its healthy middle-chain fatty acids. The main thing, though, is that you can still make Skinny Chocolate with it. One aisle over in the store, buy unsweetened cocoa powder, then mix in some plan-approved sweetener, and you'll always have affordable Skinny Chocolate on hand.

You can basically do our whole plan on these few inexpensive food items. Include some frozen berries (as they are cheaper than fresh), a piece of frozen salmon now and then (frozen fillets are much cheaper than fresh), and some green apples for more variety.

THE MEAT DILEMMA

Protein is the foundation of Trim Healthy Mama. Yes, it's true that proteins cost more than starches; but we're going to show you ways to make protein an affordable part of your grocery cart. We have to admit that white pasta, cheap fluffy white sandwich breads, ramen noodles, and packets of generic-label chips and pretzels are relatively cheap. People sometimes fill their carts with this sort of junk in the hope of getting a lot of food items without spending a ton of money. This practice might save you a dollar or two, but you haven't bought any real food. These items are essentially non-foods. They might be cheap on your bank account, but they will be expensive in the long run when it comes to your health.

In a perfect world, everybody would buy grass-fed beef and pastured eggs. The reality is, precious few can afford these forms of protein all the time. We have seen many Mamas try to limit their protein and that of their children because they cannot afford the most pure sources. Meat nights twice a week only, one egg per day max! But what do they then fill their plates with? It's not usually veggies that play a bigger role; starches take over when protein is missing. More beans, more rice, more bread, more potatoes. We are not against these foods, but when eaten in unbounded excess they are inflammatory, aging, and fattening.

So what to do, what to do?

If you know—or even are yourself—a hunter (go, girl!), your problem is solved. Wild game is the healthiest of all meat, so fill that freezer! We are blessed with sons who are excellent hunters and they provide us with enough healthy meat to last most of the year. Excuse us while we brag for a minute, but both of our oldest sons brought in five deer each this year for our families—proud Mamas we are. If your family isn't the hunting type and you truly cannot afford meat from the store, inquire into a hunter's association in your area. Many hunters kill extra deer and they are only too happy to give to families who need it. Venison is very healthy and tastes great, especially when cooked for long hours in a slow cooker.

TRICK FOR GROUND MEATS

Maybe all you can afford is the ground chuck on sale at your local Save More market. Don't worry, you can still do Trim Healthy Mama. We have a little trick to turn this ground beef (or ground turkey or ground chicken), which is likely too high in omega-6 fatty acids, into a cleaner, lean source. Toxins in meat are stored in the fat. Brown your meat, drain it, then put it in a colander and rinse it well with very hot water for a couple of minutes. This will remove most of the fat along with the toxins. If you want to be even more thorough, you can press down with a spoon or the bottom of a mug or jar to help release the fats under the hot water. Once the meat is rinsed, you are left with much cleaner, lean meat. You can use this generously in S meals, but since most of the fat has been removed, you can also use this in E or FP meals if you keep the limit at four ounces. For S purposes you can make this lean meat more "superfoodish" by adding healthy fats such as red palm oil or coconut oil.

CHICKEN TRUTHS

Don't be fooled by packaging claims on chicken. Sometimes certain brands have higher prices and claim that no hormones have been added and no antibiotics have been used. If you read the fine print on the packaging, the federal regulations prohibit use of hormones anyway. So don't spend five more bucks on that fancily worded package when the cheaper one next to it is not allowed to use hormones, either. Chicken thighs and legs are the least expensive part of the chicken and, since they contain the bones, they help to raise glycine levels in your body, which is a boon for your overall health. Big bags of frozen chicken pieces can go a long way and are much cheaper than fresh. Try our Bangin' Ranch Drums and Crispy Lickin' Chicken recipes in the "Oven Baked or Roasted Meats" chapter of the *Trim Healthy Mama Cookbook*. Or sprinkle your favorite spices on bone-in, skin-on chicken and bake until done.

FROZEN AND CANNED GOODS

Frozen and canned vegetables are often cheaper than fresh and can work on plan, but we also do want you to have plenty of fresh leafy greens. If you can eke out an extra dollar or two for organic lettuce, this is when it would really be worth it. Organic romaine is not usually priced too much higher than regular. If you can't afford it, have your salad anyway. Don't limit your greens, no matter what!

Frozen veggies are often picked at the height of freshness and snapped frozen. They are a great, cheap way to fill your diet with non-starchies. Canned forms of tomatoes, chilies, green beans, olives, artichokes, and meats can also play an inexpensive part of the plan. But we do urge you to seek out BPA-free canned goods when possible. More and more grocery stores are catching on to the dangers of bisphenol A, which is a known carcinogen, and are carrying their cheaper house-brand canned goods in BPA-free cans. Ask your local grocery store about their stance on this.

GIVE THANKS

Stress and worry can undo the most perfect, pure, and organic diet. If at this time you are not blessed with the budget to buy any of your foods in their purest forms, you do have the choice to pray for protection. Do your best but don't stress the rest. It is out of your control but in His. Be as wise and savvy as you can about sourcing pure foods, but don't obsess and destroy the joy in your journey. We have heard from thousands and thousands of Mamas whose health has miraculously turned around on Trim Healthy Mama with only regular grocery-store foods. Their blood sugars balanced, their weight dropped, and their bodies healed.

TIGHT-BUDGET IDEA MENU

Day 1

BREAKFAST—S

Strawberry Cheesecake Shake, using ¼ cup extra cottage cheese if budget does not allow for whey protein ("Shakes, Smoothies, Frappas, and Thin Thicks" chapter in the *Trim Healthy Mama Cookbook*)

LUNCH—E

Bean Boss Soup ("Quick Single Soups" chapter in the *Trim Healthy Mama Cookbook*) / Wasa or Ryvita crackers with a thin smear of butter (up to 1 teaspoon)

DINNER—S

Cabb and Saus Skillet ("Family Skillet Meals" chapter in the *Trim Healthy Mama Cookbook*) / optional deviled eggs on the side and/or a side salad with olive oil and vinegar

Day 2

BREAKFAST—S

Fried eggs with diced yellow squash

LUNCH—S

Heavy S Salad in a Jar—you can make fresh for your plate if you prefer ("Quick Single Salads" chapter in the *Trim Healthy Mama Cookbook*)

DINNER—E

Cheapskate Soup ("Family Soups" chapter in the *Trim Healthy Mama Cookbook*)

Day 3

BREAKFAST—E

Pineapple Upside Down Cake—no special ingredients version ("Quick Single Serve Cakes" chapter in the *Trim Healthy Mama Cookbook*) / Jigglegurt ("Sweet Bowls" chapter in the *Trim Healthy Mama Cookbook*)

LUNCH—S

Bread in a Mug Pizza, made with Bread in a Mug dough spread out into the size of a personal pizza crust, topped with your choice of budget-friendly toppings

("Breads and Pizza Crusts" chapter in the *Trim Healthy Mama Cookbook*) / side salad

DINNER—S

Potsticker Patties ("Extra Skillet Stuff" chapter in the *Trim Healthy Mama Cookbook*) / steamed or roasted cauliflower with butter and seasonings / side salad with oil and vinegar

Day 4

BREAKFAST—E

Cooked oatmeal / diced apple / Jigglegurt ("Sweet Bowls" chapter in the *Trim Healthy Mama Cookbook*)

LUNCH—E

Cream of Sweet Stuff Soup ("Quick Single Soups" chapter in the *Trim Healthy Mama Cookbook*)

DINNER—S

Egg Roll in a Bowl ("Family Skillet Meals" chapter in the *Trim Healthy Mama Cookbook* or you can find the recipe on Pinterest)

Day 5

BREAKFAST—FP

Large egg-white omelet with onion, spinach, and tomato and a garnish amount of grated part-skim mozzarella

LUNCH—E

Trim Healthy Pancakes ("Pancakes, Donuts, Crepes, and Waffles" chapter in the *Trim Healthy Mama Cookbook*), serving of fruit or berries, if desired

DINNER—S

Ridiculous Meatballs and Spaghetti ("Crockpot Meals" chapter in the *Trim Healthy Mama Cookbook*) / zucchini noodles

Day 6

BREAKFAST—E

Cooked oatmeal / frozen berries / Jigglegurt ("Sweet Bowls" chapter in the *Trim Healthy Mama Cookbook*)

LUNCH—S

Bread in a Mug Tuna Sandwich, the tuna mixed with diced celery and mayo, using Bread in a Mug ("Breads and Pizza Crusts" chapter in the *Trim Healthy Mama Cookbook*)

DINNER—S

BLT Frittata ("Family Skillet Meals" chapter in the *Trim Healthy Mama Cookbook*) / steamed cauliflower with butter and seasonings / side salad

Day 7

BREAKFAST—E

Bust-a-Myth Banana Cake ("Family Cakes" chapter in the *Trim Healthy Mama Cookbook*)

LUNCH—S

Large salad with canned tuna or a salmon pouch as protein and ½ an avocado

DINNER—S

Bangin' Ranch Drums ("Oven Baked or Roasted Meats" chapter in the *Trim Healthy Mama Cookbook* / buttered canned or frozen green beans

Snack Ideas for the Week

Fruit and low-fat cottage cheese or Jigglegurt ("Sweet Bowls" chapter in the *Trim Healthy Mama Cookbook*) / celery and peanut butter / boiled eggs / cheese and peanuts (peanuts are the cheapest nuts) / deli meat and cheese wrapped in lettuce / any popsicle or slushy in the "Frozen Treats" chapter in the *Trim Healthy Mama Cookbook* (since these are mainly ice, they are very budget-friendly) / Skinny Chocolate ("Candies and Bars" chapter in the *Trim Healthy Mama Cookbook*)

chapter 22

HEADS UP: WORKING MAMAS!

The title for this chapter does not mean stay-at-home moms do not work! We can vouch that, oh yes indeedy, we do. But this chapter is for our Mamas who work outside the home. Being away from your kitchen during meal and snack times has its challenges, but staying smartly on plan is very doable. While we still consider ourselves stay-at-home Mamas, these days our workload with Trim Healthy Mama sometimes has us out of the home during the day more often than we'd like. Packed lunches and snacks are often part of our life now, too. Oh, how we love to come home to our crockpots on those days!

Thousands of Mamas have had success on plan working full time outside of the home: It just takes a little prepping and a little planning. You can grab super-quick breakfasts as you run out the door, pack easy lunches and snacks the night before, and come home to simple, no-fuss meals or the aroma of a hearty meal simmering in the slow cooker. You can even still eat out for lunch sometimes using the ideas from Chapter 15, "Eating Out" (page 119); but don't leave all your meals to a restaurant. You'll have the most success if you do some prepping, too. The ideas we'll discuss here can also be very handy in helping your husband stay on plan while he is at work, if you are packing lunch for him to help him stay on plan.

GET PREPPING!

It's a great idea to use one of your days off (usually a Sunday afternoon) to prep for the upcoming workweek. Bake a chicken or two or buy a couple rotisserie chickens and separate the meat into light and dark for your various S, E, and FP needs throughout the week. Cut up lots of veggies and make your favorite versions of Salad in a Jar from the *Trim Healthy Mama Cookbook*. Try the Giant Blueberry Baked Pancake recipe ("Pancakes, Donuts, Crepes, and Waffles" chapter in the *Trim Healthy Mama Cookbook*) cut into slices and they'll be ready to go for a quick breakfast. Our Sweet Dreams Oatmeal and Crockpot Oatmeal recipes in the "Good Morning Grains" chapter of our cookbook are prepped the night before so all you have to do in the morning is eat, or heat and eat! Fix a batch of Mufflets for another breakfast option ("Good Morning Eggs" chapter in the *Trim Healthy Mama Cookbook*). They are a delicious, protein-rich cross between an omelet and a muffin and they freeze well, or you can leave them in the fridge for a few days to just grab. Prep some slow-cooker meals and put them in gallon-size zip-top bags, then into the freezer they go. You'll defrost your chosen meal in the fridge overnight, then plop it in the crockpot before you leave for work. It will cook while you are away and you'll come back to a much more stress-free evening.

The menu below uses crockpot meals for five of the seven days. For the other two days (presumably your weekend), we use two quick meals from our "Family Skillet Meals" chapter in the companion cookbook. They are quick, no-fuss meals that are sure to please the whole family.

WORKING MAMA IDEA MENU

Day 1

BREAKFAST—S

Mufflets ("Good Morning Eggs" chapter in the *Trim Healthy Mama Cookbook*)

LUNCH—S

Heavy or Deep S Salad in a Jar ("Quick Single Salads" chapter in the *Trim Healthy Mama Cookbook*)

DINNER—E

Wicked White Chili ("Crockpot Meals" chapter in the *Trim Healthy Mama Cookbook*)

Day 2

BREAKFAST—E

Giant Blueberry Baked Pancake ("Pancakes, Donuts, Crepes, and Waffles" chapter in the *Trim Healthy Mama Cookbook*) / Greek yogurt or Jigglegurt ("Sweet Bowls" chapter in the *Trim Healthy Mama Cookbook*)

LUNCH—S

Egg salad stuffed in a Joseph's pita / celery stuffed with peanut butter, or use Peanut Junkie Butter instead ("Condiments and Extras" chapter in the *Trim Healthy Mama Cookbook*)

DINNER—S

Smarty Pants Stroganoff ("Crockpot Meals" chapter in the *Trim Healthy Mama Cookbook*)

Day 3

BREAKFAST—S

Mufflets ("Good Morning Eggs" chapter in the *Trim Healthy Mama Cookbook*)

LUNCH—E

E Salad in a Jar ("Quick Single Salads" chapter in the *Trim Healthy Mama Cookbook*)

DINNER—S

Ridiculous Meatballs and Spaghetti ("Crockpot Meals" chapter in the *Trim Healthy Mama Cookbook*)

Day 4

BREAKFAST—FP

Big Boy Smoothie ("Shakes, Smoothies, Frappas, and Thin Thicks" chapter in the *Trim Healthy Mama Cookbook*)

LUNCH—E

Sprouted bread with lean meats and veggies or use Southwestern Pan Bread from the "Breads and Pizza Crusts" chapter in the *Trim Healthy Mama Cookbook* for the bread / Triple Zero Greek yogurt or Jigglegurt ("Sweet Bowls" chapter in the *Trim Healthy Mama Cookbook*)

DINNER—S

Wacha Want Mexican Chicken with grated cheese and sour cream ("Crockpot Meals" chapter in the *Trim Healthy Mama Cookbook*)

Day 5

BREAKFAST—FP

Sweet Dreams Cookie Bowl Oatmeal ("Good Morning Grains" chapter in the *Trim Healthy Mama Cookbook*)

LUNCH—S

Egg salad stuffed in a Joseph's pita /celery stuffed with peanut butter

DINNER—E

Wipe Your Mouth BBQ on sprouted rolls or bread ("Crockpot Meals" chapter in the *Trim Healthy Mama Cookbook*)

Day 6

BREAKFAST—S

Bacon and eggs

LUNCH—E

Leftover Wipe Your Mouth BBQ with brown rice and cucumber slices

DINNER - S

Reuben in a Bowl ("Family Skillet Meals" chapter in the *Trim Healthy Mama Cookbook*)

Day 7

BREAKFAST—E

Orange Creamsicle Shake ("Shakes, Smoothies, Frappas, and Thin Thicks" chapter in the *Trim Healthy Mama Cookbook*)

LUNCH—E

Personal pizza made with Perfect Pizza Crust ("Breads and Pizza Crusts" chapter in the *Trim Healthy Mama Cookbook*)

DINNER—S

Taco Time ("Family Skillet Meals" chapter in the *Trim Healthy Mama Cookbook*)

Snack Ideas for the Week

Apple and part-skim cheese stick / no-sugar-added beef jerky / Babybel cheese and a handful of nuts / Salmon Mousse and celery sticks or cucumber slices ("Crackers, Chips, and Dips" chapter in the *Trim Healthy Mama Cookbook*) / any leftovers from evening meal /deli meat slices / berries and Greek yogurt or Triple Zero Greek yogurt or Jigglegurt ("Sweet Bowls" chapter in the *Trim Healthy Mama Cookbook*) / any swirl, mousse, or pudding from the "Sweet Bowls" chapter in the *Trim Healthy Mama Cookbook*) / any chip or cracker from the "Crackers, Chips, and Dips" chapter in the *Trim Healthy Mama Cookbook*) / any frozen treat from the "Frozen Treats" chapter in the *Trim Healthy Mama Cookbook* or plan-approved store-bought ice cream such as Enlightened brand that does not contain sugar

chapter 23

HEADS UP: PREGNANT AND NURSING MAMAS!

W hat a beautiful honor to nurture new life from within your body. Whether your precious miracle is growing within you or has graduated to your arms and breasts, this special undertaking requires a new level of responsibility and dense nutrition.

The "Mama" in Trim Healthy Mama refers to all women in any season of life, but thankfully it also embraces the literal Mama—the one growing and nurturing life. Most diet plans abandon pregnant and nursing women; but we believe that if a way of eating is not sustainable during these physically demanding times, then it shouldn't stand up for the long haul, either. Pregnancy and nursing are a true litmus test for any diet. The Trim Healthy Mama Plan rises to the challenge and meets the rigorous demands. With all food groups included, and each meal strongly anchored around protein, the THM eating plan has its duckies in a row as far as solid nutrition for the growth and the healthy blossoming of both Mama and baby.

YOUR UNIQUE NEEDS

First, let us be clear: You should not try to make pregnancy a time for focusing on weight loss. Baby is more important and should be your focus rather than fretting the pounds right now. Trim Healthy Mama will help you gain a healthy amount of pregnancy weight. What it won't do is promote needless fat gain, which brings no further health benefits to you or your baby.

Both pregnancy and nursing can cause you to feel like your hunger is sometimes

OUTTA CONTROL! Some days you might be ravenous, but thankfully, some will be more settled. Both are okay, so just flow with the changes. The generous superfood fats in S meals and the blood sugar–friendly carbohydrates in E meals provide a balance of healthy, nutrient-dense fuel. Eating plentiful amounts of scrumptiously cooked non-starchy veggies, leafy green salads, or color-rich berries to round out each meal tucks you and baby soundly into a nutritional bedrock. No worries for nourishment here; but there are a few tweaks we want to give you to make your journey through these seasons even more grounded, gentle, and comforting. You'll be including some Crossovers and S Helpers along with your core S and E meals, so make sure to give those chapters a little reread.

SERENE CHATS: *Halfway through the writing of this book I was thrilled to discover I was pregnant with my eighth biological baby. Pearl wanted me to tackle the majority of this chapter, since I'm going through this with you.*

This will be my third Trim Healthy Mama pregnancy, and the positive differences between these and my other five pregnancies continue to bless my socks off. Certain issues that afflicted me in my previous pregnancies (such as chronic yeast infections) are simply not there! Nada! I wish I could tell you I no longer experience any nausea in the first trimester, but that wouldn't be true. I do have some tips, though, on how to get through that first twelve to fourteen weeks without completely making a nutritional mess of things.

Between the two of us, Pearl and I have had thirteen full-term pregnancies and nursed each of those babies. I was also able to nurse one of my adopted babies, so make that fourteen little nurslings for a combined twenty-two years of milk making. Both Pearl and I know all too well the crazy cravings, the morning sickness (make that twenty-four-hour sickness), the sleepless nights and fatigue, the insatiable nursing snackies, and the round-the-clock gorgeous little barracudas that are always at the tap. Let's tackle some of these issues.

CRAVINGS . . . CRAVINGS!!!

I get it, healthy foods you normally love when not pregnant are suddenly revolting, right? Everything makes you feel like throwing up except maybe one weird quirky thing. As long as that strange craving is healthy (not Cheetos) and not spiking to your blood-sugar levels, then have at it—for survival. This first trimester will soon pass.

In my last pregnancy I craved foods like hearty meat loaf and buttery veggies and didn't care much for fruit. In this pregnancy I can barely tolerate meat and I want to eat oranges all day. What's a girl to do with these strange cravings and aversions? Well, I have tried it both ways and I've figured something out. Completely giving in to all pregnancy whims will backfire on you.

I'm thoroughly enjoying oranges but I realize that eating them all day without enough protein is silly and hazardous to my blood-sugar levels. I'd end up back with those annoying yeast infections if I gave in completely to the cravings. Oranges may be healthy, but there is such a thing as too much of a good thing, Serene! Elevated blood-sugar levels are known to be a cause of miscarriage, pregnancy health issues, and even birth defects. As you know from previous chapters, you can get elevated blood sugars without eating actual sugar. Keeping this knowledge in mind, I enjoy one orange for a snack and make sure to eat some protein with it. Maybe I'll have another for a dessert, but shoveling orange after orange into my mouth all day long just because I'm craving them AIN'T A SMART MOVE! I've also been curbing my citrus cravings by sipping on the Singing Canary (see the recipe in our companion cookbook). I opt to leave out the essential oil drops in that recipe while I'm pregnant, just to be on the safe side. I'm working through my aversion to meat by including lots of salmon and Greek yogurt, because I can still tolerate those, and am getting protein in other ways, including by adding collagen and gelatin to my shakes, hot drinks, and whips. And of course Pristine Whey Protein Powder is a quick and easy protein source. Whole sources of protein are so important, I know, so I have not forsaken meat altogether; I'm trying to get in little amounts here and there until my regular appetite returns.

In my first couple of pregnancies I would cave in to cravings for Taco Bell in the first trimester when nothing else sounded edible. But I made a discovery. I would eat the "forbidden" meal, yet would still feel sick afterward. I would eat something healthy, and feel sick afterward. The junk food that I craved did not help the sick-

ness! The healthy food made me feel good about my pregnancy even though I still suffered with ickiness. The junk food made me feel out of control about my health and weight and worry about the baby. The good food choice helped sustain my energy but the poor choice drained me even more than the already drained feeling of the initial first trimester.

Do your best to stick to on-plan foods even if you cannot perfectly keep to meal timing, because those wild cravings for potato chips you think might help, probably won't. Those foods will just bite back all the more. Yes, the first trimester is the hardest. You will not be able to be perfect. You'll slip now and then (or more than now and then) and crave ridiculous things—and maybe give in sometimes. But don't throw your whole first trimester away even if you slip up multiple times. Endeavor to do your best in all trimesters even if you mess up. Make a healthier choice for you and your baby in your very next meal. Give yourself grace but don't throw in that towel! Things should get better after the twelve- to fourteen-week mark, and keeping to plan won't seem as daunting a task then.

SNACKING

If you have to eat before the recommended three-hour mark, that is perfectly okay; but don't graze all day. Your baby may be having a growth spurt or your milk supply may need to build up to compete with new demands, so it is natural to sometimes have to eat before three hours have passed. Waiting too long to eat during the first trimester can make nausea worse. This doesn't mean you shovel something in your mouth every half hour, but eating a protein-based snack every two to three hours does usually help.

Make sure you are always well hydrated. If it is not nausea bothering you but hunger, do a "drink" test to check for real hunger. True hunger brought on by the demands of a baby is different from mind hunger that tells you to eat just because you wanna. When hunger strikes and it is obviously too early to eat again, grab a nice glass of pure water or carbonated water laced with lemon or one of our All-Day Sipper drinks. Or try an iced or hot tea or Trimmaccino. If that doesn't do the trick and you are still truly hungry, then you do need to furnish your body and the growth of your baby and or milk supply with proper sustenance. Most of us pregnant and nursing Mamas will also want a little protein-rich snack before bed, while late-night snacking for those not nursing or pregnant is not usually necessary.

Fuel Pull snacks and desserts are excellent for providing a lighter caloric balance to these seasons of constant hunger. We preggie and milk-making Mamas need our main meals to provide solid fuel, ample protein, and concentrated nutrition, but there is room for the trimming talent of Fuel Pulls between meals and afterward for desserts. Used in this way, Fuel Pulls can be an extra tool to help control excess weight gain during pregnancy and help gently lose that weight while nursing. You can still enjoy some S and E snacks and desserts, but don't neglect these recipes from our cookbook: Tummy Tucking Ice Cream, Tummy Spa Ice Cream, Cottage Berry Whip or Collagen Berry Whip, Thin Thicks and Baby Fraps, other Fuel Pull options like Swiss Crackers, Crunkers, Mad Melbas, and Crunch Puffs from the "Crackers, Chips, and Dips" chapter, and Wonder Wraps stuffed with lean chicken and a sprinkle of Parmesan cheese. These are just a few ideas for Fuel Pull slim-friendly snacks that can help you out when the ravenous snackies of growing a baby keep knocking. But caution: If you are a Mama who struggles to put on twenty pounds during pregnancy or who can't keep weight on during nursing, limit Fuel Pull snacks and rely on denser fare. Make every snack either a Crossover or an S or an E.

SAFE WEIGHT GAIN

A nice twenty- to thirty-pound weight gain is a sensible goal if you are starting your THM pregnancy already at or close to goal weight. This amount of weight will support your baby but will help prevent pregnancy problems such as preeclampsia and high blood pressure. It also won't make it difficult for you to get back into your pre-preggie jeans. But of course we are all different: For some a thirty-five-pound pregnancy is fantastic if the usual gain is sixty pounds! Your journey will be unique and we don't want to push hard numbers on you and squish any pregnancy joy.

If you start a pregnancy well above your healthiest weight, you do not have to gain a certain number of pounds. Your weight may not climb much at all on the scale but if you nourish your pregnancy the THM way, your baby will still grow healthfully while your own body fat diminishes.

GET YOUR CROSSIES IN

If you start your pregnancy at a healthy weight, you'll want to include plenty of Crossovers as well as some core S and E meals, depending on how your body responds weight-wise. If you are not gaining enough weight, you'll need to up the frequency of those Crossovers. Some of our high-metabolism Mamas will need to make every meal in their pregnancy tandem-fueled. If the scale goes up too quickly, pull Crossies back a little but don't stop them altogether. I have at least one Crossover per day while pregnant but I don't follow any strict rules on this. Some days I cross over all day and other days I eat more S's and E's than Crossovers. I try to tune in to my body as it lets me know what it needs.

Even if you are starting your THM pregnancy significantly overweight, Crossovers can still play a part in your pregnancy. There is nothing wrong with focusing more on the core S and E meals since they offer your body all the nutrients it needs, but don't ditch Crossovers altogether. Smatter a few here and there during your week. This way your body won't feel stressed by having to always seek out more fuel once it has burned through only one main fuel in your meal. A basic suggestion is to include four Crossover meals per week even if you are carrying extra weight when starting your pregnancy. Once again, this is not a strict number; listen to and learn from your own body during your pregnancy. Nourish deeply with your fats but don't forget your lighter meals, too. Keep juggling those fuels between S and E and a few Crossies. Fuel Pull snacks are fine but we don't want our pregnant or nursing women eating many Fuel Pull meals.

If you are exclusively nursing your baby, you'll also want to include some Crossovers along with regular S and E meals. S and E meals alone do contribute to rich milk but, similar to pregnancy, nursing is a time of extra demand on your body. You don't want to stress your body by not offering both fat and carbs in the same meal a few times per week, even if you have weight to lose. Quinoa and oatmeal both promote a good milk supply, so enjoy them as pure E meals and also as Crossovers. If you are nursing but your baby has started eating some solids, Crossovers are not quite as necessary; but be sure to still enjoy a couple per week.

Remember, CROSSOVERS ARE NOT CHEATS! They are protein-centered meals with safe carb amounts and luscious fats. It is very important to stabilize your blood sugar during pregnancy. Getting pregnant and then using it as a reason to go off plan and just eat anything can be hazardous to your own body and the health of your baby. Spiking your blood-sugar levels is one of the fastest ways of aging internally and externally. While pregnant, your baby—and especially his or her brain development—can be adversely affected by dangerously high sugar levels. Cross-

overs will negate that risk yet still give you plenty of tandem fuels to gain healthy pregnancy weight.

CROSS WITH EASY-BURNING FATS

Here's a great tip for adding Crossovers without too much weight gain. Have more Crossover meals containing easy-burning fats. Coconut oil, red palm oil, butter, olive oil, and avocados are more weight-friendly than cheese, cream cheese, cream (especially the pasteurized versions), and heavy nut consumption. This is not a warning to steer clear of those other fats—just a little helpful tweak.

Enjoy liberal coconut oil or butter on your sweet potatoes instead of a cheesy Crossover. Pop a couple Skinny Chocolates in your mouth after your E meal instead of a dessert made with cream cheese. Don't make yourself miserable avoiding the fats that promote less weight loss, but do be mindful that every Crossover needn't contain them. Balance is a beautiful thing.

BEWARE OF CROSSIES IN A RUT

If you do have a weight issue while pregnant or nursing, you'll still need your pure E meals in the mix to change up the caloric load and rev your metabolism. It is not a wise approach to eat constant S meals, then splurge on a complete cheat meal, then go back to regular S meals. E foods contain important nutrients that both you and your baby need. Replacing those well-needed E meals with sugar or refined starches leaves you and your baby depleted. It is also another weight trap to go back and forth between S meals and Crossovers. Your trim will happen best when pure E meals are included. If you don't feel filled up enough after an E meal, finish your meal by blending a glass of unsweetened almond, coconut, or cashew milk with one to two tablespoons of whey protein, or one tablespoon Integral Collagen sweetened to your liking with an on-plan sweetener. You can always add cocoa to make that an easy chocolate milk—yum! Or tag on a nourishing Thin Thick found in the "Shakes, Smoothies, Frappas, and Thin Thicks" chapter of the Trim Healthy Mama Cookbook—*ain't nobody going to be hungry after one of those thickies!*

GESTATIONAL DIABETES

During pregnancy you are naturally more insulin-resistant and subsequently are more easily affected by foods that offer your body the fuel of glucose. This is a natural consequence of your body sparing sugar for the baby's rapid growth. Mamas who are already insulin resistant from the ravages of a "normal high-sugar diet" might find their prediabetes catapulted into gestational diabetes by the added insulin resistance of pregnancy. Incredibly, we've heard from so many women who had previous pregnancies with gestational diabetes, but the next time were able to avoid it and have a healthier pregnancy eating the THM way. It's all about getting your blood sugar stable in each and every meal.

If you suffer from gestational diabetes, you may have a harder time with pure E meals. If you find yourself unable to handle E meals and many Crossovers cause too much weight gain for you, try the following ideas:

1. Eat your carbs as S Helper meals. This is not a good long-term option as you are still constantly in an S fuel state and your metabolism needs change. Using S Helpers to adjust to E meals in the beginning and then smattering them into your fuel juggle is the balanced, "no-rut" approach for your particular season.

2. Use only slow-burning carbs rather than higher-glycemic ones. Choose quinoa over rice and an apple over pineapple. Our Trim Healthy Pancakes are an extremely gentle E option. Chana Dal soup should be an extremely kind E meal to your blood sugar.

3. Take advantage of Gluccie's ability to lower blood sugar. Make a Gluccie gravy to top your grain dish or sweet potato. Add a half teaspoon of Gluccie to an Orange Cream Shake to slow the rush from your added fruit. Eat a light Gluccie pudding snack before an E meal to help the glucose absorb at a slower pace. Add Gluccie to your lentil or Golden Chana Soup for thickening or make Pancake Syrup with Gluccie to cover your sprouted French toast.

4. Learn to use okra. It can be a pregnant Mama's best friend. If you are saying "Oh, gross!" hold on a minute, because okra can be fantastically delicious depending on how you use it. Okra is an amazing vegetable that helps put the brakes on accelerating blood sugar. Including it frequently can help your body respond better to carbs. It is super high in folic acid, which is important for preventing birth defects. Okra also boasts high amounts of the B complex vitamin group as well as vitamins K, A, and C, iron, calcium, manganese, and magnesium, all of which are important during pregnancy. Check out Chapter

17, "Affordable Superfoods" (page 129), for more information about okra and try some of our many recipes using it in our THM companion cookbook.

YES TO EXERCISE, NO TO OVERDOING IT

Exercise can help energize you, release stress, keep you stronger for the challenges of pregnancy, birth, and nursing, and keep you from being a couch potato which is never healthy. Of course there are many scientific reasons behind the benefits of exercise and its positive effects on pregnancy and postpartum; but our chief concern is not to promote more exercise here. It is to warn you against over-exercise in this season.

Waking up at five when you have nursed all night to fit in your "must-do" kick-boxing or spin class is counterproductive to your physical and emotional health goals. It is not respecting your body or this beautiful season. If you set the alarm for an hour of "gut-bustingness" when your body is desperate for rest, your body will feel the added stress, release catabolic cortisol, break down your muscle, slow your metabolism, and possibly store fat rather than release it.

When you are pouring so much of your body's energy reserves into supporting your baby nutritionally and physically, you really—REALLY—need to be diligent about paying attention to your body's signals to slow down. You are expending a lot and don't have room for "overexercise neurosis." Just because it is your weight-lifting Wednesday doesn't mean you need to robotically tick the box and "get 'er done" when your body and baby need you to take a nap that afternoon instead.

Many times over we have seen these very precious seasons sabotaged by the abuse of doing too much. I have been guilty of this myself. Don't be a lazy Mama who needs a good kick in her rear, but be wary of the opposite extreme of pushing your limits. Check out our Trim Healthy Mama Workins DVD if you want to exercise safely with us.

STRESSIN' OVER SWEETENERS

I am extremely comfortable using stevia during my pregnancies. In fact, I have either been pregnant or nursing for my entire Trim Healthy Mama journey. This is my third pregnancy in which I have been sweetening with stevia. I don't have a huge sweet tooth so a doonk or two of stevia in my treats or drinks does not concern me at all. I don't urge all women to do the same but after in-depth research, conversa-

tions with several doctors, and my own experience, I have total peace about it. My own midwife, who has delivered hundreds of babies, has no problems with me or any of her Mamas using stevia. She enjoys it in her own treats.

If you have concerns, please talk with your doctor or read Chapter 13, "Sweet Mama" (page 102), where we have addressed some of the issues that come up when stevia is mentioned. In the end, it must be your decision and we want you to feel comfortable and at peace in your Trim Healthy pregnancy. If you can't shake off concerns no matter what the studies, or people, say, then you can sweeten your THM life with some of the other healthy options we advise. Pregnancy is not a time to stress over issues. Use a little raw honey or coconut sugar if they fit better with your approach, but please be aware that although considered natural, higher-glycemic sweeteners like these do impact your blood sugar. We cannot in good conscience give you license to get liberal with them. It is an undisputed fact that elevated blood sugar is harmful to your pregnancy, so keep these sweeteners to smaller amounts, especially if you have any signs of gestational diabetes.

A HEALTHY SET OF COCONUTS

Breast milk is the only edible source of MCTs (middle-chain triglycerides) in nature with the exception of tropical oils or the small amounts in goat's milk. Breast milk should be rich in these immune-defending, disease-fighting, brain-feeding, and energy-rich fatty acids. Sadly, due to our modern depleted diets, studies show that breast milk is often a very poor source of MCT for a needy baby. Thankfully, that can be easily remedied by incorporating into your diet foods that are rich in MCTs, such as coconut oil and products made with its meat or milk. Another option is MCT oil itself, which is made by isolating just these middle-chain fatty acids from coconut oil and palm oils.

When a Mama's breast milk is lacking in MCTs, the baby may not be as sufficiently nourished as he or she could be and may become more vulnerable to infectious diseases and viruses. A diet lacking in MCTs causes the mammary glands to only be able to produce 3 percent lauric acid and 1 percent capric acid. Baby will miss out on the wonderful antiviral, antimicrobial, antifungal, antiprotozoal, and brain-nourishing benefits of these immune-enhancing substances.

The good news is that you can positively alter the fat composition of your breast milk. High-five to Trim Healthy nursers! We can potentially raise the percentage in *our breast milk from the meager single digits to about 18 percent MCTs by frequently supplementing with yummy goodies like Skinny Chocolate! A 1998 study published in the* American Journal of Clinical Nutrition *revealed that it is possible to shift lauric acid levels in breast milk from a low 3 percent to almost 10 percent only fourteen hours later. Women who consumed coconut oil in this study had their breast milk tested and it was found that three tablespoons of coconut oil in just one meal gave their breast milk a threefold boost! In an article entitled "Coconut Oil and Medium-Chain Triglycerides," Dr. Bruce Fife suggests that with frequent intake of coconut oil over time, it is likely a woman may be able to increase her breast milk's lauric acid levels to an incredibly health-boosting 18 percent.*

Supplementing with therapeutic-grade 100 percent MCT oil can bring up your levels of the smaller-chained capric and medium-chain caprilic acids extremely quickly and this oil does not have a coconutty taste, which is a boon sometimes. MCT oil is highly antimicrobial and antiviral and provides immediate energy, delivered faster than glucose and without sugar's detrimental effects. Start slowly with one teaspoon at a time, as it is very potent and can result in diarrhea if you use too much too soon. Your body will gradually be able to handle more with time. You can read more about MCT oil in Chapter 18, "Specialty Food Stars" (page 140). It does not replace coconut oil in your diet, but it can be a great addition.

To boost your milk supply with lauric acid (which is a slightly longer middle-chain fatty acid and a potent and powerful immune booster), dig in to virgin coconut oil or the nut itself. Our recipes for Skinny Chocolate and Skinny Chocolate Truffles will help with this in the yummiest of ways. Be liberal with treats made with shredded coconut during pregnancy and the nursing season to provide immune protection and vital brain nourishment for your baby. Coconut chips are a good addiction for a pregnant or nursing Mama to have. We have a wonderful recipe for those in the companion cookbook called Savory Crispy Addictions ("Crackers, Chips, and Dips" chapter). Cream up your hot chocolates, chais, or coffee Trimmacino-style with MCT oil or coconut oil. You can choose to cross over the superfood way by drizzling generous virgin coconut oil over a gooey, caramelized baked sweet potato—yum!

Happy baby making and milking! The best chunk of wisdom Pearl and I can give you at this time is to embrace this season with wholehearted, "dive-in-deep" gratitude and gusto. Enjoy the wild ride. It is precious and ends all too soon.

Day 1

BREAKFAST—XO

Two eggs any style on 1 piece of buttered sprouted or Artisan Sourdough toast—either store-bought or homemade (see the "Breads and Pizza Crusts" chapter in the *Trim Healthy Mama Cookbook*) / 1 whole orange / Hot Chocolate Trimmy ("Hot Drinks" chapter in the *Trim Healthy Mama Cookbook*)

LUNCH—S

Superfood-Loaded Salad ("Quick Single Salads" chapter in the *Trim Healthy Mama Cookbook*) / Beauty Milk ("More Drinks" chapter in the *Trim Healthy Mama Cookbook*)

DINNER—SH

Cilantro Lime-Burst Chicken ("Crockpot Meals" chapter in the *Trim Healthy Mama Cookbook*) / ½ cup cooked quinoa

Day 2

BREAKFAST—E

Creamy Grains ("Good Morning Grains" chapter in the *Trim Healthy Mama Cookbook*)

LUNCH—S

Cream of Mushroom Soup ("Quick Single Soups" chapter in the *Trim Healthy Mama Cookbook*) / Swiss Bread with butter ("Breads and Pizza Crusts" chapter in the *Trim Healthy Mama Cookbook*) / optional salted sliced cucumber

DINNER—XO

Cabb and Saus Skillet ("Family Skillet Meals" chapter in the *Trim Healthy Mama Cookbook*) / ¾ cup cooked quinoa

Day 3

BREAKFAST—S

Bacon and eggs / Healing Trimmy, decaf if desired ("Hot Drinks" chapter in the *Trim Healthy Mama Cookbook*)

LUNCH—E

Waldorf Cottage Cheese Salad ("Quick Single Salads" chapter in the *Trim Healthy Mama Cookbook*) / Swiss Bread with 1 teaspoon butter ("Breads and Pizza Crusts" chapter in the *Trim Healthy Mama Cookbook*)

DINNER—S

Cornbread Crusted Mexican Pie ("Oven Dishes" chapter in the *Trim Healthy Mama Cookbook*) / side salad / steamed broccoli with butter

Day 4

BREAKFAST—XO

Apple Cinnamon Crockpot Oatmeal with cream, butter, or coconut oil ("Good Morning Grains" chapter in the *Trim Healthy Mama Cookbook*) / Collagen Tea ("Hot Drinks" chapter in the *Trim Healthy Mama Cookbook*)

LUNCH—S

Leftover Cornbread Crusted Mexican Pie / side salad

DINNER—S

Crispy Lickin' Chicken ("Oven Baked or Roasted Meats" chapter in the *Trim Healthy Mama Cookbook*) / green beans / optional side salad

Day 5

BREAKFAST—E

Leftover Apple Cinnamon Crockpot Oatmeal, reheated with unsweetened almond or cashew milk / Healing Trimmy Light, decaf if desired ("Hot Drinks" chapter in the *Trim Healthy Mama Cookbook*)

LUNCH—S

Superfood-Loaded Salad ("Quick Single Salads" chapter in the *Trim Healthy Mama Cookbook*)

DINNER—XO

Sweet Potato Bar ("Oven Baked or Roasted Meats" in the *Trim Healthy Mama Cookbook*) crossed over with butter or coconut oil

Day 6

BREAKFAST—E

Trim Healthy Pancakes ("Pancakes, Donuts, Crepes, and Waffles" chapter in the *Trim Healthy Mama Cookbook*) with 0% Greek yogurt and berries or fruit / Collagen Tea ("Hot Drinks" chapter in the *Trim Healthy Mama Cookbook*)

LUNCH—XO

Egg salad made with whole eggs and full-fat mayo on 2 pieces sprouted or sourdough bread / celery stuffed with peanut butter

DINNER—S

Super Salmon Patties ("Extra Skillet Stuff" chapter in the *Trim Healthy Mama Cookbook*) / side salad / steamed and buttered yellow squash

Day 7

BREAKFAST—S

Cheese- and spinach-stuffed omelet / Healing Trimmy, decaf if desired ("Hot Drinks" chapter in the *Trim Healthy Mama Cookbook*)

LUNCH—S

Just Like Campbell's Tomato Soup ("Quick Single Soups" chapter in the *Trim Healthy Mama Cookbook*) / grilled cheese on Swiss Bread ("Breads and Pizza Crusts" chapter in the *Trim Healthy Mama Cookbook*)

DINNER—XO OR E

Wicked White Chili ("Crockpot Meals" chapter in the *Trim Healthy Mama Cookbook*) with sour cream and grated cheese if desiring a Crossover

Snack Ideas for the Week

Celery or apple with nut butters / fruit and cottage cheese / Wasa or Ryvita crackers with Laughing Cow Creamy Light Swiss cheese wedges or Laughin' Mama Cheese ("Condiments and Extras" chapter in the *Trim Healthy Mama Cookbook*) / cubed cheese and nuts / Greek yogurt and berries / BBBB Thin Thick or any other Thin Thick, shake, or smoothie ("Shakes, Smoothies, Frappas, and Thin Thicks" chapter in the *Trim Healthy Mama Cookbook*) / any single-serve muffin ("Quick Single Muffins" chapter in the *Trim Healthy Mama Cookbook*) / any muffin from the "Family Muffins" chapter in the *Trim Healthy Mama Cookbook*) / Avo Cream Pudding or Chia Pud ("Sweet Bowls" chapter in the *Trim Healthy Mama Cookbook*) / Cottage Berry Whip, Collagen Berry Whip, or Tummy Spa Ice Cream ("Frozen Treats" chapter in the *Trim Healthy Mama Cookbook*) / Skinny Chocolate, Skinny Chocolate Truffles, or Superfood Chews ("Candies and Bars" chapter in the *Trim Healthy Mama Cookbook*)

chapter 24

HEADS UP: TURTLE LOSERS!
(WITH FUEL CYCLE INFORMATION)

Do you feel like you are doing everything right yet still the pounds won't budge? Let's help you troubleshoot to make sure you are not unknowingly sabotaging yourself. But sometimes, even if you *ARE* doing everything right, your body has some healing to do and that takes time.

Stephanie and her husband have been missionaries in Mexico and Puerto Rico for the last sixteen years. She started Trim Healthy Mama after a lifetime of dieting—taking off and then putting back on the same fifty pounds. She'd suffered with a thyroid condition since the age of fourteen and PCOS since her early twenties. Not surprisingly, her metabolism was completely broken when she began THM.

In fact, once Stephanie started Trim Healthy Mama, she did not lose one pound, not even an inch, for four months! She continued on, enjoying her food, realizing she was feeling a lot better; and that was a victory. Due to her past low-carb dieting habits, she was terrified of carbs at first but slowly began tuning in to her body. She started nourishing herself with both S and E meals and, when the scale remained on the same number, reminded herself that her journey was no longer about the weight so much as the health. After the four-month mark, Stephanie ever so slowly began dropping pounds. She is now down forty pounds after close to two years on the plan. Her husband joined her and has dropped significant weight, too.

To some people, forty pounds may seem like slow loss in that length of time, but to Stephanie it is a huge accomplishment. She did it without having to starve herself or remove whole food groups as she had done her entire life. What would have happened if she'd given up mad and frustrated because the plan hadn't appeared to be working? Her only alternative would have been to go back to the diet extremes that had ruined her metabolism, or to give up and adopt an "I-don't-care-so-I-may-as-well-eat-whatever" diet and gain more weight. Stephanie is not quite at her goal weight yet, but she happily continues in the right direction and encourages other slow losers not to quit.

Take a page from Stephanie's book and hang in there. Don't quit if pounds are slow to move or won't move at all. Your journey may be painstakingly slower than others', and it is difficult to struggle while watching your friends start the plan and lose weight quickly. But your journey is your own. You can still enjoy it even if you are carrying stubborn post-menopausal, hypothyroid, or severe-insulin-resistant weight. The turtle might have been slower, but he crossed the finish line, didn't he? Hopefully, some of the tips and tweaks we'll give you here can help.

ARE YOU REALLY A TURTLE?

Let's clear something up first. Don't automatically label yourself a turtle if you are losing on average about a half pound to a pound per week. At that rate you are not a stubborn loser and probably don't need to do anything different on plan than what you are already doing.

If your weight loss stalls for a week or two, or even a month or two, don't freak out! The body often takes breaks from losing weight, especially after each twenty-pound loss or so. This also doesn't mean you are a stubborn loser; it is quite normal. Your liver has to work extra hard eliminating toxins as fat is released. Including collagen and gelatin into your diet can help it stand up under the pressure. But remember, your liver needs some down time, too! Let's not expect it to be a super-organ that never tires.

GENTLY DOES IT

If you are coming to the Trim Healthy Mama Plan from any sort of extreme diet, shift your focus from the scale for a month or two. Many Mamas arrive on THM's door bone-weary, in many cases having been diagnosed with adrenal fatigue like Adrenal Splat Pat, whom we met in Chapter 1 (see page 9). Their nerves, hormones, and metabolisms are suffering after long years of harsh treatment from obsessive calorie counting or long-term fat or carb restriction and/or overexercising.

It is possible that at first your body may even want to store as it heals. Your scale may go up just a bit since your body may want to cling to every nutrient and bit of nourishment that it's offered after having been deprived for too long. If tiny gains on the scale throw you into a tailspin, simply focus on nourishing and fueling your body these first few weeks or even months. Remember, you're fueling your metabolism. You want to help it heal, and get stoked up hot again, so no skipping meals!

Take a break from hour-long gym sessions. They truly don't help with stubborn weight since they further tax your adrenal glands. Enjoy walks in the fresh air and read Chapter 29, "Let's Talk Exercise" (page 263), in which we discuss the hazards of overexercising and how to do it in a way that is kind to your hormones.

While we absolutely do not want you to count the calories in your every bite, it isn't wise to fall off into the opposite extreme as you recover, by indulging in all Heavy-S meals overflowing with cream, nuts, and cheese. Once you find your feet firmly in the very basics of the plan, give Chapter 11, "Higher Learning" (page 90), a read. You'll want to learn to juggle your fuels with a mix of Light-, Heavy-, and Deep-S meals, balancing those with E meals and Fuel Pulls. Whatever you do, don't nix your E meals! Damaged thyroids and adrenals need healthy carbs! This foundational precept of juggling is especially important for damaged metabolisms and skewed hormones. Deep-S and Light-S meals will be kinder to you than Heavy-S meals, along with Fuel Pull desserts and snacks. Once you feel ready, also read through the part of that chapter that deals with fuel stacking (see page 92). It may be something that you need to be more careful about than others do. It's not fair, we know. We feel for you, sister; we think about you often and are pulling for you. We are researching all we can to help with your stubborn situation.

CHECK YOUR HORMONES

Stubborn weight often means imbalanced hormones. It will be important to test your hormones. We suggest that you ask your doctor for a full blood panel and include the following:

Prolactin
Insulin
Thyroid, including TSH, Free T3, and Reverse T3

(A full sex-hormone panel may be important for perimenopausal women, including estradiol, testosterone, and progesterone. Postmenopausal women will automatically be low in all three of these sex hormones but testing is still helpful if you find a doctor familiar with bioidentical hormone treatments who can help you naturally boost your sex-hormone levels back to an optimum range.)

Prolactin

High levels of this hormone can go hand in hand with extremely stubborn weight loss or weight gain, no matter what eating style is adopted or how hard you try. High prolactin levels sometimes indicate a growth on the pituitary gland, which is usually a benign condition but needs to be dealt with under a doctor's supervision. These benign tumors are quite common, with an estimated one in ten people being afflicted; but they can often be an undiagnosed reason for extremely stubborn weight. The normal levels for prolactin for a non-nursing woman are between four and thirty. Most doctors will dismiss prolactin as a problem unless levels are above one hundred, but some reproductive endocrinologists like to see a prolactin level below fifteen, given that high prolactin will also negatively impact fertility.

Nursing is another time of high prolactin levels. Prolactin is needed during this season in order to stimulate milk and suppress estrogen, which promotes regular fertility. While some women find that nursing promotes easier weight loss after giving birth, others appear to be sensitive to these high prolactin levels. Many find it frustratingly difficult to shed weight, sometimes even gaining despite their best efforts.

The relationship of prolactin to stubborn weight loss during nursing is still rather untested and it is not known whether women with this issue have excessively high prolactin during nursing or whether they are just more sensitive to the weight-loss-inhibiting aspects of this hormone. Hormone testing during nursing (especially while the body is not yet ovulating) is hit or miss, with too many variables. If you suspect you may have a pituitary tumor (which would have already manifested symptoms before nursing), you could talk to your doctor about the safety of a pituitary scan while nursing. There are some supplements and medications that may help bring down prolactin levels, but of course none is appropriate during the season of nursing as they can dry up milk supply. What's a Mama to do?

There is a school of thought that the essential amino acid tryptophan can increase prolactin levels through raising serotonin, but studies conflict. Tryptophan has many benefits in the body and is found in foods such as muscle meats and many dairy products. It stands to reason, though, that those who struggle with the weight-loss-inhibiting aspects of prolactin might not want to overdo foods high in this amino acid.

The ability of tryptophan to cross the brain barrier and give rise to prolactin only appears possible in studies through an insulin pathway—either in the presence of high carbs (which you won't be doing on THM) or through the anabolic mechanism of insulin in the form of whey protein. We are all so unique and while for most of us whey protein helps with weight loss, it might not be the perfect supplement for those really struggling with prolactin issues. If extremely stubborn weight is an issue for you during nursing or even if you are not nursing, consider that this prolactin issue could be a possible reason. If so, collagen and gelatin may be the better form of protein supplement for you. In fact, they can be the very keys that will balance tryptophan levels in your body and make them less dominant.

Animal products that are higher in tryptophan should not be shunned, but it might be a good idea to scale them back to smaller portions—say three ounces of beef or chicken on a salad instead of six ounces. An added scoop of collagen or gelatin somewhere in your meal or in a drink will give you more of the protein your body needs. Now, that's a perfect protein balance. Salmon is lower in tryptophan, so be more liberal with it. Dairy products such as Greek yogurt and cottage cheese, while so helpful to many of us, may also need to be scaled back and replaced with our gelatin-based dairy-substitute recipes. Or try our Jigglegurt recipe (found in the *Trim Healthy Mama Cookbook*), which volumizes Greek yogurt while decreasing its calories and carbs. This doesn't mean you have to forgo dairy completely, but instead of including it at every meal, try it once a day and see what happens.

These tweaks have worked for several that we have shared them with who had incredibly stubborn weight during their nursing months. We are not scientists or doctors so these are only suggestions, but we are passionate about finding solutions to nutritional problems without going to extremes. Melody is a Mama who gained fifty-five pounds with each of her pregnancies prior to discovering Trim Healthy Mama and always had great trouble taking any of that weight off during her seasons of nursing without severe calorie counting. She discovered Trim Healthy Mama and was able to get down to goal weight slowly but happily, but then got pregnant again. She had a healthy, nourishing thirty-five-pound pregnancy gain, eating the Trim Healthy Mama way all the way through her pregnancy, but then once again had trouble shedding that weight in the first year after her baby's birth. She was stuck!

We suggested she try some of these tweaks—replace her whey protein with collagen, decrease dairy and muscle meats a little, and increase glycine-rich proteins instead with cups of tea with collagen at the end of meals that were lower in meat or dairy protein. Now, just a few months later, Melody is just a few pounds away from goal weight again. She's loving her tweaked way of doing Trim Healthy Mama, is still making lots of rich milk for her still-nursing one-year-old, but is steadily losing—and is even incorporating three or four Crossovers per week!

Some people have high prolactin levels for unknown reasons even when not nursing or when pituitary growths are ruled out. The tweaks we suggest here for nursing women could be tried in these situations, even for men. Aside from glycine, the amino acid tyrosine and vitamin B_6 are both thought to help balance out high prolactin levels.

Thyroid

Interestingly, low thyroid hormones and elevated prolactin levels are often tied to one another, so addressing both of these is a smart approach. While thyroid issues can make weight loss more challenging, we have received thousands of messages from women who have found success on the THM Plan even with severe thyroid issues—so don't lose hope.

We talk a lot about not forsaking E meals; but if you have a thyroid issue, including them is especially important. Low-carb diets are notorious for suppressing levels of T3, which is the thyroid hormone your body uses for all functions. Of late there has been a backlash against low-carb diets from people with tanked thyroid levels. Some experts even encourage sufferers to indulge in refined carbs.

While thyroid hormones may indeed respond to carbs, this approach to overdoing carbs only brings destruction to the thyroid itself and in other areas of the body. Weight gain inevitably happens, which drives up insulin resistance, which drives up inflammation, which drives up a host of other diseases. Extremes are never the answer. Enjoy your healthy E meals with their safe blood-sugar zone and be vigilant about not jumping from one extreme diet to the other.

Testing for thyroid antibodies is important if you have a thyroid issue. The presence of antibodies can indicate an autoimmune condition called Hashimoto's disease. Many with this condition cannot tolerate gluten and often, but not always, dairy. Sadly, these foods become inflammatory to the body with this condition and the inflammation can prevent weight loss. Even if you don't have a known allergen to gluten or dairy, if you test positive for thyroid antibodies, you should read Chapter 26, "Heads Up: Allergen-Free Mamas!" (page 240), to gain some knowledge about how to do the plan while limiting or completely abstaining from those foods. We have come up with lots of recipes in our companion cookbook to make this doable.

Insulin

High insulin levels can be an indication of PCOS, which can be another cause for stubborn weight since it goes hand in hand with severe insulin resistance. Coming off sugar and adopting the basic principles of Trim Healthy Mama will go a long way in combating this issue, but your weight loss still may be slower than that of others.

Your blood sugar may be more sensitive to carbs at first. Use pulled-back E meals as described in Chapter 10, "Just the Numbers" (page 85), if you are having trouble keeping your numbers steady; or let Gluccie help you out with its magical ability to level blood sugar.

Chromium and inositol are considered to be excellent supplements for PCOS since they are known to help regulate high blood sugar and insulin levels. If your doctor has prescribed Metformin for your PCOS, ask him or her about taking a B_{12} supplement. Although Metformin is a prescribed drug, it is considered to be a helpful medication that has anticancer properties. It does, however, lower B_{12} levels over time.

TRY THESE TIPS FOR TURTLE WEIGHT

- Eat more okra. Read about its help for stubborn weight loss in Chapter 17, "Affordable Superfoods" (page 129). For some people, lectins in many foods cause the body to cling to fat rather than release it. Okra has a positive influence in this situation. Our companion cookbook is chock-full of recipes that contain okra that you would never be able to detect!
- Watch your Frankenfoods: Don't overdo low-carb wraps, pitas, and other packaged low-carb store-bought items. They are not perfect THM foods, just items that can make the plan more doable for some of us. If you are replacing vegetables, fruits,

and proteins with them, your weight may not appreciate it. If you have thyroid antibodies, then nix them altogether. If you can't manage a complete nix, pull back to a couple times per week.

- Change up your S meals as described in Chapter 11, "Higher Learning" (page 90), and don't overdo the Heavy-S type. Too much cheese and too many nuts may not be friendly to your weight. Focus more on pure oils, meats, and eggs as your S sources but don't completely deprive yourself of a Heavy-S meal now and then.
- Go easy on dairy if you have Hashimoto's disease or elevated prolactin.
- Put more emphasis on Fuel Pull desserts after meals rather than on Heavy-S desserts.
- Avoid grazing and gobbling (as described in Chapter 9, "Snacking Mama," on page 79). You need wise intervals between snacks and mealtimes.
- Don't undereat. One egg alone is not enough fuel for your entire morning. Don't take your calories down so far that your body thinks it is starving and holds on for dear life! Undereating is as bad for stubborn weight as overeating is.
- Don't overexcerise!
- Try an edgier fuel juggle—this means including some Fuel Pulls as full meals here and there (if you are not pregnant or nursing) but also even a Crossover or two. Some people find that if they have been doing primarily S meals, E meals, and Fuel Pulls for months and are stalled, adding a couple of Crossovers can help soothe the adrenal glands and help weight loss begin again. After a Crossover or two, you'll have had plenty of carbs; so it is best to switch to a Deep S versus Heavy S as described in Chapter 11, "Higher Learning," on page 90. Then back to some E meals. This really keeps your body guessing.

THE ONE-WEEK FUEL CYCLE

We're about to give you a tool as extra help for very stubborn weight issues. If you've been doing the plan for at least a couple of months, are not exclusively nursing, and are truly a turtle, feel free to give this a whirl. Did you catch that? Only try this after a couple months on the plan. Please don't *start* your Trim Healthy Mama journey with a Fuel Cycle!

No bones about it, this cycle is strict! We can't promise you'll feel love and joy or abounding Food Freedom during this cycle. It might be the first time you have to summon up some willpower on the plan. This is why we designed this cycle not as your mainstay but as an occasional kick-in-the-pants to turtle weight.

We are also fully aware that some of you are drawn to rules and rigidity and might cling to this cycle because it provides you with more boundaries and that little bit of misery you actually might miss with the freedom of freestyling. If this is you, you're not allowed to overdo or abuse this cycle. By that we mean doing it more than you are freestyling . . . uh-uh. That's undermining the way we want you to roll as a Trim Healthy Mama. The Fuel Cycle is too rulesy, too stricty, and too set-in-its-waysy to be your foundation.

Where it shines is not only in its ability to help you rev your metabolism but as a powerful learning tool. It helps you understand with more clarity each fuel type, since you have to spend more quality time with each one. It forces you to get creative with E, FP, and Deep-S meals where you might have been playing only with Heavy-S meals and desserts you find on Pinterest. Perhaps you've been eating only apples or oatmeal for E. If so, you're missing out on a world of other energizing foods. The Fuel Cycle makes you branch out. You can't survive happily on only apples and oatmeal for an extended period. If you don't know how to build an S meal without cheese, nuts, or sour cream, then you're going to find out!

Digging down to the core of each fuel deepens your relationship with its true character. The ultimate weight-loss power of each fuel can be experienced only through getting to know it more intimately. Acquaintanceship only takes you so far. Real friendship will take you much farther. When you've finished your Fuel Cycle, you can take away the treasures of knowledge you gained and apply them to your everyday freestyling. Your freestyling will have more power!

Prepare to Start

This will be a seven-day focused fuel juggle. You'll start with two days of Deep S. Two full E days will follow. Fuel Pull is next, two full days of that. Another Deep-S day will end your week for a full cycle. If you want to repeat for a two-week double whammy, then your last Deep-S day will end with an E dinner and then you'll have an E breakfast the next morning before continuing on with Deep S for the remainder of the next two days. Do not Fuel Cycle for more than two weeks at a time. Take off the straitjacket and go back to freestyling for a while, using your newfound tools for success.

The day before your Fuel Cycle, do not hang out in S mode. You need to nourish your thyroid and adrenals with Energizing foods before you strip them away. So have a couple of good E meals or just one E meal and a couple of E snacks, or even enjoy a Crossover (not a cheat, for goodness' sake!).

While not mandatory, it is more practical to start the Fuel Cycle week on a Sunday. This makes sure none of your Fuel Pull days hit a Saturday, which would feel miserable. Your Saturday will be fat-friendly so you can even go out to eat and have a Deep-S meal, which is much easier to achieve than with the other fuels.

Stock up on the foods you'll need throughout this week. You don't want to suddenly find you're out of leafy greens or coconut oil on Day 1 or 2 when these are a big part of the plan. So take a look at each segment of the Fuel Cycle and make sure you have the right foods for victory. A major help to you this week will be foods rich in gelatin and/or collagen supplements, since the high amounts of glycine they contain aggressively helps to push fat from your fat cells via stimulation of glucagon. The glycine they contain also helps give your energy levels a boost by hitching a ride into your body's fuel-burning furnaces called your mitochondria. Your body will release the fat and you'll be able to burn it for energy. A gelatin-rich diet paired with management of blood sugar is one of the most powerful fat-loss protocols. In the Fuel Cycle week we are pairing not only those two but also engaging in a more intense fuel juggle for a triple whammy.

You'll notice in our Fuel Cycle Idea Menu on page 225 that many of the recipes focus on these supplements. If you don't have the funds for gelatin/collagen, make sure to prepare gelatin-rich stock for your week. We have two easy recipes for that in our companion cookbook, but there are plenty of videos on YouTube showing you how to make stock from bones. You can use the stock as a base for your soups, or even just as a soothing afternoon daily broth or meal finisher. You'll also notice we're trying to slip some okra into your week. Sometimes stubborn weight can be tied to what some people call a "leaky gut" and both gelatin and okra combined can help to heal the mucosa lining of your intestines.

You have the choice to do the Fuel Cycle in one of two ways: You can go dairy-free only on your Deep-S days, or rev it up and go both gluten-free and dairy-free all week. If you do a full week including dairy and gluten and the scale does not budge, then maybe that is the litmus test to show that these may be stalling your weight loss. Try the Fuel Cycle again, excluding them fully, and see what happens. Let's be clear here before anyone thinks that gluten and dairy are second-class citizens and that the ultimate diet excludes them. Au contraire: The majority of us do just fine; in fact, we thrive on a diet that contains healthy sources of them. But for some, they can cause an inflammatory response that slows weight loss or stops it altogether.

Days 1 and 2 (Deep S)

Make sure to read Chapter 11, "Higher Learning" (page 90), for an explanation of a Deep-S meal, which is a little different from a regular S. You'll be cutting out dairy, nuts and seeds, store-bought low-carb breads (Frankenfoods), and any non-superfood fats like Ranch dressing or mayo. Sorry, we're even taking out our beloved Baking Blend because of the little bit of almond meal it contains. Avocados are out just for this week. The only dairy allowed is one tablespoon of Parmesan or pecorino-romano cheese used as a garnish (omit if you have a dairy allergy). You can use one tablespoon of cream in your coffee but for a greater boost to weight loss try the Trimmaccino recipe, which you can find in our companion cookbook.

The only exceptions to this no-nut rule will be unsweetened almond, flax, or cashew milk, since they are so watered down (avoid canned coconut milk during Deep S because it has a higher carb content). Up to one tablespoon of pressed peanut flour can go in a smoothie or another recipe. But we do want to encourage you to focus on the true Deep-S foods, which are your pure superfood oils, the healthiest butter, meat, and eggs, and (preferably organic) greens, greens, greens! This doesn't mean you can't do a Fuel Cycle if you are a Drive Thru Sue and never buy organic anything. Just do your best.

Leafy greens are the lowest in carbs of all non-starchy veggies so we really want you to concentrate on packing them in on your Deep-S days. Other non-starchy veggies can also be used on Deep-S days except for peas, tomatoes, onions, and most winter squash.

Enjoy our All-Day Sippers if desired with your meals.

Days 3 and 4 (E)

This will be the same as regular E freestyling meals except we want you to change it up and try some new E fuel sources. If you've been eating only apples and oatmeal for E meals, try other fresh fruits (not just berries). Include soaked beans and lentils, sweet potatoes, or other root veggies such as cooked carrots and parsnips. Perhaps you should try your

E meals gluten-free if you have a thyroid issue. Try quinoa, which does not contain gluten and boasts a bunch of health benefits.

Days 5 and 6 (FP)

Don't forget, we want to force you out of the comfy feathered nest by pulling away the Frankenfoods this week. No store-bought low-carb wraps or pitas. You may have been overdoing these, so try the recipe for Wonder Wraps in our companion cookbook instead. Told you we'd be forcing you to branch out. Okay, that was our suggestion; we know we really just freaked some of you out if these "Personal Choice" Items are your mainstay. We'll relent just a little bit and say "dramatically reduce them!" If you have to have a Frankenfood on a Fuel Pull day just to get by, you have not failed. Keep going to the end.

Day 7 (Deep S again)

You'll do Deep S again all day unless you wish to repeat the Fuel Cycle, in which case you'll end the day with a thyroid-boosting E meal and awaken to an E breakfast the following morning, then continue on with Deep S.

The following menu excludes all gluten and dairy with the exception of whey protein. We do not mean for the following gluten- and dairy-free menu to be considered the ultimate way to do the Fuel Cycle. It is just the hardest way to do it, so we wanted to help out those who have fewer options and truly have to be gluten- and dairy-free.

FUEL CYCLE IDEA MENU

Day 1—DEEP S

BREAKFAST

Fried eggs in butter or coconut oil / Trimmaccino Rich ("Hot Drinks" chapter in the *Trim Healthy Mama Cookbook*)

LUNCH

Deep S Salad in a Jar, made fresh for your plate if you prefer ("Quick Single Salads" chapter in the *Trim Healthy Mama Cookbook*)

DINNER

Crispy Salmon Siesta ("Quick Single Skillet Meals" chapter in the *Trim Healthy Mama Cookbook*) / side salad with superfood oils

Day 2—DEEP S

BREAKFAST

Fields of Green Omcake ("Good Morning Eggs" chapter of the *Trim Healthy Mama Cookbook*) / Trimmaccino Rich ("Hot Drinks" chapter in the *Trim Healthy Mama Cookbook*)

LUNCH

Soothe Your Soul Soup made with cabbage ("Quick Single Soups" chapter in the *Trim Healthy Mama Cookbook*); add Superfood Chocolate Chews if still hungry ("Candies and Bars" chapter in the *Trim Healthy Mama Cookbook*)

DINNER

Baked chicken with skin / dairy-free version of Collagen Creamed Spinach ("Sides" chapter in the *Trim Healthy Mama Cookbook*) / side salad with superfood oils

Day 3—E

BREAKFAST

Creamy Grains ("Good Morning Grains" chapter in the *Trim Healthy Mama Cookbook*)

LUNCH

Sweet potato with 1 teaspoon butter or superfood oil / can or pouch of tuna / salad or cucumbers spritzed with vinegar

DINNER

Golden Chana Soup or Lentil Soup ("Family Soups" chapter in the *Trim Healthy Mama Cookbook*)

Day 4—E

BREAKFAST

Sweet Dreams Apple Cinnamon Oatmeal Bowl ("Good Morning Grains" chapter in the *Trim Healthy Mama Cookbook*)

LUNCH

E Salad in a Jar (nix cottage cheese if doing cycle dairy-free); you can make the salad fresh for your plate if you want ("Quick Single Salads" chapter in the *Trim Healthy Mama Cookbook*) / Grapefruit Slushy ("Frozen Treats" chapter in the *Trim Healthy Mama Cookbook*)

DINNER

Blackened Chicken with Mango and Black Beans ("Family Skillet Meals" chapter in the *Trim Healthy Mama Cookbook*)

Day 5—FP

BREAKFAST

Large egg-white scramble with lots of sautéed non-starchy veggies / a Healing Trimmy Light ("Hot Drinks" chapter in the *Trim Healthy Mama Cookbook*)

LUNCH

Wonder Wraps ("Breads and Pizza Crusts" chapter of the *Trim Healthy Mama Cookbook*) stuffed with diced cucumber, tuna with a light vinaigrette / Beauty Milk ("More Drinks" chapter in the *Trim Healthy Mama Cookbook*)

DINNER

Popeye's Power Soup ("Family Soups" chapter in the *Trim Healthy Mama Cookbook*) / Glycine Glory Pudding ("Sweet Bowls" chapter in the *Trim Healthy Mama Cookbook*)

Day 6—FP

BREAKFAST

Choco Secret Big Boy ("Shakes, Smoothies Frappas, and Thin Thicks" chapter in the *Trim Healthy Mama Cookbook*)

LUNCH

Large Fuel Pull salad loaded with fresh greens and moistened with lots of luscious diced tomatoes and cucumbers plus balsamic vinegar, spritzed with MCT or olive oil and tossed with 3 to 4 ounces of seasoned chicken breast / Lemon Pucker Gummies ("Candies and Bars" chapter in the *Trim Healthy Mama Cookbook*)

DINNER

Fussless Fuel Pull Quiche (use dairy-free version if desired; "Oven Dishes" chapter in the *Trim Healthy Mama Cookbook*) / Troodles ("Sides" chapter in the *Trim Healthy Mama Cookbook*) / Tummy Spa Ice Cream ("Frozen Treats" chapter in the *Trim Healthy Mama Cookbook*)

Day 7—DEEP S

BREAKFAST

Turkey or venison sausage (or bacon) with sautéed mushrooms or spinach with generous amounts of superfood oil or butter / a Healing Trimmy ("Hot Drinks" chapter in the *Trim Healthy Mama Cookbook*)

LUNCH

Deep S Salad in a Jar made fresh for your plate if you prefer ("Quick Single Salads" chapter in the *Trim Healthy Mama Cookbook*) / Beauty Milk ("More Drinks" chapter in the *Trim Healthy Mama Cookbook*)

DINNER

Cilantro Lime-Burst Chicken Thighs ("Crockpot Meals" chapter in the *Trim Healthy Mama Cookbook*) / Deep S side salad / Hot Chocolate Trimmy ("Hot Drinks" chapter in the *Trim Healthy Mama Cookbook*)

Note: If you are continuing your Fuel Cycle for another week, have an E meal for dinner: Wicked White Chili minus the yogurt ("Crockpot Meals" chapter in the *Trim Healthy Mama Cookbook*). You will also want to have an E breakfast the following morning and then continue with the normal order of things for the remainder of the Fuel Cycle.

Snack Ideas with Deep-S Fuels

Leftover chicken reheated by sautéing with butter or superfood oils and spices / Skinny Chocolate, Skinny Truffles, Gummies, or Superfood Chocolate Chews ("Candies and Bars" chapter in the *Trim Healthy Mama Cookbook*) / any of the Trimmaccino Rich drinks ("Hot Drinks" chapter in the *Trim Healthy Mama Cookbook*) / Kale Chips ("Crackers, Chips, and Dips" chapter in the *Trim Healthy Mama Cookbook*)

Snack Ideas with E Fuels

Fruit with Beauty Milk for added protein ("More Drinks" chapter in the *Trim Healthy Mama Cookbook*) / leftover small or ½ sweet potato / leftover Creamy Grains ("Good Morning Grains" chapter in the *Trim Healthy Mama Cookbook*)

Fuel Pull Snack Ideas (also suitable for E and Deep-S days, except nix berries for Deep S)

Lean meat jerky with no sugar / berries (but not for Deep-S days) / any Secret Big Boy, Frappa, or Thin Thick ("Shakes, Smoothies, Frappas, and Thin Thicks" chapter in the *Trim Healthy Mama Cookbook*) / FP versions of NoGurt, Collagen Berry Whip, Gluccie Puddings, or Glycine Glory Puddings ("Sweet Bowls" chapter in the *Trim Healthy Mama Cookbook*) / Tummy Spa Ice Cream, Tummy Tucking Ice Cream, or Lemon Cream Ice Pops ("Frozen Treats" chapter in the *Trim Healthy Mama Cookbook*) / Purist Primer ("Quick Single Soups" in the *Trim Healthy Mama Cookbook*) / Banana Meringue ("Brownies and Cookies" chapter in the *Trim Healthy Mama Cookbook*) / Crunch Puffs ("Crackers, Chips, and Dips" chapter in the *Trim Healthy Mama Cookbook*; the tiny amount of Baking Blend is not enough to cause issues)

chapter 25

HEADS UP: VEGETARIANS!
(OR VEGETARIANS IN TRANSITION)

I f you relate to Raw Green Colleen or even Whole Grain Jane, whom you met back in Chapter 1, perhaps you've shunned meat completely or just tried to cut back thinking that was a healthy approach. Yet here we are telling you to go ahead and eat burgers and chicken wings. Huh?! Your head is spinning at the liberal way in which we include animal foods in THM meals. We both spent more than a decade as vegans, so we understand the mind adjustment needed when making the decision to return to an omnivore diet. Yes, it is possible to do the plan as a vegetarian (including eggs and dairy), but if you decide to take the plunge back into eating some meat, we have some tips. It is common for vegetarian meals to be centered predominantly on grain and fruit. For this reason, despite the fact that many eat a plant-based diet to help control weight, it often bites back. Many Mamas have made the switch back to animal foods with us and haven't regretted it for a minute. Watch how your body shrinks in sizes even if your scale doesn't move much. This is the power of animal protein! Hang in there, vegetarians. We have tips for you, too!

START BACK SLOWLY

If you want to start including some meat again, you don't have to jump into the plan with a T-bone steak! Adding animal-based protein back into your diet more gradually in the form of wild-caught salmon, whitefish, omega-3 eggs, and raw homemade kefir can be a more gentle approach. You can start including red meat slowly by adding chopped mushrooms as half of your ground beef or venison. Mushrooms are potent cancer fighters and immune boosters and they just might make the transition to red meat psychologically easier.

If you can't (or simply don't want to) eat enough meat or dairy in a meal to get enough protein, there are other ways around this. Gelatin and collagen are animal-based proteins that offer you incredible health and slimming benefits without you having to chew on hunks of meat. You can even put these supplements in fruit smoothies and your taste buds will never know this supportive protein is going to work its regenerating power on your body. What does this look like in a practical sense? You can load up on non-starchy veggies, add your carb or your fat for S or E, perhaps try to get in a little animal protein, even if it is only one or two ounces, then finish your meal with a hot or cold drink that includes a loaded scoop or two of gelatin or collagen.

Another way to get protein in your meals is with whey protein. Use a full scoop of our Pristine Whey Protein Powder in your breakfast smoothie or, if the food contains another protein source, such as cottage cheese, use half a scoop. Don't rely on these supplements for the bulk of your protein needs, as we want you to vary your protein sources with whole foods; but they can be great helpers.

You sure don't have to eat meat at every meal. Consider other wonderful protein sources like Greek yogurt or cottage cheese. Bean and lentil soups are not as high in protein as other animal-based options are, but if they are eaten for just a few meals each week, your overall protein level should still be ample enough. Keeping those in your diet can help you not feel too extreme about your return to animal foods. The wise choice of throwing a few scoops of gelatin into a large pot of bean-based soup will easily amp up the protein content and aid your health at the same time.

GREENS GALORE

Be careful not to switch over into an extreme. If you previously included lots of greens in your vegetarian diet, don't suddenly pull them out and focus entirely on meat and dairy. Not only is that an imbalanced approach, your digestive system will get very grumpy. Forgetting your greens and focusing only on dense animal foods is not the Trim Healthy way. You can still enjoy large salads every day; in fact please do! Simply top them with a few ounces of fish, chicken, or eggs and an on-plan dressing. And remember, if you don't always want to put meat on them, finish your meal with Beauty Milk, Collagen Tea, or a Healing Trimmy—all of which contain gelatin, which fills you with the important amino acids your body needs (and the recipes can be found in our companion cookbook). Eating lots of greens will help your body make the adjustment back to animal-based foods an easier and healthier one.

It is possible that no matter how many greens you include or how much water you drink, you still might have a few days of bathroom issues when changing up your diet to include more animal protein. Putting this more bluntly, you may suffer from some constipation—"Help . . . I can't go!" Ugh, nothing feels as bad as that! Your body is used to eating one way and now it must learn to adjust to another.

Consider taking a magnesium supplement at night before bed to help with this. This mineral calms the body and soothes the nerves, but here's the really great thing: It makes certain you "go." You know what we mean, right? We Mamas need to "go" to be happy!

This magnesium-before-bed habit is not just for those transitioning from a vegetarian diet. It can help all sorts of Mamas on plan with this issue. Magnesium is inexpensive. In citrate form it is a little pricier but in oxide form it is dirt cheap. Usually three to five tablets will do the trick—each magnesium oxide or citrate tablet is about 250 mg. Any more than that may cause diarrhea.

JUICING REPLACEMENT

If you were in the habit of daily juicing, try Earth Milk Sip (check out a free video of us making it on our website) or check the All-Day Sippers in the *Trim Healthy Mama Cookbook*. This drink will cleanse, alkalize, and detoxify your body while keeping your blood sugar in check. If you are determined to continue to juice, replace the carrot and apple concoctions with mild green juices from bases of celery, cucumber, and lettuce with a dash of stevia for sweetness. Apple and carrot juices are notorious for spiking blood sugar, which can undo any health benefits the juice might offer. You can add stronger greens such as kale and parsley to top them off.

ADD SOOTHING COOKED VEGGIES

If you were like Raw Green Colleen from Chapter 1, and constantly consumed raw veggies thinking they were the hierarchy of all foods, open your mind to cooking some of them and adding fats such as butter. In this form, broccoli, cauliflower, and cabbage can soothe and help heal an inflamed digestive tract and cause less bloating than when they are consumed raw. Nutritional profiles of many veggies are actually enhanced by gentle cooking. The tough cellulose wall of greens like kale and cabbage needs to be broken down to release their nutrients and not be quite as harsh on the intestines. No one wants to be a gassy Mama—been there. Certain vegetables have nutritional profiles that are only enhanced by cooking. The powerful cancer fighter lycopene is released in far greater amounts when tomatoes are cooked. Health-boosting carotenoids in broccoli are found in higher concentrations when this veggie is cooked versus raw.

ADAMANT VEGETARIANS

"Serene and Pearl, I'm just not going to do it! I have my reasons for my vegetarianism and you can't talk me out of them!" Okay, so meat is completely out for you. You'll need to rely more on eggs and dairy, and hopefully some fish? If not fish, you can still do the plan by including eggs and dairy and a few helpers like gelatin, collagen, and whey protein. We don't encourage a lot of soy, but fermented soy such as tempeh and miso can be healthful additions to your diet along with sprouted tofu.

Soy becomes a problem when it is too frequently a part of the diet. Soy milk, soy cheese, soy crumbles, soy sausage, soy yogurt ... be very careful about how much soy you are consuming, especially if you have hormonal imbalances. We'd also prefer you stay away from soy protein powders. Sprouted tofu, however, has a much more easily absorbed nutritional profile than regular tofu. It is higher in protein than regular tofu, too, which is a boon for vegetarians needing to get in more protein. The sprouting process makes it easily digested by the body and it offers more vitamins and minerals than regular tofu.

When we stopped being vegans after years of eating tofu for so many of our meals and began to eat meat, we didn't touch tofu for a long time since we had overdone it and felt we really needed that break. Now, about eight years later, we are enjoying some sprouted tofu again, but always in moderation. You can find some tasty and fun recipes for it in the *Trim Healthy Mama Cookbook;* the Chicken Fried Tofu is a big hit with our children.

VEGANISM

If you're a staunch vegan . . . we gotta be honest here, it will be challenging to make the plan work for you as written, but you can certainly take the basic premise and merge it with your own eating philosophy. The understanding that balanced blood sugar is foundational to health is crucial and can help prevent a vegan diet from becoming a blood-sugar monster. Vegan diets that overdo dried fruits, fruit juice, maple syrup, and starches are hazardous to one's health.

As a vegan, you can liven up your culinary world with many Trim Healthy Mama desserts. Gluccie can thicken delicious puddings made with almond milk and stevia, and you'll fall in love with the recipes for Tummy Tucking Ice Cream and Tummy Spa Ice Cream in our companion cookbook. Gluccie can also thicken up vegan soups and go a long way to balance higher blood-sugar levels that sometimes come with a vegan diet.

VEGETARIAN IDEA MENU

The sample menu below uses no meat. If you enjoy fish, you're going to have a lot more choices; but we wanted to do this menu the hardest way to help give ideas to our ardent vegetarians.

Day 1

BREAKFAST—S

Shake Gone Nuts including 1 tablespoon peanut butter ("Shakes, Smoothies, Frappas, and Thin Thicks" chapter in the *Trim Healthy Mama Cookbook*)

LUNCH—E

Waldorf Cottage Cheese Salad ("Quick Single Salads" chapter in the *Trim Healthy Mama Cookbook*)

DINNER—S

Spinach and Sausage Quiche, but nix the sausage ("Oven Dishes" chapter in the *Trim Healthy Mama Cookbook*) / large side salad

Day 2

BREAKFAST—E

Sweet Dreams Peachy Cream Oatmeal ("Good Morning Grains" chapter in the *Trim Healthy Mama Cookbook*)

LUNCH—S

Superfood-Loaded Salad with boiled eggs ("Quick Single Salads" chapter in the *Trim Healthy Mama Cookbook*)

DINNER—S

Creamy Pearlchiladas Bake using sprouted tofu in place of chicken ("Oven Dishes" chapter in the *Trim Healthy Mama Cookbook*) / side salad

Day 3

BREAKFAST—E

Trim Healthy Pancakes ("Pancakes, Donuts, Crepes, and Waffles" chapter in the *Trim Healthy Mama Cookbook*) / 0% Greek yogurt and berries

LUNCH—S

Cheesy Dream Soup ("Quick Single Soups" chapter in the *Trim Healthy Mama Cookbook*) / Swiss Bread with butter ("Breads and Pizza Crusts" chapter in the *Trim Healthy Mama Cookbook*)

DINNER—E

Meatless version of Sweet Potato Bar using Greek yogurt, cottage cheese, or tempeh for protein ("Oven Baked or Roasted Meats" chapter in the *Trim Healthy Mama Cookbook*)

Day 4

BREAKFAST—S

Mufflets, meatless version ("Good Morning Eggs" chapter in the *Trim Healthy Mama Cookbook*) / coffee and cream

LUNCH—E

E Salad in a Jar made fresh on your plate if you prefer ("Quick Single Salads" chapter in the *Trim Healthy Mama Cookbook*) / Beauty Milk or Easy Chocolate Milk ("More Drinks" chapter in the *Trim Healthy Mama Cookbook*)

DINNER—S

Tomato Chicken Bisque, using sprouted tofu or tempeh in place of chicken ("Family Soups" chapter in the *Trim Healthy Mama Cookbook*) / Swiss Bread with butter ("Breads and Pizza Crusts" chapter in the *Trim Healthy Mama Cookbook*) / small side salad

Day 5

BREAKFAST—FP

Fat-Stripping Frappa ("Shakes, Smoothies, Frappas, and Thin Thicks" chapter in the *Trim Healthy Mama Cookbook*)

LUNCH—S

Grilled cheese on Swiss Bread ("Breads and Pizza Crusts" chapter in the *Trim Healthy Mama Cookbook*) / Berrylicious Thin Thick ("Shakes, Smoothies, Frappas, and Thin Thicks" chapter in the *Trim Healthy Mama Cookbook*)

DINNER—E

Lentil Soup ("Family Soups" chapter in the *Trim Healthy Mama Cookbook*) / optional slice of sprouted or sourdough toast with a light smear of butter / side salad with lean dressing

Day 6

BREAKFAST—E

Sweet Dreams PB and J Oatmeal ("Good Morning Grains" chapter in the *Trim Healthy Mama Cookbook*)

LUNCH—S

Spiced Eggy Noodles ("Quick Single Skillet Meals" chapter in the *Trim Healthy Mama Cookbook*)

DINNER—S

Popeye's Power Soup, chicken-free version ("Family Soups" chapter in the *Trim Healthy Mama Cookbook*) with grated cheese and Swiss Bread ("Breads and Pizza Crusts" chapter in the *Trim Healthy Mama Cookbook*)

Day 7

BREAKFAST—E

Chocolate Monkey Crepes ("Pancakes, Donuts, Crepes, and Waffles" chapter in the *Trim Healthy Mama Cookbook*)

LUNCH—S

Loaded Crunkers or Swiss Crackers or Mad Melbas with avocado, tomato, and thinly sliced cheese ("Crackers, Chips, and Dips" chapter in the *Trim Healthy Mama Cookbook*) / any Thin Thick ("Shakes, Smoothies, Frappas, and Thin Thicks" chapter in the *Trim Healthy Mama Cookbook*)

DINNER—S

Loaded Spaghetti Squash Casserole, meatless option ("Oven Dishes" chapter in the *Trim Healthy Mama Cookbook*) / Light and Lovely Coleslaw ("Sides" chapter in the *Trim Healthy Mama Cookbook*) / Choco Chip Baby Frap containing ½ scoop of whey protein and 1 scoop of collagen to give enough protein for your meal ("Shakes, Smoothies, Frappas, and Thin Thicks" chapter in the *Trim Healthy Mama Cookbook*)

Snack Ideas for the Week

Celery and peanut butter / fruit and a part-skim mozzarella cheese stick or fruit with cottage cheese / a handful or two of nuts / lettuce wraps with mayo, cheese, and pickles with tea made with a scoop of collagen / hard-boiled eggs / any cracker or chip from the "Crackers, Chips, and Dips" chapter in the *Trim Healthy Mama Cookbook* /any sweet treat made from "Sweet Treats" in the *Trim Healthy Mama Cookbook* / any drink made from "Beverages" in the *Trim Healthy Mama Cookbook*

chapter 26
HEADS UP: ALLERGEN-FREE MAMAS!

The difference between Trim Healthy Mama and many other plans out there is that you can customize this one for your own challenges. You may have to leave out a food or two that others get to enjoy, but you'll still have plenty of "can haves." Even with multiple allergies you're still likely to be able to enjoy meat, fish, healthy fats such as oils and butter (or ghee or coconut oil), fruit, lush greens, certain grains such as quinoa, rice, and buckwheat—and not too many people are allergic to sweet potatoes. Focus happy thoughts on your own friendly-food list and learn to thrive in your unique Trim Healthy Mama pasture.

When you think about it, many people live on a very insular diet with just a handful of staples that they rotate. Chicken nuggets, fries, burgers, cereals, pasta, crackers, a lettuce leaf or two, an occasional slice of tomato, processed cheese, ketchup, sugar, and the occasional banana. That is pretty common for a standard American diet. Compare that to your healthy list. Who has it better, even if you do have to be gluten- or dairy-free?

Think of all the wonderful meal creations you can make living in a land of plenty. Our problems are all relative when you think of what some people in Third World countries in extreme poverty get to choose from. When you have options to eat other than just rice or beans, you are blessed! It is up to you whether you'll see your food restrictions as a wonderful challenge or as a burden that robs your daily joy. Your challenges can open up a whole new world of exciting foods and culinary adventures that those with iron stomachs will never be inspired to try.

SENSITIVITY VERSUS ALLERGY

Having a food sensitivity doesn't necessarily mean you'll have to remove the culprit food for life. Sometimes it is the processing of a food that causes inflammation and reaction. Some people find that when they replace the processed, refined, or pasteurized offenders with raw pastured dairy or cultured/fermented ancient versus hybridized grains, their body can tolerate them quite nicely.

In other instances it is just the overdoing of certain foods that causes problems for those of us with sensitive stomachs. High fiber and fermented foods can easily turn from helpful to hurtful if we don't tune in to our own unique and necessary stopping points. Even the healthiest foods like kefir, sauerkraut, broccoli, cabbage, flaxseeds, nuts, and Gluccie can cause us trouble if we eat too much of them or do not give ourselves natural rests from them. Just as exercise and sunshine can quickly turn from healthy to harmful, so too can certain ultra-healthy foods if we don't use caution. If your tummy is throwing a fit, ask yourself, "Am I overdoing something?" then simply give that food a time-out. When you go back to it, take it more gently and in smaller amounts.

It is super-trendy to go gluten-free these days but fewer than one person in one hundred has true celiac disease, which is an inherited autoimmune disorder. People with gluten sensitivity often suffer from annoying gastrointestinal (GI) symptoms or sometimes develop strange skin rashes, but this is very different from celiac disease, in which gluten actually destroys intestinal tissue and can even be a life-threatening ailment.

Obviously, most people who decide to go gluten-free are not true celiacs. We all need to ask ourselves if we truly do have gluten intolerance or if we are just joining the gluten-despising in crowd. Gluten is a protein, not a manmade toxic chemical. God put it in certain grains for a reason. Man messed with grains such as modern wheat to push gluten to unnatural levels so bread could have that soft, fluffy texture. Avoiding modern wheat varieties and eating grains that are still untampered with should not pose such GI stress. Of course, after years of gluten abuse some of us need to take a complete break from gluten grains to allow our bodies a time of healing before introducing healthier varieties.

True life-threatening food allergies are another story and cannot be experimented with. In these cases offending foods need to stay completely out of the picture. Those with Hashimoto's disease (an autoimmune thyroid condition) often need to be much more careful about including foods containing gluten and dairy no matter the source. The school of thought is that those with Hashimoto's also usually suffer from a leaky gut (this theory is debated by some but is the current school of thought). Gluten passes through the damaged intestinal walls and enters the bloodstream. This is when the trouble starts. The molecular structure of gliadin, which is the protein portion of gluten, closely resembles that of the thyroid gland. When the gluten protein infiltrates the bloodstream, the body goes on a high threat alert. It attacks not only this protein but thyroid cells as well.

It appears to be unknown whether the link between Hashimoto's disease and a leaky gut is always present. There may be cases in which a person suffers from Hashimoto's but has an intact intestinal lining and, in this scenario, gluten would not pose such a problem. However, we hear from many women with autoimmune thyroid issues who seem to do much better completely avoiding gluten and often dairy, too. See Chapter 17, "Affordable Superfoods" (page 129), for how okra may help with leaky gut.

GLUTEN-FREE FRIENDLY

Gluten-free is easy-peasy as a Trim Healthy Mama. No, you won't be eating the Franken—oops, Personal Choice—low-carb wraps and pitas that many other Trim Healthy Mamas enjoy; but look on the bright side, that can be a good thing because they can be too easily overdone. You will be eating most of our bread and muffin recipes, which are naturally gluten-free. Trim Healthy Mama Baking Blend is certified gluten-free, which means pizza crusts, breads, muffins, pancakes, and cookies won't be left off your plate. Grocery shelves are lined with new gluten-free products, but many of these do your waistline no favors due to their high-carb or -calorie content. Now you can avoid gluten and slim down at the same time.

LIFE BEYOND DAIRY

Some of us thrive on cultured dairy products such as Greek yogurt and cottage cheese. All that lean protein helps our bodies shed unnecessary weight, and the more we have of the stuff, the more we lose. That may not be true in every case. If you have Hashimoto's disease or other issues, dairy and you may not play well together. Sometimes dairy can cause inflammation, weight gain, gut problems, and even some strange skin issues. At first glance some of the recipes we talk about, such as Cheeseburger Pie, may have you doubting Trim Healthy Mama can work for you. It absolutely can. We have included many dairy-free recipes in our companion cookbook. Try our dairy-free Hello Cheese recipe to fill your life with cheesiness once again. Suffering without yogurt? Many call our NoGurt recipe even better than the real thing! Desserts won't be a problem, either. Skinny Chocolate is completely dairy-free. Ice Cream? You betcha. Try Tummy Spa Ice Cream, Tummy Tucking Ice Cream, or Polar Bear Soft Serve (if you can tolerate whey protein) found in the "Frozen Treats" chapter in the *Trim Healthy Mama Cookbook*.

NUTTY PROBLEMS

Perhaps you are allergic to certain nuts and wonder what on earth you'll eat on a plan like Trim Healthy Mama, which is nut-friendly. We mention almond milk frequently, but if you have an allergy to almonds, there are plenty of alternatives: Cashew, coconut, or flaxseed milk in unsweetened form will be wonderful replacements. Don't overlook the ease of our Foundation Milk recipe, which is a superhealthy option and very budget friendly (see the "More Drinks" chapter in the *Trim Healthy Mama Cookbook*).

Choose seeds like sunflower or pumpkin seeds over nuts for snacks if you have allergies. Our Baking Blend does have a small amount of almond flour in it so if you have an allergy to almonds, you can get great baking results using an equal mix of our THM oat fiber and flax meal. There are the rare few people who cannot tolerate coconut in any form, even coconut oil. Try cooking with red palm oil or butter. Light sautéing with extra-virgin olive oil or grapeseed oil should be okay sometimes, too.

SUNNY SIDE OF EGGLESS

Just like with grain and dairy, the source of your eggs may be triggering your sensitivity. Battery cage–raised hens that are fed high-gluten grains and an imbalanced fatty acid ratio can result in many needless egg intolerances. Eggs from pastured hens may make all the difference in your tolerance to them.

If your body is currently uneasy with eggs, take a break for a month or two before you switch to healthier egg sources. This will help allow your system to heal from the prior inflammation so your test on adding healthier eggs back into your diet will be more accurate.

Here is a helpful egg substitute for baking needs:

1 tablespoon ground flaxseeds or chia seeds
3 tablespoons water
1 teaspoon Apple Cider Vinegar (optional)
Mix, then let gel for a few minutes before adding to recipe (this mixture replaces one egg).

Final note: Along with adding okra to your diet to help heal sensitivities, also be mindful to supplement with gelatin or make your own bone stock, as this can soothe an inflamed, impaired gut as well. We created a drink that includes both of those healers specifically to help with gut problems and food sensitivities. Check out our Sensitive Big Boy smoothie in the "Shakes, Smoothies, Frappas, and Thin Thicks" chapter in the *Trim Healthy Mama Cookbook*.

ALLERGEN-FREE IDEA MENU

The following menu is completely free of gluten, dairy, soy, and eggs, given that those are the four most common food offenders. We have not taken out all nuts, but peanuts are not part of it since they are the most common nut allergy. Most dairy-intolerant people can still add Pristine Whey Protein Powder since it is naturally lactose-free, but some people do have an allergy to the dairy protein itself. For this reason we have not included it in this menu.

Day 1

BREAKFAST—E

Creamy Grains made with quinoa and blueberries ("Good Morning Grains" chapter in the *Trim Healthy Mama Cookbook*)

LUNCH—FP

Tuscan Tomato Soup ("Quick Single Soups" chapter) with Swiss Bread ("Breads and Pizza Crusts" chapter in the *Trim Healthy Mama Cookbook*) and 1 teaspoon ghee (this is tolerated better by most dairy-free folk than butter) or plan-approved oil

DINNER—S

Taco Salad ("Family Salads" chapter in the *Trim Healthy Mama Cookbook*) with grated Hello Cheese ("Condiments and Extras" chapter in the *Trim Healthy Mama Cookbook*)

Day 2

BREAKFAST—FP

Sensitive Big Boy ("Shakes, Smoothies, Frappas, and Thin Thicks" chapter in the *Trim Healthy Mama Cookbook*)

LUNCH—S

Loaded Crunkers (egg-white-free version) ("Crackers, Chips, and Dips" chapter in the *Trim Healthy Mama Cookbook*) with avocado, sliced Hello Cheese ("Condiments and Extras" chapter in the *Trim Healthy Mama Cookbook*), tomato, and natural deli meat / Beauty Milk ("More Drinks" chapter in the *Trim Healthy Mama Cookbook*)

DINNER—S

Tomato Chicken Bisque ("Family Soups" chapter in the *Trim Healthy Mama Cookbook*) / side salad

Day 3

BREAKFAST—S

Sautéed sausage, tomato, and onion scramble (add matchstick sliced radishes if desired) / a Healing Trimmy ("Hot Drinks" chapter in the *Trim Healthy Mama Cookbook*)

LUNCH—S

Superfood-Loaded Salad—S ("Quick Single Salads" chapter in the *Trim Healthy Mama Cookbook*)

DINNER—E

Sweet Potato Bar ("Oven-Baked or Roasted Meats" chapter in the *Trim Healthy Mama Cookbook*) but omit Greek yogurt and include grated Hello Cheese ("Condiments and Extras" chapter in the *Trim Healthy Mama Cookbook*)

Day 4

BREAKFAST—S

Breakfast-size Chia Pud ("Sweet Bowls" chapter in the *Trim Healthy Mama Cookbook*) / tea with an added scoop of collagen

LUNCH—FP OR S

Cheesy Dream Soup ("Quick Single Soups" chapter in the *Trim Healthy Mama Cookbook*) with Crunkers topped with optional ghee or virgin coconut oil to swing into S mode ("Crackers, Chips, and Dips" chapter in the *Trim Healthy Mama Cookbook*)

DINNER—E

Wipe Your Mouth BBQ ("Crockpot Meals" chapter in the *Trim Healthy Mama Cookbook*) with quinoa / Light and Lovely Coleslaw ("Sides" chapter in the *Trim Healthy Mama Cookbook*)

Day 5

BREAKFAST—E

Sweet Dreams Apple Cinnamon Oatmeal using a scoop of Integral Collagen in place of Pristine Whey Protein ("Good Morning Grains" chapter in the *Trim Healthy Mama Cookbook*)

LUNCH—FP

Creamless Creamy Chicken ("Quick Single Skillet Meals" chapter in the *Trim Healthy Mama Cookbook*) using Laughin' Mama Cheese ("Condiments and Extras" chapter in the *Trim Healthy Mama Cookbook*) / sliced cucumber sprinkled with high-mineral salt

DINNER—S

Cashew Chicken ("Family Skillet Meals" chapter in the *Trim Healthy Mama Cookbook*) / side salad

Day 6

BREAKFAST—S

Berries and NoGurt ("Sweet Bowls" chapter in the *Trim Healthy Mama Cookbook*)

LUNCH—S

Crispy Salmon Siesta ("Quick Single Skillet Meals" chapter in the *Trim Healthy Mama Cookbook*) / salad with avocado, tomato, and Tangy and Sweet Vinaigrette ("Condiments and Extras" chapter in the *Trim Healthy Mama Cookbook*)

DINNER—S

Enchilada Wonder Casserole, dairy-free version ("Oven Dishes" chapter in the *Trim Healthy Mama Cookbook*)

Day 7

BREAKFAST—E

Banana Bread Crockpot Oatmeal ("Good Morning Grains" chapter in the *Trim Healthy Mama Cookbook*)

LUNCH—S

Slim Sloppy Joes in crisp romaine hearts ("Family Skillet Meals" chapter in the *Trim Healthy Mama Cookbook*)

DINNER—S

Lemon Herb Drummies—S ("Crockpot Meals" chapter in the *Trim Healthy Mama Cookbook*)

Snack Ideas for the Week

Cut fruit with Collagen Tea or any light Trimmy for protein ("Hot Drinks" chapter in the *Trim Healthy Mama Cookbook*) or NoCream Cheese Berry Spread ("Condiments and Extras" chapter in the *Trim Healthy Mama Cookbook*) / hummus and crudités / crispy nuts (peanut-free) with small cubes of Hello Cheese ("Condiments and Extras" chapter in the *Trim Healthy Mama Cookbook*) / Crunkers or Crispy Addictions or Kale Chips ("Crackers, Chips, and Dips" chapter in the *Trim Healthy Mama Cookbook*) / Skinny Chocolate, Skinny Chocolate Truffles, or Gummies ("Candies and Bars" chapter in the *Trim Healthy Mama Cookbook*) / Green Fries ("Sides" chapter in the *Trim Healthy Mama Cookbook*) / berries and NoGurt ("Sweet Bowls" chapter in the *Trim Healthy Mama Cookbook*) / Beauty Milk ("More Drinks" chapter) / Avo Cream or Chia Pud ("Sweet Bowls" chapter in the *Trim Healthy Mama Cookbook*) / Sensitive Big Boy ("Shakes, Smoothies, Frappas, and Thin Thicks" chapter in the *Trim Healthy Mama Cookbook*) / Tummy Spa Ice Cream or any dairy-free option from the "Frozen Treats" chapter in the *Trim Healthy Mama Cookbook*

chapter 27

HEADS UP: MAINTENANCE MAMAS!

Y ou are not allowed to reach goal weight without a huge shout-out and happy dance from us. High-five, Mama!!! You plodded faithfully along and here you are the victor over excess pounds and a droopy, tired old self. You made it to the finish line and we are cheering, throwing confetti, and shaking pom-poms for you in the stands.

But what now? Do you really want this to be your finish line? For sure you need to stop with the losing weight part, but why go back to your old ways when they led you to that hopeless place where you began? It's fun to be an energetic Trim Healthy Mama who radiates a healthy glow and does not have to sacrifice tasty treats or hearty meals or suffer through crazy hours in the gym. Don't stop now! You can't be or feel healthy without controlling blood sugar, and the Crossover meal will now be your tool to help achieve this while curbing weight loss.

LET THE MAINTENANCE JOURNEY BEGIN!

The most rewarding and longest part of your Trim Healthy Mama adventure is about to begin. Join us here in awesome maintenance land. We've been enjoying ourselves here for many years now, reveling no longer over the shedding of pounds but over the enjoyment of energy and graceful ease we feel while aging with vitality and wits sustained.

Accept your beautiful, unique body type and don't keep adding unhealthy additional weight-loss goals by never being satisfied with your personal healthy weight. Not everyone should try to be a size six or even a size eight. One Mama might be healthy at a size two and another showing way too many bones and completely miserable at size eight.

Many Mamas might be just perfect at a size twelve. We all have different skeletal frames and muscle distributions. Don't be overly judgmental of your body type by continuing to make weight loss your goal when in fact you have already arrived.

If you don't know when to stop losing weight, ask a trusted friend to tell you when you are looking too skinny. By trusted we mean make sure this friend has your best interests in mind and is not telling you to stop just because she wants to feel better about any weight issues she may have herself. How does your husband feel about you always wanting to lose another five pounds? He may be much happier keeping a little more of you around. Choose a healthy versus skinny weight for yourself. We cannot tell you what that is or have you do math equations or charts to work it out. It will be vastly different for each person with too many variables to fit into a "you-should-weigh-this" box.

The weight-loss part of your journey was just the doorknob you opened into sustained and enjoyable health. Even though we hope you enjoyed every day that you were heading in the right direction toward "goal weight," you are now finally at the prime weight and size for your body to feel unencumbered and ready to fly. Your health has been improving along the way, but now your body no longer has to be burdened with the stress and inflammation from excess weight. This new maintenance season is your time to soar into health and reap the benefits of your commitment.

THE ART OF MAINTENANCE

Every maintenance journey will look different. You will learn to make little tweaks as you listen to your body and study how you personally respond to the addition of more Crossover meals. We call this special season "The Art of Maintenance" because it is a bona fide art to truly learn about "you" and your body's unique needs rather than following details designed for someone else. It's not the tools that make a charming masterpiece but the time and the understanding of how to wield those tools in your favor. If you pay attention, you can know your body better than any diet author who was not born in your skin. Just as learning the weight-loss principles of this plan took some time and practice, so too will this part of your journey. Tuning in will be your most useful key for being a successful Maintenance Mama.

While we're going to teach you here how to healthfully stop losing weight by adding in the right amount of Crossovers for you, we can't promise you won't keep shrinking. In fact we'd be liars if we told you your size will stay the same along with the number on your scale. The shrink kept slowly happening to us and over and over again we hear the same from other Trim Healthy Mamas who are now at goal weight. Little by little they keep getting smaller. Once you reach a healthy weight on the scale, your body still has other ideas of its own. You may be the same weight you were in your twenties or thirties but end up a size or two smaller. Obviously you won't keep shrinking until you disappear, but all that healthy protein ensures a denser muscle profile with less fluffy fat on your body. Well, that is the science; but this incredible shrinking effect is still a THM phenomenon that remains a bit of a mystery.

EASE INTO CROSSOVERS

Try incorporating three to four Crossover meals per week to start with and watch how your body responds. If you notice the pounds creeping back, then just pull back a little and introduce Crossovers at a slower pace, letting your metabolism adjust. Some Maintenance Mamas find that their body can only ever handle one or two Crossovers per week. These folks are not doing anything wrong. They are simply listening to their unique body makeup or season of life. If you are postmenopausal, thyroid deficient, or just designed to burn fuel more slowly than others, then you may find your Crossover quota to be much less than those who might be younger, hormonally well balanced, or very active with a high metabolism. Don't compare your special path to somebody else's and lose the joy and beauty of your own.

Both of us found that when we first reached goal weight, we did extremely well maintaining weight with just three or four Crossies per week. That lasted a year or two. As the years went on, though, we both found we had to start including more Crossovers to sustain a healthful weight. Years of healthy protein-centered meals that juggled fuels of both fats and carbs continued to rev our metabolisms to the point where we both need about one or more Crossovers a day now or we get too thin.

Some Mamas reach goal weight and immediately find their body can easily burn up three or more Crossies per week and they still lose weight. Within just a few weeks of playing around with Crossovers in maintenance they realize they have to include at least one Crossover per day or even have to make all their meals tandem-fueled in this manner. If this is you, then rejoice and embrace your own body's needs. Don't think for a second that eating this many Crossovers is any less on plan than strictly freestyling S and E. If your body embraces them, Crossovers should be at the core of your Trim Healthy Mama maintenance plan. True Crossovers stay the course of your Trim Healthy Mama health goals. They are designed to never spike your blood sugar and are antiaging, anti-inflammatory, and anti–carb binging. You are every bit a Trim Healthy Mama even if you never purposely eat an E or S again in your life.

DON'T STRESS IT

Even if you are able to predominantly live on Crossies and keep your trim, you don't have to get too religious about this, either. You'll be fine with some true single-fueled meals here and there. Going out to a restaurant and ordering grilled and buttered wild salmon with steamed broccoli and a luscious side salad with creamy dressing or olive oil would be a super-healthy option for you even if it is a true S meal. Sometimes finding healthy-carb options when dining out can be a real challenge and you sure don't want to eat the white, devitalized dinner rolls just to add some glucose fuel to your fat fuel. Don't think you have to carry a slice or two of sprouted bread in your purse just to make sure you "cross over."

S meals are going to happen naturally, as are E meals and, yes, even a Fuel Pull here and there. You might just be craving Greek yogurt and scrumptious plump raspberries for a snack: That is a yummy Fuel Pull and your body won't fade away to nothing just by including some Fuel Pull snacks occasionally. Don't be concerned with the religiosity of maintenance. Just be alert and attentive to how your body is reacting and what it is really needing. If you begin losing weight swiftly, again be mindful to keep your diet extra rich in Crossies but don't become imprisoned by them.

A fired-up metabolism is beneficial for many functions of the body and not for weight loss alone. The occasional natural juggle of an S meal here and E meal there just throws a wild curveball into your new Crossie life and keeps your metabolism on its toes.

PROTECT THE INTEGRITY OF YOUR CROSSIES

Now that you are not actively seeking weight loss, don't give in to the temptation to just eat whole foods any ol' way and think of this blanket strategy as Crossing Over. A true

Crossover never jumps over the safe E boundaries for starchy carbs or high-energy fruits. Many healthy foods can be unhealthy when eaten in excess. This is very true for carb sources that can throw your whole body off balance when not respected. The inclusion of carbs is paramount to health, but this doesn't mean you go for second and third helpings of rice casserole or eat piece after piece . . . after piece of sprouted toast with butter. Eat your two sane pieces of bread, then have second helpings of veggies and protein if you are still hungry. Don't opt for a large buttered popcorn at the movies and call it a Crossover—'cause it ain't! That's a cheat. Movie theaters don't use healthy oils and most of us don't eat safe Crossover portions of popcorn from a big movie-theater popcorn bucket. You are welcome to enjoy it and call it what it is, but don't call it a Crossover, okay?

Weight may not be such a huge deal anymore, but even skinny people feel like death warmed up when their bodies are continually crashing from roller-coastering blood-sugar levels. So keep tabs on your definition of this healing and nourishing meal so you don't ruin your "goal weight" or lose your healthy glow.

GUARD AGAINST CONSTANT CHEATING

There is a lot more to Trim Healthy Mama than this "trim" business. The *healthy* word is smack dab in the center of this title. Be careful not to slide back to old ways and cheat on junk more liberally now that your pants fit nicely and you don't feel as much motivation to stay on plan. By now you know that you can have the freedom for an occasional completely embraced and enjoyed cheat meal, but the inclusion of too many will not only slide you backward (or upward on the scale) quicker than you realize but will also tear down your renewed energy and radiant luster.

If you wake up one morning and realize you have cheated for two weeks straight, you have gained back a few pounds, and you basically feel crummy—don't let shame take over. Don't stay there in the brambles. We love the Bible story in Luke 15 in which the good shepherd leaves the ninety-nine sheep to rescue the one stuck in the thorns. Our heavenly Father wants to rescue you from your mess but you have to allow Him, you have to accept His grace. His grace and forgiveness are so much bigger than what we have for ourselves, but we need to learn from His great grace and apply it to our own mess-ups, too. It's clear from the scriptures that good health is a biblical blessing: 3 John 1:2 says, "Beloved, I wish above all things that you prosper and be in health, even as thy soul prospers."

Deuteronomy 30:19 challenges us, "I have set before you life and death, blessing and cursing, therefore choose life that you and your descendants may live." This verse has both spiritual and physical applications. We have this choice every morning as we start a new day and, thankfully, His mercies are new every morning; so if we messed up yesterday, our slate is once more clean. We have this choice before every meal. Will we choose life or death for our bodies for breakfast, for lunch, for dinner? Allow Him to gently untangle you from thorny thickets and guide you back to healthy green pastures, which is where He wants you! Remind yourself of this choice and then choose life!

WHERE'S MY MAINTENANCE MENU?

We didn't include a menu for our Maintenance Mamas for two reasons. First, as we explained earlier, every Maintenance Mama will need to do things a little differently to suit her unique requirements. There is no one-size-fits-all. The second reason is that we already designed a menu for our pregnant and nursing Mamas that includes ample Crossovers, so head over to Chapter 23, "Heads Up: Pregnant and Nursing Mamas!" (page 199), to check it out.

While you are over there in the preggies and nursing chapter, take a read of a couple of paragraphs on crossing over with more easy-burning S fuels than heavy S fuels (see pages 203–205). This concept will help many Maintenance Mamas who have trouble including Crossovers if they ramp up the scale too quickly. Strategically placed Deep Crossovers can actually instigate weight loss in thyroid-deficient Mamas or those who are stuck, stuck, stuck on a plateau of quicksand! So heads up: If you are struggling with Crossovers, learn how to prepare this "deep" variety properly and see if your body smiles on it.

chapter 28
THE GUY CHAPTER

So we've been wondering, should we write this chapter directly to the rare guy who might pick up this book, or do we write it to the woman who loves and cherishes this guy? Hmm . . .

Decision made. Since the species of male who could make it this far into a Mama book is probably rare to the point of being on the "endangered" list, we'll write to his woman. But if you do happen to be that EXCEPTIONAL guy reading these words, a belated welcome to you and sorry we've called you Mama throughout the whole book. We hope you won't need several years of counseling from that now.

In all seriousness, though, this plan works spectacularly for men. We wrote it for Mamas simply because we are Mamas, but the way sugar affects our bodies is not gender specific.

A man who had lost forty pounds on the Trim Healthy Mama Plan to reach a healthy goal weight came up to us at an event at which we were speaking. He had a great analogy for men and shared it with us. He said, "I think of your plan this way. I use gas for my car and diesel for my truck. I don't put them both in the same engine if I want my vehicle to work. Picturing S and E meals as either gas or diesel helped me get down to a healthy weight."

MAN FOOD APPROVED

If we as women find the idea of constant rabbit-food meals so unappealing that it causes us to want to go out and gobble a Big Mac, our guy feels that to the nth degree times ten. Men can really sink their teeth into this way of eating. They love the heartiness of the food. Steak, chili, meat loaf, and pizza: This foursome of man foods that often make up most guys' diets can easily be THMified.

NO DAINTY PORTIONS

Men LOVE to be filled up. Ever notice fast-food TV ads directed to men? They're all about filling them up with gigantic portions. As long as those large portions are THMified, your man can find his trim, too.

If you need direction on how much to feed your male, then refresh yourself with the story of Goldilocks and the Three Bears. There was a baby-size portion, a mama-size portion, and then a papa-size portion. Papa's bowl had a lot more porridge. It was not "just right" for Goldilocks.

Unless you are a very high-metabolism woman who can eat circles around your guy and still stay trim, he's usually going to need to eat quite a bit more than you do to stay satisfied and happy. The simple reason for this is he is created with more muscle so he requires more fuel to burn. Our own husbands often eat twice as much as we do at mealtimes.

That means when it comes to the number guidelines we've given you, don't get so finicky about them when it comes to your man. A medium-size sweet potato is just right for you in an E meal. Your guy might need a large. Don't forget, though, that it is important to also fill him up on protein and non-starchy veggies so he doesn't have to carb out to get filled up. If he needs to lose weight, the main thing that matters will be that he is basically separating his S and E meals and eating the right carbs—those gentle ones we suggest rather than spikers like white dinner rolls and white pasta. But even if some Crossovers occur here and there, men have a better chance of losing weight by including more Crossovers than many of us women do.

We have a greater percentage of essential fat in our bodies than men and less natural muscle, so we do need to pay more attention to the actual safe boundaries suggested when it comes to carbs. Your guy might want a couple large bowls of chili while one satisfies you. Don't call him a hog in your mind. He's just being a guy. Before you stay up all night worrying that his S chili turned into a raging Crossover from too many helpings that included beans, he's really just upsizing into guy portions. A true Crossover for him looks more crossed than yours. So don't look at him crossly! The fact that he is eating healthier even if weight is not shedding fast is fantastic!

Men who have Type 2 diabetes or severe insulin resistance need to stay much closer to the forty-five-gram carb safety net we advise. They'll need to have more starchy veggies and protein on their plates if they need to fill up more.

We've had some fun stereotyping here, but if your guy naturally has a slower metabolism or a smaller appetite, don't think him less of a man. Just as a few women can outeat some men, some men don't have the huge appetites we've been describing. No biggie—it takes all types to make up this world. Your grocery budget will thank you for that.

HE WON'T PLAY NICE

What if your guy is not interested in joining you on this journey? He's very happy with his potato chips and sodas and, even though he may have glaring health and weight issues, he doesn't want to change. What now? Nag, nag, nag, and put stress on your relationship?

Our advice is to let him know that you want to do this, you'd love for him to join you, but it is up to him. A few suggestions so this goes better in your favor. You may not want to say something like, "All of us girls from the book club have decided it's time we all get skinny together, so we're reading *Trim Healthy Mama Plan.* I want to fit back into my size-eight skirts and you need to get back into your size-thirty-two jeans. Sara was over the other day and I showed her our wedding pics and she mentioned you were so cute back then."

Ouch. First, your guy does not want to be skinny. He wants to be lean, and the last thing he wants to do is join you and your girlfriends at a tape-measuring-body-parts party.

How about something like this: "I want to feel more energetic for myself and for you and the children. I'd love to try cooking some more healthy meals and actually take a sane approach to getting trim this time. I'd appreciate your feedback on some recipes I want to try and I'll do my best not to be offended if you don't like my first attempts. Of course, I'd love for you to join me in this but that would be your decision."

If he's not thrilled about it, do this for yourself first. Let your progress speak volumes, eat your yummy cheesecake in front of him—don't be obnoxious about it, but there's nothing wrong with a little "mmm-this-is-good" reverse psychology. The fact that you are enjoying your food, reclaiming your waistline, and not making this plan compulsory for him might start to make it appealing over time. Since Trim Healthy Mama meals are so man- and family-friendly, even if he is only eating your main meal at night, this alone may cause him to see enough results that he may want to go all in.

If you want a tried-and-true male-friendly recipe as his first taste of THM, try the Cheeseburger Pie. You can find that on our website or in our companion cookbook and pair it with his favorite non-starchy veggie of choice drizzled with lots of fats.

We both had our own husbands down so many rabbit trails with diet fads, they were more than twice burned and extremely gun-shy about starting yet another crazy diet. We both ate the THM way for a full year on our own before our husbands decided to jump fully on board with us. Once they realized the food was not weird and completely tofuafied, and that they could eat plenty of it, including desserts, they sheepishly came into the fold and have been happy here ever since. (Not to say they don't do their fair share of cheating, though, too.)

SKINNY JIMMY

Maybe you have the kind of husband who constantly needs to put on five pounds and appears to lose weight through mere breathing. The challenge here is to find a blood sugar–friendly approach to weight gain for him. Maybe he can eat all the empty carbs he wants like donuts, white bread, chips, and Twinkies yet he still needs to put on weight. Even though you may not see the ravages of these destructive foods surface as fat on his body, the internal inflammation and damage on a cellular level is still happening. Spiking blood sugar and eating devitalized toxic foods speeds up the aging process and initiates disease. It may even be one of the reasons for his inability to gain weight as he is undernourished.

We suggest protein-centered Crossovers at every meal, prepared with healthy fats and served with blood-sugar-safe carbs. In very challenging cases, his Crossovers may need to include butter sliced as thick as cheese on whole-grain bread or rice at every meal along with hefty protein sources, and the inclusion of a tablespoon or two of raw honey. Don't pull out white potatoes from his Crossovers. Feed him like you would a wiry, growing teenage boy, as he probably has a similar constant metabolism burn going on in his body.

He doesn't need the sugary sodas and Doritos to keep his weight on. If he's open to it, try keeping peanut butter–based treats, sweetened with raw honey, on hand for him to eat right before bed. That might be one of the worst things for your weight but the best thing for his. Keeping nutritious, high-protein Crossover treats available at all times will help prevent him from reaching for empty carbs such as corn chips. Of course . . . he may not give a rip about what we suggest, but hey, at least we tried.

PART FOUR

trim healthy and beyond

chapter 29
LET'S TALK EXERCISE

No guns-blazing, kick-in-the-pants motivational "Get stuck in, gals!" speeches to start this chapter. Hopefully you will be relieved and even intrigued to know why there will be none of that "push harder" talk from us here.

Many Mamas starting out on a new eating plan are already overwhelmed by new foods, recipes, concepts, and knowledge. Adding a bunch of physical training on top is almost a cruel joke. Not everyone starts Trim Healthy Mama with excess energy to burn, all hyped up to go sweat and burn in the gym. Hey, let's get real: Most of us don't. At first you may barely have the energy to be in a good mood let alone bust your guts in an hour-long workout. Here's a piece of advice that you may not have expected from authors of a health book: DON'T!

Don't what?

Don't start exercising yet!

Again we urge you to listen to that sane and simple voice that aims to not complicate your already complicated and weary self. PLEASE DON'T add exercise training at first if you don't have the energy! And PLEASE DON'T add new exercise routines if you are already a little baffled amid the learning curve of the Trim Healthy Mama eating plan!

For now our advice is to relax and get the eating thang down—at least for the first few weeks or even a couple months. Weight loss from Trim Healthy Mama can happen with or without exercise. In fact, you will get better health and weight-loss results by not exercising at first if you are truly run down already.

Allow your body some time to heal and become nourished. Let it begin to flourish. Exercising on top of true exhaustion is a stressor that will turn off weight loss as your body slips into survival mode. In time, as you fuel your body correctly, your energy levels will rise. As your blood-sugar levels stabilize and your cells become truly nourished with whole foods and both S and E fuels, you'll start to feel perky enough that the thought of vigorously moving your body doesn't sound so crazy anymore.

But let's be clear about something. When we talk about exercise here we are talking about training the body in ways that are different from everyday healthy movement. When we say "take it easy and don't exercise" we are not telling you to sit on a sofa all day and maybe take a stroll to and from your car and back to your house or around your living room. A sedentary life only breeds more exhaustion and demise to your body. You've got to get some fresh air and get that blood of yours moving through your body to keep you feeling alive. Please do take lovely and lively walks. We don't consider walks to be physical training sessions—they are just enjoying the two legs God put underneath you.

WHEN YOU'RE READY

There is going to come a time, we promise you, when you will want to start moving your new energetic self more vigorously. When this moment happens for you or if you are already there, actual physical training is a wise and well-needed next step. But major caution sign—hold up for a minute—the type of training you choose for your body at this point can either boost or bring down your health and shape.

Please do not suffer through long training sessions that exhaust your adrenals and raise cortisol levels. Don't overtrain or wake up at five to fit in your hour on the elliptical machine when you hardly slept the night before. You might be able to flex more muscle after lots of brutal exercise, but your hormones may not be able to handle it. As Mamas our lives are demanding, and we know that stressing our adrenals will sabotage our weight loss, not boost it. Over and over again we see women unable to shed stubborn pounds simply because they are exercising too much. Our suggestion is that you keep training sessions to no longer than a half hour (of course natural activities like walking in the fresh air, dancing, and hiking are exempt from that).

Here at THM we not only shout "FOOD FREEDOM" but we also raise the battle cry for "BOOT CAMP FREEDOM." We have to stand up and say no to these body-punishing, push-the-limits exercise notions that not only wreck our hormonal health and rob our luster for life but actually make miserable slaves out of us. Many Mamas are beaten-down prisoners to a religion of exercise that says if you don't clock in your quota of hours per week of hard labor you are a fatty and a failure. We say no! We say move and make it fun! Move so you feel like celebrating life afterward and not falling on the floor like a dead cockroach. We have only one life to live. Let's not make it a tormented existence. Exercise training should be fast and fun and practical. It shouldn't feel compulsory but should be done out of the overflow of a zest for life.

Just as we went down so many diet dead ends, we also got caught up in the many exercise fads over the years (especially Serene). There is so much conflicting and confusing information out there about how a woman should exercise. After following much of it, Serene had to end up taking off several months from any vigorous exercise at all to heal her body from damage of unwise exercising. After several years of burying ourselves in study about safe and effective exercise, we created an exercise system for ourselves and other Mamas like us—busy Mamas who want to heal our bodies rather than tear them down.

We called these sessions Trim Healthy Mama Workins. We coined them Workins because of our foundational belief that working out should never be attempted unless you are first working your insides—safely firing your deep core muscles. Healing or developing a strong inner core before adding a whole bunch of circus moves is part of our simple, sane approach to health.

We designed Trim Healthy Mama Workins to be devoid of long, boring, time-wasting and injurious movement. The sessions are fast, effective, and designed to sculpt a fit feminine physique. This is a countercultural idea to the voice of the modern fitness industry.

DISTORTED FEMALE IMAGE

Have you noticed the culturally accepted new fit female image is "hard," "ripped," and "shredded" beyond feminine soft lines? Models with rippling six-packs are splashed repeatedly on the covers of women's magazines. It's the new norm, but it is truly normal? While the portrayal of a healthy woman has changed over the decades, in recent years the example of female fitness portrayed by media is heading in a new and extreme direction. "Guns" have replaced toned biceps. The new "hot" or "sexy" is the ripple of ab muscles beneath tight skin rather than a healthy, trim waistline.

Getting your blood pumping and working up a sweat is good for you. However, this is a vastly different thing from many of the brutal workouts that are all the rage these days

Muscles are great. We want to keep them as we age for hundreds of reasons, but our natural muscle distribution is different from men's. Our natural fat stores are vastly different from those of our male counterparts. Why are so many trying to reverse this natural distinction?

As females, we have 12 percent essential fat in our bodies to support our reproductive organs, brain, bone marrow, spinal cord, and complete nervous system. Compare that percentage to men, who have only 3 percent essential fat. We also NEED nonessential fat—the fat that lies just below the skin layer and helps protect our bodies from injury and cold. It also provides us with a great source of energy and allows us to sit on something other than a tailbone.

A healthy amount of fat on a woman is not repugnant. Shredding fat much below 18 to 20 percent can wreak havoc on a female body. Our fat deposits communicate with our hormones. Too little fat and our hormones sense we are in a life-or-death state. This reduces fertility and upsets the entire endocrine balance. Yes, let's seek the trim—but the shred? That goes against our natural design! It's also dangerous.

SMART MOVES

Just because we don't want to shed off all of our female fat layers doesn't mean we aren't gonna get deep into effective moves that not only burn fat to healthy levels but also shape and strengthen a woman's body where it needs it the most. Trim Healthy Mama Workins will give you a dynamic and productive workout but yet they are safely modified for all the ages and stages of a woman's life, even the vulnerable pregnancy and delicate core-healing season of the postpartum months.

We train the "bummy" big time! (Oops, excuse us, we didn't mean BIG, like make it chunky; but it really should have some oomph, which not only looks nice but, more important, is the healing and preventative key to pelvic-floor disorders.) We train the whole back line of the body, restoring a healthy posture that is the foundation in losing the tummy pooch and reconnecting a diastasis recti (a split down the middle that makes our "innards" become "outards").

We keep it real—maybe way too real, as we lanky sisters are not coordinated and don't even attempt to pull off "professional." We shot these Workins in one of our own living rooms with all the mess, children, and chaos. We didn't bother cleaning up for you (much) because that would be fake and we wanted you to know that this is something you can fit into your mess and your own busy, crazy life. We do most of the seven Workins in our pj's or grungies and don't show any midriffs or cleavage, because you don't want to see that and neither does your family. The other reason is because we have had a bunch of babies and don't have any desire to bare the belly or boobs, know what we mean?

THE FEMININE FIT DIFFERENCE

Of course, you don't need our Workins to start to enjoy and get the benefit of exercise. You can do anything you want to do that floats your boat. Just make sure that whatever training program you choose does not exhaust your precious and delicate hormonal interplay and tear apart your inner, feminine core.

Here are some motivational fitness quotes we found all over Pinterest recently. They're being repinned tens of thousands of times.

> "I don't glisten or smile when I work out. I sweat, grunt, and curse."
> "I am not afraid to sweat. Not afraid to tear. Not afraid to bleed. I am only afraid to quit."
> "Warning: . . . [this blank spot was the name of a popular exercise strategy, which we will not mention] may cause fatigue, nausea, vomiting, and an increased risk of becoming a bad . . . [short word for donkey that starts with *a*]."

Enough is enough! When we stumbled on the above quotes (and hundreds more just like them) we cringed at the brutish attitude they expect a woman must adopt to be fit and strong. Yes, women are equal to men in terms of worth, rights, and value, but we are also gloriously different. This needs to be celebrated, not distorted!

We are designed uniquely as God's female creation. Why not inspire one another to enhance our femininity by allowing our natural shape to be revealed in a beautiful balance of fitness and softness? Fall back in love with the idea of having a fit, feminine, wonderful but imperfect body rather than a shredded, hard physique that is never quite good enough for impossible standards. Here are some new Pinteresty sayings from us that we wish were more the vogue.

"I not only smile during my Workins . . . I also laugh, joke, and have enough energy left over to play with my children or love on my husband."

"I'm afraid to not listen to my body. Afraid to strip away my feminine curves. Afraid to make a religion out of exercise. Afraid to take it all too seriously."

KEEP YOUR JOY

Whether you have fun with our Workins, design your own exercise program, or enjoy other safe and femininity-enhancing fitness programs, keep the joy of movement as your banner. Don't let exercise become the dirge of a "treadmill-captive time-clocker." Exercise should never become a means of punishing your body for the previous night's popcorn splurge at the movies. Let the beauty of movement bring healing, not hurt, to your new healthy FREE you. Laugh out loud as you progress at your own pace in fitness, and, most important, don't take it all too seriously. Go ahead and do a silly jig, move for the mere pleasure of being alive. In fact, if you're not going to do a silly jig on your own, work in with us and we're going to force you to. We make big fools of ourselves in a part of our Workins that we call the Hot Tater Crazy Dance. But this kind of carefree spirit is better for your body and mind than all this serious structured gym-bound plodding. Life has enough of its own misery without adding more to it on purpose.

Note: If you need a break from our crazy selves, as your workout buddies we suggest you try some of Suzanne Bowen's exercise DVDs. She is a great friend of ours (married to our cousin) and is a professional trainer so, unlike us, she actually makes exercising look good and graceful. We love her approach to female fitness because she takes a similar philosophy to our own. Her BarreAmped workouts are short but effective and she protects your inner core. Check out her BarreAmped workouts at www.suzannebowenfitness.com.

chapter 30
LET'S TALK SKIN

Whatever you put onto your skin becomes a part of you. Your skin is like a sponge. Think about it. Nicotine patches, birth control patches, and hormonal replacement creams are all actual medications that are absorbed through the skin and make huge impacts on the body.

Our skin is also our largest detox organ. It is meant to be a place where toxins come out, not go in. Therefore skin creams and deodorants can be a dangerous onslaught of toxic chemicals, even if they say "natural" on the bottle.

We suggest you watch out for the following harmful ingredients in most hair and skin products:

Parabens
Phthalates
EDTA (ethylenediaminetetraacetic acid)
Propylene glycol
Synthetic colorings
Ureas
Vegetable oils

It takes years for some of these chemicals to break down once they are absorbed through your skin. Deodorants are applied right next to your lymph system under your arm. It makes no sense for you (or your teenage son or daughter) to put a bunch of toxins there day after day. Antiperspirants contain aluminum—a known carcinogen. Why would we do this to ourselves?

Not to be stinky, most of us answer.

Let's find a better way.

If you're doing the Trim Healthy Mama Plan, you're already on your way to healthier skin. Preventing blood-sugar spikes is more important than any skin cream you will purchase. Dr. Nicholas Perricone, the world-renowned dermatologist, talks about how inflammation is the destroyer of skin. In his book *Ageless Face, Ageless Mind,* he explains how sugar and high-glycemic carbohydrates cause rapid inflammation on a cellular level. These elevated blood-sugar levels cause chemical reactions that create free radicals and attack the lipid bilayer membranes of our cells. The result is premature aging of our skin. This phenomenon is called glycation, and it causes irreversible cross links between adjoining collagen molecules, which translates as deep wrinkles and loss of skin elasticity.

The collagen-rich foods and supplements we encourage in your diet are known skin healers and beautifiers. As we age, our bodies make less collagen, which is what gives our skin firmness; the loss of collagen results in sagging and wrinkles. Gelatin-rich natural foods such as stock or meats with skin and bones, or the supplements we recommend, go into your bloodstream and from there to your connective tissues, including your skin. They stimulate additional collagen production, which results in a reduction of lines and wrinkles. That's not just a nice little hopeful theory. A study published in 2009 in the *Bioscience, Biotechnology, and Biochemistry* journal examined the effects of eating gelatin on skin that was repeatedly exposed to ultraviolet light. The mice in the study were separated into three groups. Mice exposed to the light without the gelatin had a 53 percent average decrease in the collagen content of their skin, compared with the mice that received no ultraviolet light exposure at all. Incredibly, the mice that were fed gelatin and exposed to the light not only had no collagen decrease at all, but they also actually had an average collagen increase of 17 percent! So let's dig into this wonder food for our skin's sake!

WHAT SHOULD YOU PUT ON YOUR SKIN?

Now you know how to eat for healthy toned skin, but what to use on it? How about adopting the idea that whatever you put on your skin should not be anything that you would not actually be able to eat? Sure, that is a lofty goal; but we can all take baby steps toward that even if we don't perfectly make it. The fewer toxins we absorb, the greater our chance for vibrant health! Even many so-called "natural" products contain chemicals such as parabens. Just because something is packaged with earthy-looking colors and you buy it in a health store does not mean it is free of toxins. You certainly don't have to purchase only our Trim Healthy products, but do seek out skin-care items (and makeup if possible) that are free from the list we mentioned on page 269. In sticking with the "keep it sane" approach we want you to take, don't start obsessing over the purity of everything you put on your skin. A whole bunch of worry and fretting is going to be worse for you than putting on a moisturizer with less-than-stellar ingredients. Just try to make wiser, more informed choices each time you purchase your personal products.

THE TRIM HEALTHY NATURALS LINE

We have another crazy story to share. Five years ago Kathleen, a close friend of ours who lives nearby, handed us a cream that she had concocted in her kitchen. She'd infused all the herbs herself into a base of soothing aloe vera and pure essential oils. We opened the jar and it smelled like oranges! All she said was, "Try it for a week then tell me what you think—it's actually edible!"

Since that day, we have not used any other skin care cream. That was Kathleen's first product, which she named Orange Silk Hydrating Cream. It hydrates and soothes our skin like nothing else, is perfect under makeup, and performed miracles on many of our family members' problem skin areas. It healed a stubborn skin condition on Pearl's husband's hands that nothing else worked on, and Serene was finally happy about a cream she could use that fit her purist standards. We were so thrilled with it we couldn't help but talk about it in our first book. We were not associated with the cream in any financial way. We simply wholeheartedly believed in such a pure product and wanted other people to experience it as well.

We told Kath to put up a website in case she got any orders and so she did, not really believing much would happen with it. Well, in the same way that the Trim Healthy Mama word spread organically from Mama to Mama, Kath's creams began to catch on. She began to receive testimonials from people using her cream. It was like nothing they'd ever used and, despite the purity, was actually affordable! Her customers became devotedly loyal. Many of their very troublesome skin conditions resolved and they told their friends. Kath soon had trouble keeping up with the orders. Her husband had to quit his job and come help her full time!

In early 2014 Kath did the same thing to us but this time with a deodorant she had created that was actually healthful rather than harmful. "Try it for a week and tell me what you think."

We'd both tried many deodorants from health food stores, but let's just say they hadn't been that successful for us. The old underarm sniff check was rarely successful. Serene, determined not to put aluminum anywhere near her underarms, had even tried making her own homemade deodorant concoctions. They were extremely messy and hit-or-miss in effectiveness. We didn't have high hopes for Kath's experiment due to this history, and we told her so.

Incredibly, it worked, on both of us. We all put our heads together to come up with a name for it—the Hippie Stick. Kath launched it to her customers, and the response was overwhelming. She and her husband realized they had grown out of their home business when they found themselves having to make Hippie Sticks until three in the morning and then get up again at six to start again.

We were thrilled and excited when Kath and her husband suggested we partner up and create a full line of natural skin-care products.

The Trim Healthy Naturals skin and personal care line was born!

We couldn't be prouder and more excited to bring you these products. We still have Kath working hard behind the scenes, but this time she is using her herbal wizardry to come up with new amazing products rather than packaging Hippie Sticks until she's blurry-eyed. One of our greatest loves is brainstorming with her about how to come up with more truly natural products. We've worked with her on a pure shampoo for well over a year now, and we're very excited to see the idea soon to become a reality. Trim Healthy Makeup? No, we don't have that ready yet; but you'd better believe we're working on it!

If you have dry, aging skin, give the original Orange Silk Hydrating Cream a go for both face and body. The coconut cream is a popular choice for oily skin. You can go to www .trimhealthymama.com and then click on Trim Healthy Naturals to find these original products plus many more skin-care and personal items we have had the honor of being able to have a voice in creating with her.

chapter 31
BALANCE IS BEAUTIFUL

You've almost made it to the end of the book, and if we've taught you anything, we hope you have it seared into your mind that it is only this balance, this decision to keep a sane approach, that enables a long-term, happy, and healthy journey of Food Freedom.

Our whole mission, the passion that drives us to take the time away from our busy, large families to write this book, is there right on the front cover: "KEEP IT SIMPLE! KEEP IT SANE!" We refuse to get trapped in the depressing fetters of food nitpicking. It is too easy to go from this nitpicking to a state of food looniness. At this point you might as well just live in a bubble, because you start believing so many foods are "bad, bad, bad" and, what do you know, latest research says there are even scary, evil villains in regular whole foods that are out to GET YA!

We don't want to bash other diets. We certainly don't want to hold ourselves up as the girls who know all there is to know about nutrition. We will be ever learning, studying, and, hopefully, gaining more precious treasures of knowledge as we go on. As we mentioned in the beginning of the book, each type of diet has gems of truth that we can all learn from. We can offer respect to other approaches but we need to draw a line in the sand when it comes to damaging extremes.

So we are going to come full circle now. We started this book mentioning all the conflicting and confusing information out there regarding diet and we must end it returning to that maze for just a little while before we step back out into the sunshine with you again.

We are often asked about new diet theories and what we think about certain foods that are suddenly slapped with a "bad" label. We want to take this opportunity to officially share our thoughts on some current diet trends. We don't want you to get caught up in unstable tangents, fads, and rabbit trails that will too easily rob your joy. You're going to have to protect your balance. It's getting even crazier out there, Mamas! Your Food Freedom approach will continually be threatened by a host of new diet theories, new studies, and new scares. We want to arm you with some knowledge to help you keep it sane going forward.

In order to see if some of these latest extremes can stand up to good old common sense and simple science, we need to take a closer look at them, shake them up a little, and see what's left standing. But no hurt feelings if you skip this part. Fair warning: We are going to get study heavy on you for a bit. If you don't care to delve deeper here with us, we'll meet you on the last page of the book to say good-bye. You have all the info you need for a successful Trim Healthy Mama journey right now. But if you are one who opens your e-mail inbox every morning to be ever more concerned and confused about what you read regarding food and diet, follow along here with us and save your sane.

UNSTABLE WISDOM

As you know, we don't have a bunch of degrees after our name and we doubt we'd blow anyone away on an IQ test. But it doesn't take a bunch of degrees to see when the big picture is lost in the overanalyzing. Man's wisdom gets so befuddling and confusing sometimes. This is depicted in the biblical story of the Tower of Babel. The designers and builders of the tower were the smartest in the land but they were so filled with their own intellect and aspirations to reach the sky that they were hampered by their own hands. They ended up babbling a bunch of nonsense and the tower was never finished.

The mind of mere man is puny compared with the one who created the universe with the power of His voice alone. His perfect nutritional balance is outlined in the blueprint He gave us. The Bible is sound and doesn't change with the trends and times. Even if you don't read the Bible or care to believe in an intelligent Creator, you still must agree that the Bible doesn't go through the cyclic changes of dietary fads that we circle through these days. It does not vilify whole food groups but embraces them all as gifts. Man is often in error: Things that are known to be true for decades are found to be false with one new study hitting the media waves. There has to be something more grounding we can lean on than dogmas, theories, and studies.

WHAT'S NEW IN THE BEFUDDLING WORLD OF DIETS?

If you haven't already heard about some of these latest diet theories we're going to mention here, we doubt it will be long before you do. Sensationalist food judging sites are all the rage. The new trendy food words on the Internet are *beware* and *avoid.* Surf the Web and you'll be swamped with top-tens for everything that has recently been found to be bad. Which food's turn is it this week to be nasty and dangerous?

Have you heard of PUFAs? These are the natural polyunsaturated fatty acids that are abundant in superfoods like eggs and salmon. PUFAs are not the result of pollution or any manmade, toxic sludge. God created salmon to contain liberal amount of these fatty acids. We are not kidding when we say there are some new diet theories gaining much popularity teaching that they are bad for us. Extraordinarily healthy foods like salmon are being labeled as harmful and dieters are being warned to avoid them. Did we mention things are getting crazy?

Lectins and phytates are two more new bad kids on the block. They occur naturally in many foods but have tainted the good name of grains, beans, and nuts to the point that it will be a miracle if their reputation ever recovers.

The stone throwing does not stop there. Fermented or aged foods such as cheeses, vinegars, and cultured milks (kefir, for example) have historically been the cornerstone foods of civilizations but are recently disdained for the fact that they contain free glutamic acid. MSG is the synthesized form of this acid but many believe the free form is just as harmful even though it is found naturally in many whole foods, such as ripe tomatoes. Funny that human breast milk has some of the highest levels of free glutamic acid of all foods. Would God really create a milk to nourish babies full of the harms of MSG?

Our beloved bone stock (used for centuries) and gelatinous supplements are scorned by some because they will make foods taste too good and we'll overeat! What? Yep.

Coconut oil made from dried coconut called copra is another new "nasty" no-no. Oh, and we'd better not leave out the mycotoxins in coffee; they're apparently damaging to humans, except for a certain brand that costs almost as much as your phone bill each month to obtain. Aflatoxins on peanuts . . . the list of baddies go on and on.

Notice something? We are not talking about foods laden with synthetic chemical toxins here. This is the stuff that is grown in the soil, caught in the ocean, or raised on a farm and has nourished people for millennia. If you buy in to all the new "evils" of foods it would not be possible to sit down and enjoy a healthy whole-foods meal without worrying about diseases forming after every swallowed morsel.

A few phytates in a handful of almonds that you didn't soak for twelve hours, a few lectins in a Mediterranean tomato and eggplant salad, a teensy bit of aflatoxin in a spread of peanut butter, some PUFAs in a delicious wild-caught piece of salmon . . . our amazing bodies are well equipped to deal with these naturally formed properties that are on or in real food. Unless you have true sensitivities or allergies to these foods, it doesn't make sense to stress about them.

We are not meant to live in a sterile bubble, our food in little morsels of perfection with every particle censored. We were made to live in a world of bacteria and funguses. Just put your fingernails under a microscope and let's get real. Yes, we're a bit heated up on this subject; but somebody needs to stand up against the joy robbers.

In fact, it is our belief that this obsessive worry and food perfectionism may threaten to weaken the human race! Not just because of the worry, which might be a huge factor, but because consuming a little bit of those so-called nasties like PUFAs in wild salmon is actually meant to happen. It's only common sense that nasties are in foods because we are meant to ingest them, that they are somehow part of the perfect symbiotic symphony of balance that makes up a truly "divine masterpiece" diet.

Remember, a little bit of bacteria strengthens the immune system and a bit of dirt to play in makes for a healthier child. Science has finally realized using antibacterial soap too often is actually harmful for us. Last decade everybody was carrying hand sanitizer around until studies showed oversanitizing yourself in this manner harms your immune system. We need a little of everything natural to balance out the whole picture, certain germs included.

Sure, there are things to sensibly avoid but they are a simple list of easy villains to recognize (aside from allergens and religious beliefs). It's best to avoid refined sugar, refined grains, GMOs when possible, BPA canned goods when possible, fake chemicalized cheese, soda, drugs, cigarettes, too much alcohol, most preservatives and chemicals, yak mucus, paint thinners, dinosaur urine . . . okay, now we're being silly. But common sense tells us what to avoid. You don't need a list from us.

You might have a couple more (or fewer) items on your own list, but none of us need food-scare sensationalists warning us against God-given foods like beans, grains, nuts, meat, dairy, butter, eggs, coffee, tea, or cooked foods. Some of us thrive on these foods, some of us find we have to pull back on certain types. We're all different. But this doesn't mean they must be out for everyone and slapped with a BAD label. Enough is enough!

THAT DRATTED MEAT AGAIN!

Did you know that poor old meat is on the chopping block again, meaning chop it right out of your diet? In the 1980s and '90s meat was considered by many to be a baddie because of its saturated fat. Science vindicated meat when it became known that hydrogenated vegetable fats messed with by man's fancy tweaks were the real problem when it comes to heart disease. Just when meat was enjoying a brief reprieve, its name had to get sullied once again, and this time, not just red meat but all of it—fish, venison, turkey, and chicken. They are all in the naughty seat again.

What is so bad about these animal foods now, you ask? It is the amino acid methionine that meat (and other animal products) contains. Yep, a naturally occurring innocent little amino acid that is essential to the body and actually helps to keep us full of vigor is recently considered to be a vicious exterminator programmed to snuff out the human race!

METHIONINE TROUBLES

All this kerfuffle about methionine is due to some studies done on mice. A 2005 study published in *Aging Cell* backed up what other studies had reflected: Mice with the lowest levels of methionine lived the longest. Certain amino acids, including methionine, help to raise IGF-1 levels. IGF-1 stands for insulin-like growth factor and it measures growth hormone in the body. Growth hormone itself is associated with youthfulness, supple skin, more energy, better muscle tone, and more. But the mice in these research studies that had lower levels of IGF-1 and subsequently lower levels of methionine lived longer than the ones with higher IGF-1. Time for a new diet theory: Suppress methionine in the body, and ban all meat!

The Real Story

Not so fast. First things first. Feeding a bunch of box-bound mice some kibble with mega doses of methionine that may have been derived synthetically is very different from a normal real-world lifestyle. Without all the other antioxidants and counterbalancing nutrients that come with a balanced whole-foods diet, this situation is not a fair assessment of the way methionine or IGF-1s work.

While it is true that mice deprived of IGF-1 lived longer, it is also true that they quickly lost their vigor and health. In the studies, the mice became more feeble and crippled and showed senility. Abundant IGF-1 sustains youth, and it impedes atrophy and aging by enhancing neuronal and muscle growth and repair.

The theory behind suppressing methionine is that by decreasing IGF-1 levels you increase the voice of stress-resistance genes and therefore increase your lifespan. In simple terms, your body recognizes that it is extremely stressed with low levels of IGF-1 and awakens your stress-resistance genes to start screaming: NO! I WANT TO LIVE! I AM GOING TO FIGHT THIS STRESSFUL LACK OF IGF-1.

This restriction does work to lengthen life in rodents but not because methionine or IGF-1 are scoundrels. It works because they are greatly needed for a flourishing body and their lack in your body initiates a defensive battle for survival.

Would You Believe Exercise Causes Cancer?

Levels of IGF-1 are highest in the young and agile, and we age in correlation to its diminishing levels. Exercise induces IGF-1 release. Does this mean we should also avoid all exercise in order to live longer? Of course not. We were made to move. We don't have to bust a gut to be fit, but we sure shouldn't shun exercise altogether. Don't call us crazy, people are actually teaching this doctine! Avoiding most forms of exercise except only the concentric contractions of some lifting moves is part of a new protocol preached from those who shy away from IGF-1. Yes folks, it is getting this crazy! When just the simple act of eating and moving gets this deeply discombobulated, someone needs to shout "Stop!"

Another theory close to this one goes like this: The wonderful fulfillment of being nourished with sufficient food and calories releases IGF-1. Starving decreases it. So if we can starve ourselves more or miserably reduce the size of our plate, we can release those stress-resistance genes and live longer. Yep, the fountain of youth is starvation, people!!!

We might live a painful, gloomy existence plagued with early aging on all levels, but hey, we might add another five years to our life. This thinking has more followers than you can imagine and is the foundation behind intermittent fasting and severe calorie restriction and other similar plans.

Be a Balancer, Not a Hater

The commonsense key to all of this is once again BALANCE. Let's include the other balancing nutrients, hormones, or mechanisms that work synergistically alongside methionine to bring healthy wholeness. If methionine and IGF-1 cause the sun to rise, then let's find the harmonizing counterbalance that makes it set. There are hormones that help sustain a pregnancy and others that stimulate birth. Insulin causes our fat cells to store, and glucagon causes our fat cells to release. This is the reason we don't eat a bunch of carbs alone: If we did, insulin would go into a fat-storing rampage. So do we throw our hands up and shove insulin into the baddie sack? No, it is a crucial hormone for our survival! By adding protein to our meals, glucagon is released and fat has a harder time sticking to our thighs. In a similar, sane manner, let's get methionine under control without ditching foods containing it altogether.

Glycine, the Methionine Antidote

The wisdom BALANCE speaks shows that the answer for a long, healthy life lies not in the reduction of essential nutrients but in the inclusion of their "seesaw" nutrients. The amino acid glycine is the perfect antidote for methionine and high IGF-1. A more recent 2011 study published in *The FASEB Journal* (published by the Federation of American Societies for Experimental Biology) showed that when rats are supplemented with glycine they experience the same life extensions as those with methionine-restricted diets. Makes sense, since glycine is the vehicle for clearance of excess methionine in the body.

As a Trim Healthy Mama, you'll get your protein from a balance of both glycine-rich protein sources and methionine-rich protein sources. That means you can enjoy steak, chicken breasts, and cottage cheese, which are rich in methionine; but it is also important to eat meat cooked with the bones and to include gelatin-rich foods so you get enough glycine. This is not hard to achieve, not something you have to make a spreadsheet for and obsess over. Who doesn't like chicken wings or chocolate pudding made with gelatin? You've got some lovely glycine right there!

These new diet approaches that are terrified of methionine might be extreme but they are doing one thing right—promoting a harder look at the way we all get our protein. In olden days or even just across the seas in less-industrialized nations, diets were and are naturally rich in this important amino acid. People didn't think the bones and skins of animals (where glycine is abundant) as gross. They didn't meticulously remove these "nasties" before cooking. They threw them all in the pot or frying pan. Soups were simmered with meat that was still on the bone. Fish-head soup and chicken-feet stock have nourished whole civilizations! Sounds nasty to most of us, but that is only because we are not used to it. Today most meats sold in grocery stores are packaged with this new meticulous pickiness in mind. Sadly, nearly everything seems to be boneless or skinless these days.

As we mentioned in Chapter 2, "The Basics" (page 16), when we described the crucial role of protein on plan, you can still heartily enjoy skinless boneless chicken breasts and canned tuna; but don't forget your meat on the bone and your homemade gelatin-rich stock or collagen or gelatin supplements. Oh, what a beautiful balance!

Easy Ways to Restore Glycine

If your budget is too tight for the glycine-rich supplements we recommend (see page 143) and you don't have excess time to make purist bone stock from scratch, you can still easily get glycine in your diet. You don't have to resort to fish heads and chicken feet (although you're welcome to; many of our purist Mamas go gaga over that sort of thing).

Check out our recipe for Drive Thru Sue Bone Stock in our companion cookbook. Make Super Salmon Patties using canned salmon with skin and bones included. Don't let your brain say "yuk" before trying these patties found on our website or in the cookbook. They are a family favorite around here. Process the salmon in a food processor if you are icked out mashing it with a fork. Enjoy Salmon Mousse found in the companion cookbook for a snack with cucumber slices. Buy bags of quartered chicken legs and enjoy Crispy Lickin' Chicken ("Oven Baked or Roasted Meats" chapter in the *Trim Healthy Mama Cookbook*). Strapped for time? Pick up some rotisserie chickens, and enjoy some skin on your drumstick! Notice that jelly that forms around the rotisserie chickens when they cool? That is wonderful gelatin in all its healthful glory, chock-full of glycine! It was released because the chickens were cooked with all their bones and skin, enriching the meat with glycine.

Extra Helpers for Balancing Methionine

One of methionine's jobs in your body is methylation. This function is extremely important for cellular communication and the governing of gene expression in your body. It maintains and repairs existing tissue and supports the building up of new healthy tissue. When methionine fails in this task of methylation it produces instead homocysteine, which is a burdensome by-product that can contribute to cardiovascular disease, inflammation, and the rise of cancers. Folate found in foods like lentils, legumes, okra, dark leafy greens, broccoli, asparagus, avocados, oranges, egg yolks, and liver assists methionine in performing this important task.

Vitamin B_{12} found only in animal products, and of lesser importance B_6, also found in muscle meats, as well as niacin in foods like sweet potatoes and riboflavin in almonds and Parmesan cheese, also helps methylation succeed. Choline, provided in egg yolks, and betaine, made in your body from choline or provided through foods like spinach, help as well. All of those foods are abundant in your THM diet, so no worries—but do branch out and include some of these if you've been stuck in a food rut.

Lowering Animal Protein Is Not the Answer

Methionine avoiders who cut out meat altogether because they haven't yet relaxed into the natural healthy balance of including seesaw amino acids can create more problems for themselves. Many vegetarian foods still contain methionine, though not as much as meat does. Vegetarian sources of protein do not provide vitamin B_{12}, which is essential for methylation. This broken methylation pathway creates greater homocysteine problems and attenuates the dark side of methionine. Animal protein foods rich in methionine and vitamin B_{12} are healthy choices for complete methylation.

A Better Way to Turn On Longevity Genes

Rather than resorting to severe calorie restriction, exercise restriction, and meat restriction to increase longevity—try hormesis!

Hormesis is the process by which a very small dose of something that the body views as slightly harmful triggers the longevity mechanism of stress-resistance genes. Catechins and polyphenols are labeled potent antioxidants, but they are actually slightly toxic to our cells so they activate this "hermetic effect." They increase the "voice" of antioxidant genes and in that way they act as antioxidants.

Mamas, let's dig into catechin- and polyphenol-rich foods like green tea found in recipes like our Earth Milk Sip, dark chocolate, turmeric (hooray for the Singing Canary recipe), blueberries and other deeply pigmented berries, and red wine. (Maybe we shouldn't dig too excessively into wine or it won't be in the good-girl category.) Sprinkle the herb rosemary on your grilled and baked meats. Consider using essential oils, especially orange, lemon, and grapefruit, which are rich in these substances that create hormesis in the body. Vanilla also has a hermetic effect, which is just another reason to celebrate healthy desserts on plan.

MOVE OVER METHIONINE, IT'S TRYPTOPHAN'S TURN

Tryptophan is kin to methionine in that it belongs to the family of nine essential amino acids that our body cannot manufacture and needs to get in adequate supply from our diet. We are talking about the form found in whole foods here, not the supplement.

Tryptophan-rich foods are on the hot seat because tryptophan is a precursor to serotonin production and lately serotonin is getting a very bad rap. Serotonin is a brain biochemical that promotes restful sleep, happy emotions, and satiety. The lack of it leads to depression, anxiety, insomnia, sugar cravings, and the impulse to eat yet another brownie. But, of course, it has its dark side. Apparently serotonin can be blamed for a myriad of ailments including hypothyroidism, inflammation, cancer, aging, and the overall demise of your health. People who follow this theory say "down with serotonin and down with estrogen, too!" When estrogen levels rise, then serotonin levels follow suit.

The problem with demonizing estrogen is once again imbalance. While excessive estrogen, just like excessive anything, is unhealthy, insufficient estrogen is equally detrimental. Progesterone is not healthier than estrogen, just as glycine is not healthier than methionine or tryptophan. Dopamine is not a better brain neurotransmitter than serotonin. It is just the imbalance of one without the counterbalance of the other that causes issues.

Hooray for Glycine Again!

Once again it is glycine to the rescue when it comes to balancing excessive levels of tryptophan, serotonin, and estrogen. As with any hormone or transmitter in the body, when these three are too high in the body they can do some damage. It is true that excessive levels of these can stimulate more cortisol, overexcite cells, and suppress the thyroid, but when balanced by glycine, their good points can shine rather than allowing their dark sides to take over. Gelatin-rich foods, which contain glycine, have many antistress actions. Glycine calms cells and inhibits tumor necrosis factor and prostaglandins, two things you don't want excited in your body. Glycine helps the liver detoxify your body of harmful estrogens, which are the ones that tend to dominate.

Tryptophan Science Clears the Air

Along with muscle meats and certain dairy products like aged or cultured cheeses, there is a long list of other foods that contain tryptophan. Bananas, chocolate, a host of veggies, grains, legumes, nuts, and seeds are all rich in this amino acid. A diet becomes extremely limited if you try to limit tryptophan. But that doesn't deter some new diets. There are a few foods low in tryptophan, so dieters are encouraged to consume them over and over again and basically ditch the rest of God's provision to us. They limit meat yet encourage high amounts of milk as their core protein choice. Apparently, they have their reasons why the tryptophan in this form of dairy is okay.

The science of how tryptophan is absorbed makes their worry over high-protein, tryptophan-rich foods like meat unnecessary. If blood-sugar levels are kept stable, there will not be an excessive tryptophan rise. The only efficient way to absorb tryptophan into the brain and induce a drastic rise in serotonin is through high carbs or other strong insulin pathways. This means a high-protein meal centered around animal protein, without a bunch of carbs, is not effective alone in dramatically changing serotonin levels in the brain.

Your Trim Healthy Mama meals always safely anchored around ample protein do not promote excessive serotonin rises. But we absolutely need some of this good serotonin stuff, so E meals, with their gentle carbohydrates always balanced with protein (that hopefully frequently includes glycine), help sustain happy levels of serotonin in the brain.

You Gotta Love Serotonin

Serotonin is an antidote to premenstrual syndrome (PMS). As estrogen drops before and during your period, it is common for many during PMS to experience a drop in serotonin, which is the trigger behind all those high-carb cravings. When estrogen levels rise once again after your period, serotonin naturally rises along with it and all that "lack-of-serotonin grumpiness" and "give-me-chocolate-or-I'll-scream disorder" settles down. Carbohydrates are used to make serotonin and, sadly, simple sugars are the quick fix for many women. Imagine PMS exacerbated by a low-tryptophan diet—shudder.

To get safe sources of tryptophan during your low-serotonin PMS days, enjoy the recipe for Skinny Chocolate in the *Trim Healthy Mama Cookbook* or find the many creative versions on Pinterest that Trim Healthy Mamas have come up with. Chocolate is a rich source of tryptophan but the high sugar that usually accompanies it can undo its merits. Exercise is another way to increase serotonin when you're feeling grumpy and lousy, but as we advise in Chapter 29, "Let's Talk Exercise" (page 263), don't overdo it. Finding a little sunshine and bathing in its golden rays for a few minutes also gives a healthy serotonin lift. We can't forget about sufficient sleep, which gives a natural boost to this happy brain chemical without the impending blues.

Supplementing with whey protein is another excellent and safe way of getting the "happies" from serotonin when feeling a little depleted. The alpha-lactalbumin in whey is very rich in tryptophan and tips the ratio of plasma tryptophan to the other neutral amino acids in favor of tryptophan's absorption without a lot of competition.

But a caution about whey for those who are nursing and CANNOT drop weight no matter what you do (possibly due to high levels of prolactin) or for those with hyper-prolactinemia for other reasons. In these cases you may be very sensitive to serotonin and anything that works hand in hand with prolactin production. You may wish to avoid whey if you have this issue and choose to use only collagen or gelatin as a protein supplement. Check out Chapter 24, "Heads Up: Turtle Losers!" (page 214), and our special diet suggestions for those with overly elevated prolactin levels.

Contradicting Protocols

Many followers of low-tryptophan or tryptophan-cautious plans also advise abundant fructose—that is, lots of orange juice and the embracing of generous amounts of sugar, even table sugar. These are apparently included to soothe the adrenals.

Looking at the science, it is clear that spiking blood-sugar levels promotes excessive serotonin levels and this carries a bitter backlash! The excessive release of serotonin can deplete the balanced levels of this happy hormone in the long term and leads to an increased rate of depression in diabetics.

All of this "sugar-spiking" talk now leads us to warn you of another diet trend that embraces large amounts of sugar under the guise of healing the adrenals.

DOUBLE CHOC ICE CREAM SUNDAES ARE BACK

While the low-carb diet craze gave the world a lot of much-needed knowledge about the overdoing of carbohydrates, it also did some damage. Many dieters are still confused and left trying to piece the jigsaw puzzle called balance back together. Not only did low-carbism falsely accuse an entire macronutrient of being unnecessary and make it take the blame for everyone's ailments, it desecrated the common sense of balance. This carb-dismissing extreme has contributed to body imbalances in the form of wrecked thyroids and burned-out adrenals.

When this realization hit the dieting world, instead of adding back healthy carb choices there was a frenzy to go in the complete opposite direction. In an effort to heal thyroids and restore adrenals, there is a new trend to eat nightly ice cream before bed, drink generous glasses of juice and milk, eat more fruit than veggies (in fact, vegetables are considered second-class citizens), and even scarf down a candy bar without guilt. Sadly, this is the new "healthy thyroid and adrenal-nurturing diet" followed in some extreme camps.

The Thyroid: Another Victim of Excess Blood Sugar

If one of the remedies for thyroid sluggishness is sugar, then Americans should have thyroids that work like purring Ferraris. Instead, according to the American Association of Clinical Endocrinologists, twenty-seven million Americans are burdened with thyroid dysfunction. Subclinical hypothyroidism is estimated to affect an additional twenty-four million Americans. It is sobering to think that more than fifty million Americans are inflicted with some form of thyroid disorder.

Refined sugar and blood sugar–spiking carbs are not the answer for the thyroid gland just like they are not the answer for the adrenal gland. Thyroid problems are 90 percent autoimmune in nature. Sugar battles against your white blood cells and makes them ineffective against battling toxins for five hours after a sugar spike. This destroys your natural immune defense. Research shows that thyroid disorders are more prevalent in diabetics and those suffering with obesity and metabolic syndrome.

Both extremes of low- and high-carb diets have booby traps waiting in the wings to strangle the thyroid. Studies reveal that the repeated insulin spikes that lead to insulin resistance destroy the thyroid gland in people with autoimmune thyroid issues. On the other hand, insulin is needed for the conversion of the inactive T4 hormone into the active T3 hormone. While our T4 hormone does have use in the body, T3 is approximately four times more potent than T4. We need robust T3 levels so we're going to have to eat some carbs to get them. But . . . diets high in sugar and the chronic inflammation they promote stop the conversion of T4 to T3. Do you see the conundrum here? We need carbs for a well-working thyroid but excessive carbs cause the thyroid to break down. There has to be a sensible middle ground.

Going Too Low in Glucose Fuel Promotes Reverse T3

There is another key player in all this thyroid madness called reverse T3 (rT3). It is synthesized from T4. It binds to thyroid receptors and blocks the action of T3. BOO!!! This means it lowers the metabolism and promotes fat storage. It is not the hormone someone who is trying to lose weight wants to have in charge.

Diets too low in glucose (for too long), commonly known as low-carb diets, have proven to inactivate the wonderful T3 hormone and give rise to overly high levels of rT3. The body recognizes there is not enough energy being consumed to furnish the brain and slows down the metabolism and many other bodily processes to conserve this vital nutrient. Remember, T3 is something you want. And rT3 is something you don't want.

The biggest take-home point in thyroid health is to avoid drastic blood-sugar fluctuations. This means stay away from high sugar "spikers" but don't get stuck in S ruts, either. Keep those E meals a regular at your Trim Healthy Table and throw in a few Crossovers or S helpers as your weight-loss journey permits.

Again and again it comes down to that beautiful seven letter word: BALANCE. Seven speaks of perfection. But remember your perfect balance might be different from someone else's. A Mama who swings kettlebells and nurses a set of twins will need more glucose nourishment than a sedentary office worker who is postmenopausal. Listen to your body and remember that healthy gentle carbs are an integral fuel to keep juggling in your

Trim Healthy Mama lifestyle. For more info on thyroid health and important thyroid testing, check out Chapter 24, "Heads Up: Turtle Losers!" (page 214).

SUGAR TO HEAL YOUR ADRENALS?

The new approach of using simple sugars like fruit juice, table sugar, honey, and refined carbs to soothe the adrenals makes no sense to us. Yes, there is truth to the underlying principle that carbs are needed for well-functioning adrenals, but the extreme approach that is all over the blogosphere right now is what doesn't make sense. We've really tried to wrap our minds around it . . . to give the idea a fair chance. But after months of study on it the facts are still the facts. High blood-sugar levels deplete cortisol levels and burn out the adrenals. That is one of the main jobs of the adrenal gland and cortisol: to balance blood sugar. Indicators of adrenal fatigue are usually seen in tandem with glucose intolerance and insulin resistance in lab testing.

No matter what any modern backlash fad is teaching, wisdom, science, and common sense still scream the danger of refined sugar and the excessive consumption of carbohydrates. Suggestions like ice cream and glasses of fruit juice for thyroid and adrenal health simply don't hold water in the big picture. Spiking of blood sugar is one of the reasons adrenals are so weak these days. Using high sugar to repair what it already broke? How is that a healthful remedy? Inflicting the adrenals and thyroid again with the same treatment that helped send them down for the count is just plain cruel to them.

The "sugar rush" and flood of hyperactive energy from a high-sugar spike is not necessarily desirable sugar energy but more likely a desperate adrenaline surge in response to the crisis. You are actually experiencing an adrenaline rush. Dr. William Tamborlane of the Yale Center for Clinical Investigation at Yale University reported on research showing that children had much higher levels of adrenaline after they were given sugar. He correlates their hyperactive behavior not to the energy from blood sugar itself but to these higher adrenaline surges. This clearly reveals that a surge of stress hormones is consequentially leached from the adrenals with every blood-sugar spike.

This dire situation that the adrenals are faced with under a high-sugar load can be made very clear with the following four common steps.

STEP 1: You guzzle a large glass of orange juice or down a hearty bowl of ice cream. NOW YOU HAVE HIGH BLOOD SUGAR!

STEP 2: Insulin surges to clean up the stressful situation of your spiking blood sugar. High blood sugar is destructive at a cellular level and the body responds to this emergency. Your body, intelligently realizing the toxic situation of high blood sugar, sends high doses of insulin and cleans it up overzealously, bringing it super-low, safe from the prior stressful high.

NOW YOU HAVE LOW BLOOD SUGAR!

STEP 3: Low blood sugar is another emergency and the adrenals, our primary stress glands, respond with urgency. Adrenaline starts to pump, causing the liver to convert stored glucose and release it into the bloodstream in an effort to bring the blood sugar out of the dangerous dumps. Epinephrine, norepinephrine, and cortisol are crucial stress hormones delivered to try to fix the stressful situation.

STEP 4: The body, now in a traumatic state of low blood sugar, craves a high sugary meal to provide energy for the brain, and this vicious cycle repeats.

Repeating this situation over again with nearly every meal burns out your adrenals. During adrenal fatigue, when adrenal hormone levels are already compromised, it becomes extremely difficult to maintain blood-sugar levels.

If you relate to Adrenal Mess Jess, whom we met back in Chapter 1, nourish your adrenals back to strength with lots of rest, drink the Singing Canary, and do not leave E meals out of your fuel juggle. But don't fall back into the vicious cycle of those four steps. Sensible servings of sweet potatoes, ancient grains, whole fruit, and legumes are healers. These not only contain necessary glucose to soothe your adrenals but also offer it in a much gentler way to your body. Shoving more sugar fuel than your body can handle to try and nurture your adrenals is like eating dynamite. Soon something's gonna blow . . . maybe the buttons on your pants or your clean bill of health.

FINDING RESPECTFUL BALANCE WITH LECTINS AND PHYTATES

Lectins and phytates are two more newly convicted felons that need some defense. It used to be butter and coffee, but now it is the "Loser Lectins" and "Foul Phytates" that people are being trained to avoid like the plague. If you are a Drive Thru Sue you may not give a rip whether your food contains them or not. But these terrible two have really dealt a heavy burden to the purist who sometimes lies awake at night wondering whether her oatmeal's overnight soak will be enough to destroy their evil powers.

Let's take a look at both of these so-called menaces and see whether their bite is truly as bad as their bark.

Loser Lectins?

Recent diets that tout that all grains are bad for us (something to do with Caveman Grok) point to lectins as one of the reasons. Lectins are proteins that are designed to withstand digestion and not be broken down by the intestines. One of lectin's purposes is to naturally repel pests from the plants they are within. All plants contain defense mechanisms designed to protect them from animals, bacteria, and fungi. Many have multiple systems in place and lectins are only one of these defenses that some health gurus are magnifying for now.

What's wrong with lectins? Umm ... pretty much everything, according to lectin-avoidance diets. They are thought to cause leaky gut, autoimmune issues, fibromyalgia, arthritis, stubborn weight issues ... the list goes on and on.

If you buy into all that, you essentially have to believe that God created food to harm us. Lectins are not manmade; they are in foods that God called good and they have always been in these foods. They are not a new menace.

Another name for lectins is glycoproteins. These proteins eventually find their way into cell walls in your body. Your body actually uses these glycoproteins on the outside of your cells for important messaging and signaling. Glycoproteins are an amazing and necessary bodily mechanism!

In the big picture lectins aren't losers, they are underestimated cool dudes that are necessary for a myriad of life-sustaining functions. For instance, lectins break down the membranes of hurtful invaders like cancer cells and help reduce the risk and growth of many deadly cancers. Lectins attack the membranes of fungi, bacteria, and viruses in the body and have been reported to be effective even against the HIV-1 retrovirus.

A 1997 study done on rats cited in the *British Journal of Nutrition* (rats again ... we know ... yawn) determined that the biggest problem with lectins comes when people eat an insufficiently varied diet. In one study, rats put on a varied diet showed significantly less damage from the inclusion of lectins than rats fed a continuous soy protein diet with the inclusion of lectins.

Eating a balanced healthy whole-foods diet prepared the right way is a more sensible answer than eliminating whole food groups in fear of lectins. The problem with lectins is not the healthy balance in which they occur with natural whole food but the extreme concentration of them that comes from processed and finagled modern foods. This is where the balance of something healthy becomes toxic and disturbing to the flourishing environment of the body.

Carbohydrates aren't villains, but the overconsumption of refined ones can be very dangerous. The kiss of sunshine is the sparkle of health, but too much of this good thing leads to sunstroke and poisoning. Likewise we just need to harness the right balance of lectins by avoiding modern junk and using some traditional food preparations that naturally lower their concentration. Don't hate lectins; just respect their limits.

Lectins are found in all food, so avoiding grains for the fear of lectins does not really help you. The lectins in grains and beans can be mostly deactivated by boiling them for fifteen minutes, but some lectins in veggies cannot be cooked out. Dairy products, nuts and seeds, and many fruits and veggies carry their own fair share of lectins, the highest levels being among the nightshade family such as tomatoes, eggplants, potatoes, bell peppers, chile peppers, and goji berries. Kale chips are a trendy health food and we love them, too; but they are probably more tainted with lectins than a well-prepared (soured or sprouted) whole-grain bread would be.

Don't give up the kale or the healthfully prepared grains for lectin's sake, though, as you would then have to give up most yummy spices, which also contain lectins. Oh, and you'd have to put chocolate and coffee on your elimination list while you are at it. All plants contain these defense mechanisms and we can trust our God who created us to eat them to also have equipped our bodies to DEAL!

Healthy Ways to Avoid Excessive Lectins

Do opt for sprouted, soaked, or fermented grains and beans, as these methods decrease the lectins in many of these particular foods. Modern hybridized wheat is an exception: Sprouting is not able to cause a significant reduction of lectins in this form of grain.

Do choose ancient grains such as einkorn, emmer, spelt, rye, farro, kamut, quinoa, and barley instead of modern hybridized wheat.

Do enjoy homemade gelatin-rich stock or supplement your diet with Just Gelatin or Integral Collagen that nurture the mucosa lining of the intestines and prevent negative lectin issues of the gut. There is a correlation between celiac disease and lowered levels of glycine, which is a potent amino acid in bone broth and gelatin supplements.

It is interesting that celiac disease is on the rise in our modern world, where the ancient practices of eating glycine-rich cuts of meat on the bone and making homemade stock are forgotten.

Do try to fall in love with okra, which has the ability to bind with lectins and make them harmless to the intestinal cells. Okra is a BFF of anyone with leaky gut or severe gastrointestinal issues.

Healthy Lectin Level Don'ts

Don't eat regular "wheat" bread from the grocery store. Modern wheat is hybridized to be way higher in gluten so is therefore higher in lectins.

Don't overdo store-bought Frankenfood low-carb wraps that are enriched with the lectin-rich bran of various grains to raise the fiber high enough to lower net carbs in a normally carbohydrate-rich item. While they are an option on plan, they should not be a part of every meal. Boiling destroys more lectins than baking and since these products are neither boiled, sprouted, nor fermented, their lectin levels will still be high.

Avoid when possible, or at least don't overdo, GMO foods like nonorganic corn. GMO foods have been modified for greater pest resistance, which consequentially heightens lectin levels above natural order. In saying this, if you want a little corn in your E-style Wicked White Chili and you can't afford the organic kind, don't stess, because the stress will harm ya just as much as the lectins will. You'll survive! Corn is not a big player in the Trim Healthy Mama life.

Foul Phytates?

Are phytates like those pesky tonsils that no one appreciated in the 1960s and '70s? They just got in the road and got infected, so "off with their heads?" Or could it be that they have a purpose? This will be our last discussion about imbalanced diets and then we are sooo done; hopefully we'll never have to speak of all this craziness again.

Phytates are mostly located on the outside of the germ in grains and their purpose is to nourish the plant embryo with phosphorus so it can germinate and flourish. Phytates are considered to be part of the "nasties" group, but let's bring in balance for the final time. In the human body phytates do have a purpose! They bind with metals in your body and they are very skillful in their line of work. Yay for phytates! Metals won't be nearly as harmful to you when phytates are around. But they also get name-called the "antinutrient" because they can bind to nutrients within your meal and prevent their absorption by your body. Boo for phytates, you foul things you!

Actually, this ability to bind with metals enables them to also eliminate some nasties from your body like the bad kind of cholesterol and triglycerides. Phytates in the human body are a potent and powerful antioxidant. They perform this talent by preventing ions such as iron and zinc from donating electrons that then become peroxides. Eventually this leads to dysfunctional lipids and excessive cholesterol levels. When viewed through a bigger lens, phytates are not as foul as their first mudsling suggests.

In a robust balanced diet the mineral pull of phytates is negligible. In Third World countries with extreme poverty, where people survive on rice, corn, or beans alone with nothing else to furnish the body, phytates are a bigger issue. Rather than blaming phytates for a lack of nutrition, it's more obviously the sad exclusion of other necessary nutrient-rich foods that is to blame.

We want you to be fully nourished, so encouraging you to prepare phytate-rich foods in more traditional fashions to help remove excess phytates makes some sense. But if you are a Drive Thru Sue and feel like giving up Your Trim Healthy Mama Plan because you can't imagine soaking your oats the night before, then don't throw in your towel. You aren't gonna die from unsoaked oatmeal or unsoaked lentil soup.

Here is a little feature that could make us even love a little bit of phytate from time to time (Serene the purist is almost choking as we type). Phytates also bind with amylase, which is the enzyme responsible for breaking down carbohydrates. When grains and tubers have their phytates attached, their insulin response is reduced by 50 percent. Whoa. You ain't foul no mo', phytates! But Serene wants to tell you to try to soak and sprout as much as possible to keep the natural balance in check.

DO YOUR BEST, DON'T SWEAT THE REST

Let's not make eating become something so difficult that regular folks are robbed of the satisfaction of knowing that they can attain a healthy diet without nitpicking up a storm or draining their last penny to do it. Where is their beacon of hope for a healthier life when all they read on the Internet are constant top-ten lists of what to avoid? It sounds impossible and miserable, so it causes many to simply give up. We need to make feasible healthy food choices and let God take care of the rest.

It is sad that natural food has now become a thing to fear. Eating should be a simple joy, not a source of anxiety. We have seen Drive Thru Sues who have never, ever stepped foot into a health food market have their health revolutionized, watch their inflammation markers go way down, get off all their medications, and find their Trim Healthy Mama "glow" through regular foods. If you keep away from the basic junk we listed earlier, then you are doing better than those who eat packaged organic high-glycemic food from the health food store.

Let's leave loonyville far behind and bask in the land of Food Freedom, where we always keep it simple and sane. We EAT, DRINK, and are MERRY without fearing the monsters in God-given foods.

Rant is officially OVA! Phew.

chapter 32

GET CONNECTED!

We're so excited that you are taking this journey of Food Freedom and sanity with us. Encouragement and community will help you stay on track. Many Mamas have started local Trim Healthy Mama groups in homes and in churches. You can meet up with other Mamas doing the plan, exchange recipes, share victories and challenges, and be one another's support systems. We soon hope to have study guides for groups to do together, but for now women are just sharing their personal experiences with one another and having a blast.

You'll also have wonderful support online at our website, www.trimhealthymama.com. There we have resources and teaching tools such as printable, searchable recipes, lots of cooking and question-and-answer videos by yours truly, additional menu ideas (along with a personal menu builder), helpful articles, support groups with official THM guides, and much more—all to help you streamline your Trim Healthy Mama journey.

But we need to stress again (otherwise we'll feel like salesy gals peddling wares and won't be able to live with ourselves): You don't HAVE to have a website membership for this plan to work. We are also launching a coaching program for those who want more personalized help and accountability, but you don't need a coach, either, unless you want one (many have begged us to get that program going as they long for one-on-one help).

The pages in this book will equip you with all the knowledge you need to be a Trim Healthy Mama. It was never our intention to go write a book and leave out important information so we could get thousands of people to give us some of their hard-earned money every month via a website. Repulsive! Mamas kept asking us for more Trim Healthy Mama in their lives. They wanted the extra resources, so we have worked hard on providing this for them.

Having said that, all the extra-fun help on the subscription side of our website has been priced at less than buying one cup of coffee per week—so enjoy it if you have a little bit of budget wiggle room or find a great certified Trim Healthy Mama coach in your area or online who can help you with your own unique challenges (once that program is up and running).

You can also find plenty of free support at our official Trim Healthy Mama Facebook page and in our Facebook groups, where Mamas discuss the plan and cheer one another on all day. These groups literally exploded on their own. They are safe, peaceful, encouraging places where Mamas can feel accepted and encouraged whether they are Drive Thru Sues or purists. There are plenty of other groups on the Internet where people debate issues all day, but we find that sort of thing tiresome and a big old joy buster. If we as sisters can call a truce with our differences—hey, there's hope for a group of women coming together and actually getting along. Other Mamas obviously feel the same way. These groups quickly became the size of cities, hundreds of thousands of women all talking about the way they do the plan without getting in one another's faces and all hot under the collar if they choose to take a different approach. Unheard of? Miracles do happen! Our amazing volunteer brigade of Trim Healthy Mama admins have been an incredible help on the Facebook groups.

After a while, though, it was evident we could no longer keep up with the volume of discussions posted in the main Trim Healthy Mama groups, especially the biggest one. The wall feed began moving too quickly. We essentially outgrew Facebook! Many posts from Trim Healthy Mama newbies got lost as soon as they were posted amid the high volume. We ended up having to move many of the official groups over to the website to control the pace of the Facebook groups' growth a little more and try to curtail the population.

The Facebook groups are still awesome places to hang out; you'll be inspired, find new recipes, and learn a thing or two from other women doing the plan. But despite our efforts to curtail growth, they are still large. So please don't feel hurt if your question gets missed or your response gets no comments. Posting a picture always helps gets some traction in the large groups; or find a local, smaller unofficial Trim Healthy Mama Facebook group where you can interact on a more personal level.

You can sign up for our free Trim Healthy Living Ezine at our website. That will come to your inbox every couple of months and contain articles from us, new recipes, tips, testimonials, and inspirational interviews with other Mamas doing the plan.

If you want to see and hear more from us two crazy sisters, we'll post up free videos on our YouTube channel every so often. We'll also be making many of the recipes from the *Trim Healthy Mama Cookbook* and other new recipes we come up with and be releasing those on the subscription side of our website. We'll also take your questions and answer them there, too, on video. In addition, check out our new radio show. Podcasts of that are available to listen to on our website.

We want to hear from you. Don't wait until you hit goal weight to share your story and your pictures with us. You're going to have many victories along the way and we want to celebrate them with you. We want to do a happy dance when you drop your first ten pounds . . . when you find yourself no longer a slave to sugar . . . when you have not lost anything on the scale for a month but you suddenly fit into the next size down . . . when you take that hike you never thought possible with the rest of your family . . . when your wedding ring fits again! Yeah . . . bring them on! Hearing from you makes all of this worth it for us.

Love you, Mamas!
See you soon,
Serene and Pearl

THE MEAL RECAP

THE SATISFYING (S) MEAL

1. More fat, less carbs (anchored with protein)
2. Keep grains, sweet potatoes, and most fruits away from S meals

Build an S Meal
- Choose your protein (lean or fatty meat or fish, whole eggs and egg whites).
- Add fats as desired.
- Add optional Fuel Pull foods like non-starchy veggies, berries, and certain forms of cultured dairy.

TIPS
- Good fats can also include egg yolks, butter, red meat, coconut oil, and red palm oil, in addition to extra-virgin olive oil, nuts, and avocados.
- Non-starchy veggies can be any vegetable that is not a root vegetable (such as potato, sweet potato, or carrot) or corn.
- Nuts are also allowed in moderation.

S-Friendly Meats: All meats and fish, both fatty or lean (grass-fed is best but not mandatory)
S-Friendly Eggs: Whole eggs and egg whites

S-Friendly Dairy: Heavy cream; half-and-half; butter; all cheeses; sour cream; double-fermented kefir; both full-fat and reduced-fat forms of cottage cheese, ricotta cheese, feta cheese, and paneer; plain Greek yogurt, both 0% (stick to half cup as dessert or full cup for main protein) and full-fat Greek yogurt; Laughing Cow Creamy Light Swiss cheese wedges (for non-purists)

S-Friendly Veggies: All non-starchy veggies. Don't go overboard with tomatoes, onions, peas, butternut squash, and acorn squash (small amounts of raw or cooked carrots can squeeze in here and there).

S-Friendly Fruit: Up to 1 cup of all kinds of berries (except blueberries—keep those to ½ cup); lemons and limes

S-Friendly Nuts and Seeds: Raw or roasted seeds or nuts in moderation, nut butters without sugar in moderation, nut and seed flours in moderation

S-Friendly Condiments: Most cold-pressed oils, mayo, mustard, horseradish, vinegar, salad dressings with 2 grams of carbs or less, olives, nutritional yeast, all broth and stock prepared without sugar, spices and seasonings, unsweetened cocoa powders, sugar-free ketchup, sugar-free hot sauce

S-Friendly Grains and Beans: Keep these foods away from your S meals, with the exception of very small garnish amounts to be used occasionally.

S-Friendly Healthy Specialty Items: Pristine Whey Protein Powder (www.trimhealthymama.com), Integral Collagen (www.trimhealthymama.com), Just Gelatin (www.trimhealthymama.com), Trim Healthy Mama Baking Blend (www.trimhealthymama.com), Pressed Peanut Flour (www.trimhealthymama.com), Gluccie (www.trimhealthymama.com), plan-approved sweeteners (www.trimhealthymama.com), Not-Naughty-Noodles or Not-Naughty-Rice (www.trimhealthymama.com), stevia-sweetened chocolate or a square or two of 85% dark chocolate, 100% cacao baker's chocolate, unsweetened nut milks such as almond, cashew, coconut, or flaxseed

S-Friendly "Personal Choice" Items: Joseph's low-carb pita or lavash bread, low-carb tortillas, fat-free Reddi-wip, Laughing Cow Creamy Light Swiss cheese wedges, Dreamfields pasta (limit to once a week)

THE ENERGIZING (E) MEAL

1. More healthy carbs, less fat (anchored with protein)
2. Your carbs include fruit, sweet potatoes, beans/legumes, and gentle whole grains like oatmeal or quinoa.

Build an E Meal
- Choose your lean protein.
- Add your carb (fruit, gentle whole grains, beans/legumes, or sweet potatoes).
- Add minimal fat (roughly 1 teaspoon); nuts and seeds are only used in garnish amounts.
- Add optional Fuel Pull foods like non-starchy veggies and berries and optional lean dairy.

TIPS
- Keep carbs to palm-size portions.
- MCT oil has the lowest amount of calories, so occasionally you can use 2 teaspoons with your E meal.
- Don't make corn your go-to grain.

E-Friendly Meat: All lean meats, chicken breast, tuna packed in water, salmon (look for less than 5 grams of fat), all other fish (not fried), venison, turkey breast, lean ground turkey or chicken (96% to 99% lean), lean deli meats (natural brands are best), ground meats with higher fat levels can be browned, drained, then rinsed well with hot water and used in E meals in up to four-ounce portions

E-Friendly Egg Sources: Egg whites

E-Friendly Dairy: 0% plain Greek yogurt, low-fat or nonfat regular plain yogurt, plain low-fat or nonfat kefir, 1% cottage cheese (2% should be fine for purists who cannot find a suitable 1%), low-fat ricotta cheese (up to ¼ cup), skim mozzarella cheese (in small amounts), reduced-fat or 2% hard cheeses (small sprinkles only)

E-Friendly Grains: Brown rice (up to ¾ cup cooked serving), quinoa (up to ¾ cup cooked serving), whole barley (up to ¾ cup cooked serving), farro (up to ¾ cup cooked serving), oatmeal (up to 1¼ cups cooked serving), whole-grain bread in sprouted, artisan sourdough, or dark rye form (2-piece servings); sprouted tortilla (1 large tortilla); sprouted whole-grain flours; sprouted whole-grain pasta; 4 Light Rye, Fiber, or Flax Seed Wasa crackers or 2 to 3 Multi-Grain, Hearty, Sourdough, or Whole Grain Wasa crackers (most Ryvita crackers are E-friendly, too); popcorn (4 to 5 cups of popped kernels spritzed with 1 teaspoon fat); baked blue corn chips

E-Friendly Fruit: All fruits in moderate quantities, e.g., 1 apple, 1 orange, 1 peach, 1 generous slice of cantaloupe; all berries in liberal quantities

E-Friendly Beans and Legumes: All beans and legumes including lentils and split peas—stick to 1 cup densely packed cooked, but more can be eaten when liquid is involved, i.e., chili or lentil soup

E-Friendly Veggies: All veggies except potatoes; enjoy sweet potatoes (1 medium) and carrots, both raw and cooked

E-Friendly Oils: 1 teaspoon oil (exception of occasional 2 teaspoons MCT oil)

E-Friendly Nuts: Limit nuts to garnish amounts or 1 teaspoon nut butters

E-Friendly Condiments: Mustard, horseradish, hot sauce, low-fat dressings, mayo (up to 1 teaspoon), soy sauce/tamari/Bragg Liquid Aminos/Coconut Aminos, all vinegars, all spices without sugar, unsweetened cocoa powder, nutritional yeast, all skimmed stock and broth (prepared without sugar)

E-Friendly Healthy Specialty Items: Pristine Whey Protein Powder (www.trimhealthymama.com), Integral Collagen (www.trimhealthymama.com), Just Gelatin (www.trimhealthymama.com), Pressed Peanut Flour (www.trimhealthymama.com), Gluccie (www.trimhealthymama.com), plan-approved sweeteners (www.trimhealthymama.com), Trim Healthy Mama Baking Blend (www.trimhealthymama.com), Not-Naughty-Noodles and Not-Naughty-Rice (www.trimhealthymama.com), unsweetened nut milks (avoid coconut milk for E meals)

E-Friendly "Personal Choice" Items: Joseph's low-carb pita or lavash bread (fruit, beans, or sweet potatoes will be needed for a proper E meal), low-carb tortillas (fruit, beans, or sweet potatoes will be needed for a proper E meal), fat-free Reddi-wip, Laughing Cow Creamy Light Swiss cheese wedges, Dreamfields pasta (limit to once a week, another carb source will be needed), light Progresso soups (another carb source will be needed)

FUEL PULLS

These are lighter foods that round out your plates and make your S and E meals complete (although they can be occasional full meals). They have low amounts of both fats and carbs.

Build a Fuel Pull Meal
- Choose your lean protein; limit meat to 3 to 4 ounces.
- Add minimal fat (roughly 1 teaspoon).
- Add other Fuel Pulls to your plate: generous non-starchy veggies, moderate berries, and optional lean dairy.

TIPS
1. Limit nuts to garnish amounts or 1 teaspoon nut butters.
2. Examples of non-starchy veggies: asparagus, broccoli, cabbage, cauliflower, cucumber, eggplant, mushrooms, jicama, okra, tomatoes, yellow squash, zucchini, sugar snap peas, okra, onions, green onions, leeks, parsley, all leafy greens, radishes, spaghetti squash, pumpkin, chestnuts, baby Chinese corn
3. Fuel Pulls shine as slimming snacks and desserts and help you avoid accidental Crossovers.

Fuel Pull–Friendly Meat: All lean meats, chicken breast, tuna packed in water, salmon (look for less than 5 grams of fat), all other fish (not fried), venison, turkey breast, lean ground turkey or chicken (96% to 99% lean), lean deli meats (natural brands are best), ground meats with higher fat levels can be browned, drained, then rinsed well with hot water and used in FP meals in up to 3- to 4-ounce portions

Fuel Pull–Friendly Egg Sources: Egg whites

Fuel Pull–Friendly Dairy: 0% plain Greek yogurt, double-fermented nonfat kefir, 1% cottage cheese, low-fat ricotta cheese (up to ¼ cup), skim mozzarella cheese (in small amounts), reduced-fat 2% hard cheeses (small sprinkles only)

Fuel Pull–Friendly Veggies: All non-starchy veggies. Avoid potatoes, corn, sweet potatoes, and turnips.

Fuel Pull–Friendly Fruit: Up to 1 cup of all kinds of berries, lemons, and limes can be used, but keep blueberries to ½ cup.

Fuel Pull–Friendly Grains and Beans: 2 Light Rye, Fiber, or Flax Seed Wasa crackers or 2 Sesame Ryvita crackers; up to ¼ cup beans or oats occasionally (not in every Fuel Pull meal)

Fuel Pull–Friendly Oils: 1 teaspoon oil (exception of occasional 2 teaspoons MCT oil)

Fuel Pull–Friendly Condiments: Mustard, horseradish sauce, hot sauce, low-fat dressings, mayo (up to 1 teaspoon), soy sauce/tamari/Bragg Liquid Aminos/Coconut Aminos, all vinegars, all sugar-free spices, unsweetened cocoa powder, skimmed broth or stock prepared without sugar

Fuel Pull–Friendly Healthy Specialty Items: Pristine Whey Protein Powder (www.trimhealthymama.com), Integral Collagen (www.trimhealthymama .com), Just Gelatin (www.trimhealthymama.com), Gluccie (www.trimhealthy mama.com), plan-approved sweeteners (www.trimhealthymama.com), Trim Healthy Mama Baking Blend (www.trimhealthymama.com), Pressed Peanut Flour (www.trimhealthymama.com), Not-Naughty-Noodles and Not-Naughty-Rice (www.trimhealthymama.com), unsweetened nut milks (avoid coconut milk for FP)

Fuel Pull–Friendly Personal Choice Items: Joseph's low-carb pita or lavash bread, low-carb tortillas, fat-free Reddi-wip, Laughing Cow Creamy Light Swiss cheese wedges, light Progresso soups (avoid chowder versions)

CROSSOVERS (XO)

Crossovers merge the two fuels of fats and carbs for healthy tandem fueling. They keep to the E guidelines of carbs and add as many fats as desired.

Build a Crossover Meal
- Choose your protein (lean or fatty meat or fish, whole eggs and egg whites, or certain cultured dairy products).
- Add fats as desired (even if your protein source contains fat, other fats can be added).

- Add your carb in E-meal-safe amounts (fruit, gentle whole grains, beans/legumes, or sweet potatoes).
- Add optional Fuel Pull foods to your plate (non-starchy veggies, berries, and cultured dairy).

TIPS

1. People with extremely high metabolisms and healthy growing children will do well with mostly Crossover meals.

2. Pregnant and nursing women, as well as Maintenance Mamas, will benefit from including some Crossover meals.

S HELPERS (SH)

Add a little carb to your S meal for pleasure's sake, but not enough that it becomes a Crossover.

TIP

People who may not be used to eating meals with lower amounts of carbs, or people who suffer with hypoglycemia, may at first need S Helpers to help their bodies gently adapt to the pure S meal.

Same Foods List as S Meals (with these additional options)
⅓ to ½ cup quinoa
¼ cup brown rice
⅓ to ½ cup oatmeal
⅓ to ½ cup beans or lentils
½ piece of fruit like an apple or orange
½ medium sweet potato
1 piece of whole-grain sprouted, dark rye, or artisan sourdough toast
½ sprouted wrap or tortilla

index

VALIANT | JODY HOUSER | PERE PÉREZ
MARGUERITE SAUVAGE | COLLEEN DORAN

#1

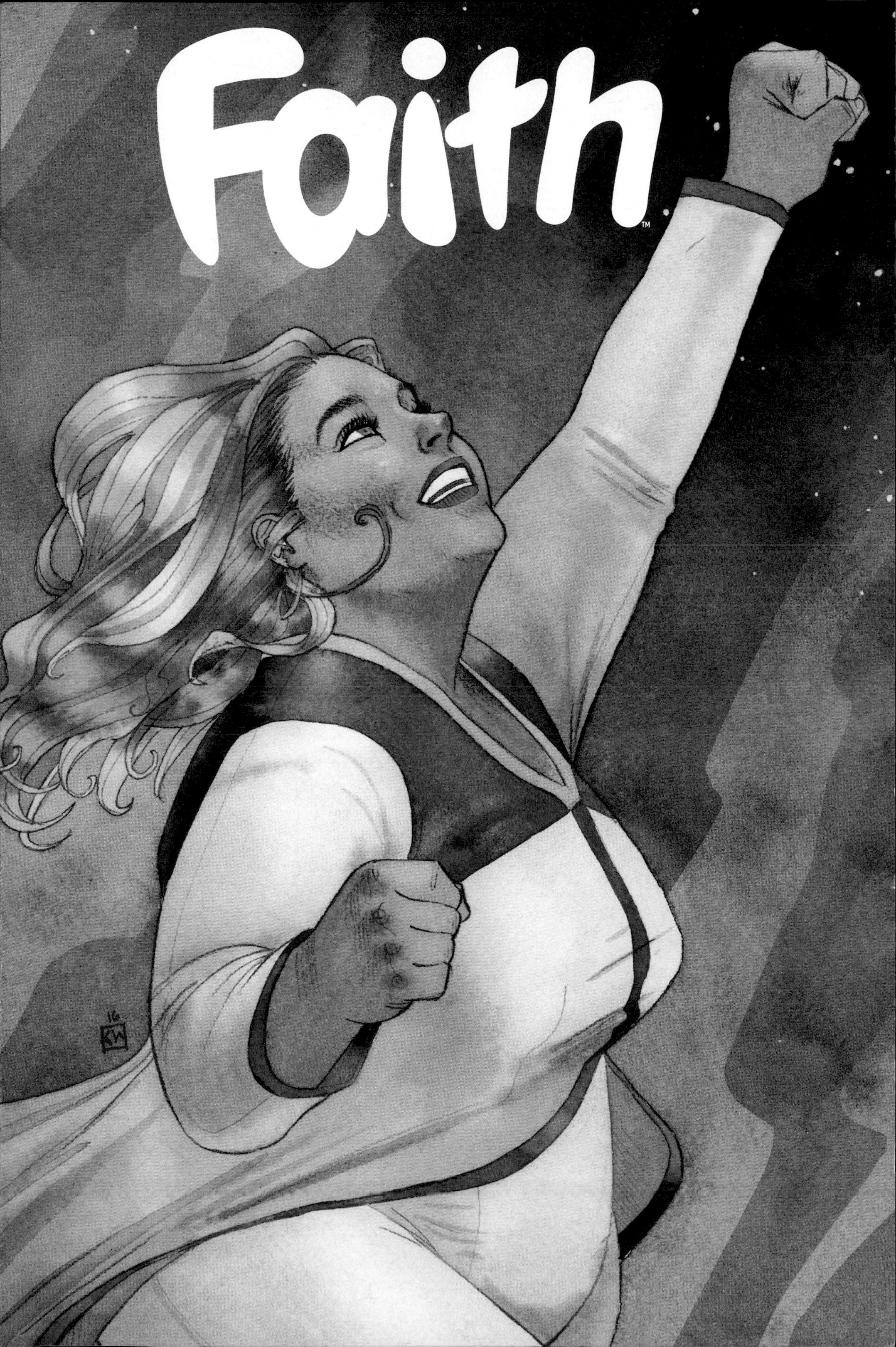

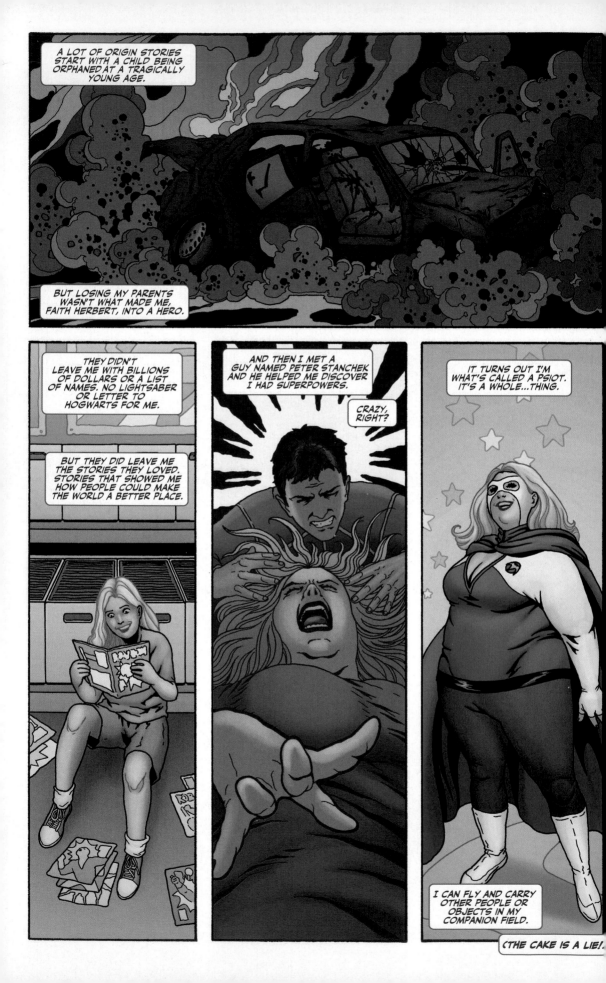

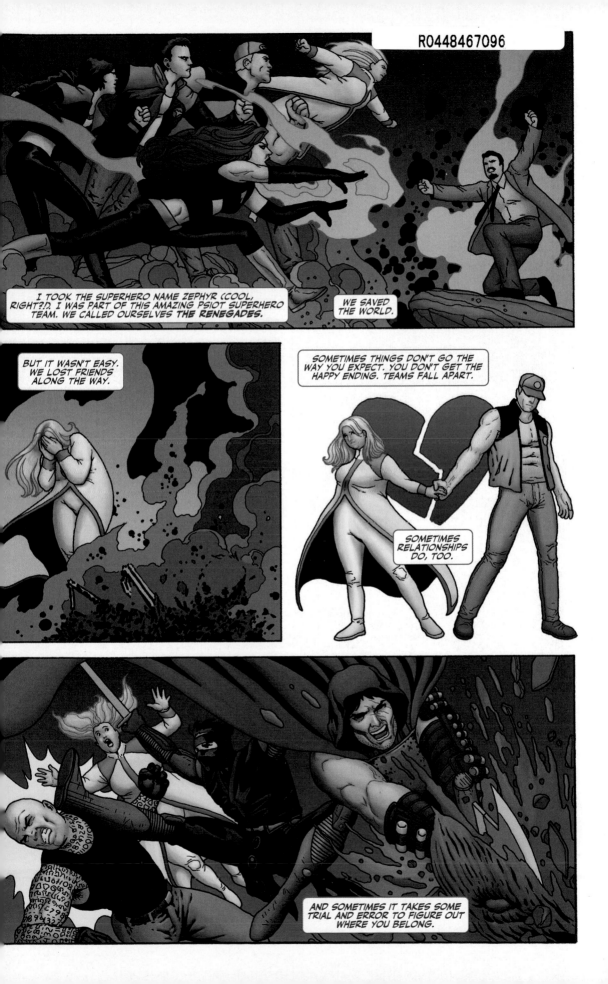

I TOOK THE SUPERHERO NAME ZEPHYR (COOL, RIGHT?). I WAS PART OF THIS AMAZING PSIOT SUPERHERO TEAM. WE CALLED OURSELVES THE RENEGADES.

WE SAVED THE WORLD.

BUT IT WASN'T EASY. WE LOST FRIENDS ALONG THE WAY.

SOMETIMES THINGS DON'T GO THE WAY YOU EXPECT. YOU DON'T GET THE HAPPY ENDING. TEAMS FALL APART.

SOMETIMES RELATIONSHIPS DO, TOO.

AND SOMETIMES IT TAKES SOME TRIAL AND ERROR TO FIGURE OUT WHERE YOU BELONG.

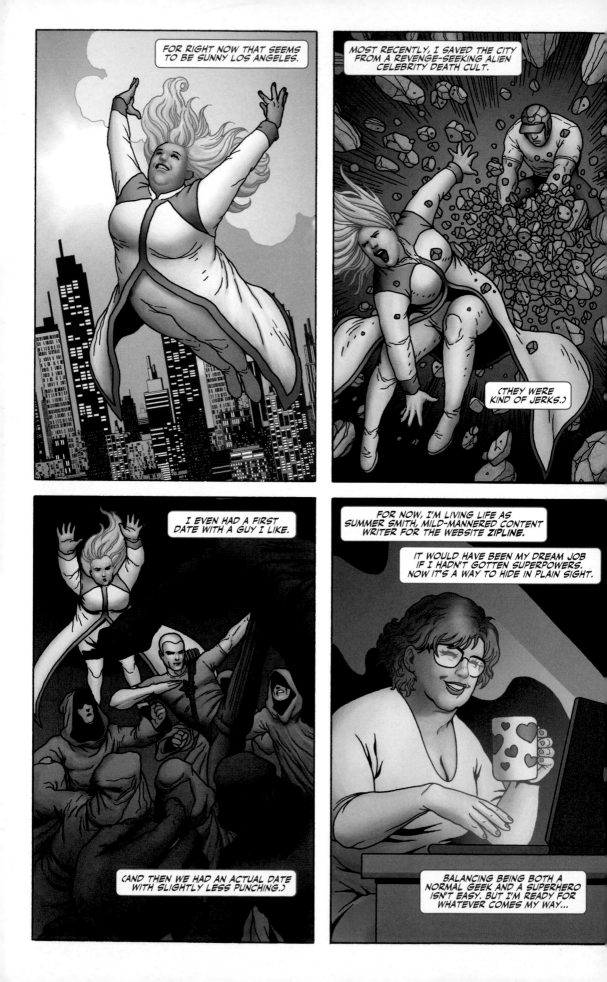

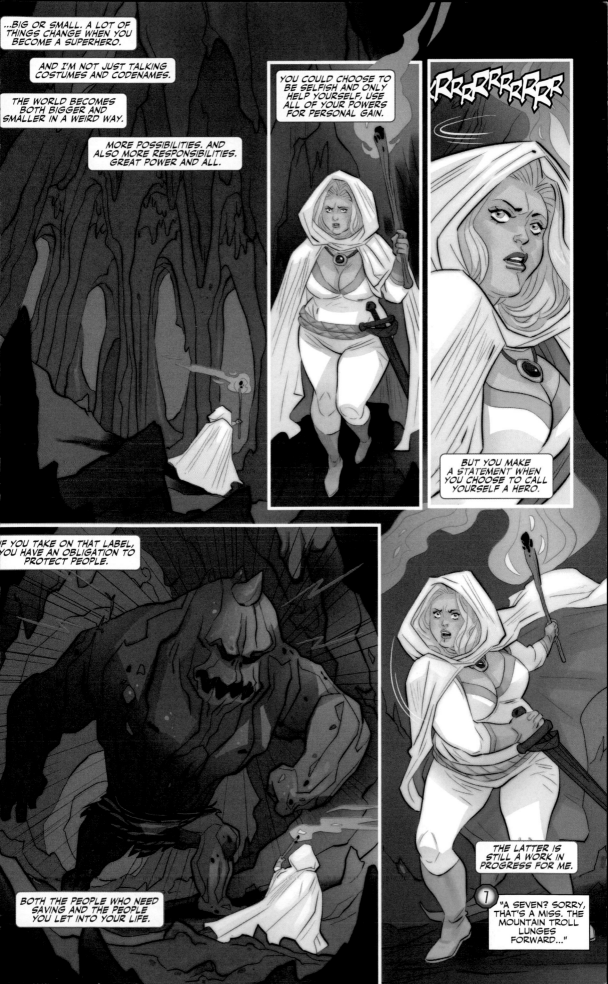

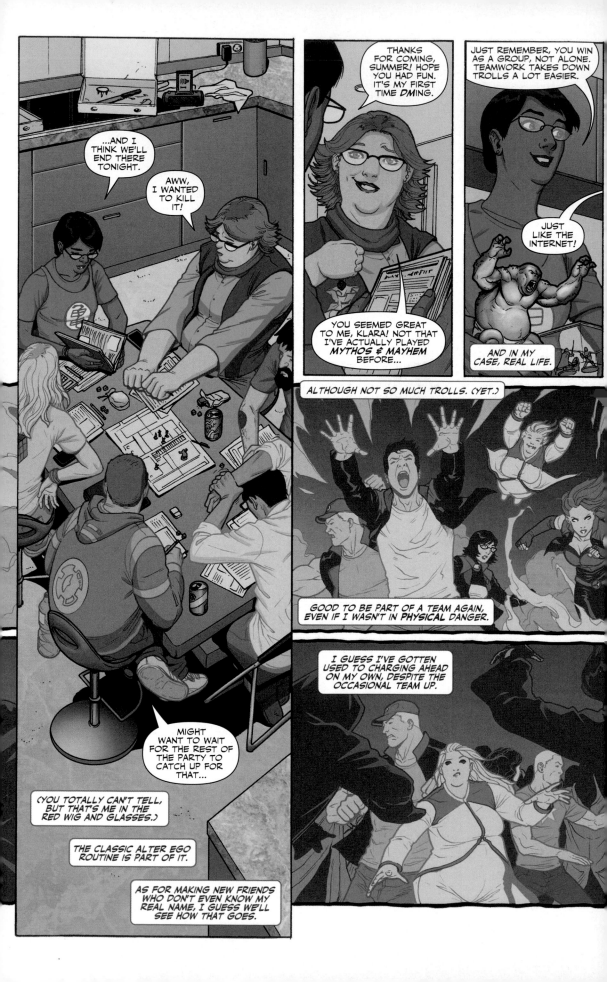

...AND I THINK WE'LL END THERE TONIGHT.

AWW, I WANTED TO KILL IT!

MIGHT WANT TO WAIT FOR THE REST OF THE PARTY TO CATCH UP FOR THAT...

(YOU TOTALLY CAN'T TELL, BUT THAT'S ME IN THE RED WIG AND GLASSES.)

THE CLASSIC ALTER EGO ROUTINE IS PART OF IT.

AS FOR MAKING NEW FRIENDS WHO DON'T EVEN KNOW MY REAL NAME, I GUESS WE'LL SEE HOW THAT GOES.

THANKS FOR COMING, SUMMER! HOPE YOU HAD FUN. IT'S MY FIRST TIME DMING.

YOU SEEMED GREAT TO ME, KLARA! NOT THAT I'VE ACTUALLY PLAYED MYTHOS & MAYHEM BEFORE...

JUST REMEMBER, YOU WIN AS A GROUP, NOT ALONE. TEAMWORK TAKES DOWN TROLLS A LOT EASIER.

JUST LIKE THE INTERNET!

AND IN MY CASE, REAL LIFE.

ALTHOUGH NOT SO MUCH TROLLS. (YET.)

GOOD TO BE PART OF A TEAM AGAIN, EVEN IF I WASN'T IN PHYSICAL DANGER.

I GUESS I'VE GOTTEN USED TO CHARGING AHEAD ON MY OWN, DESPITE THE OCCASIONAL TEAM UP.

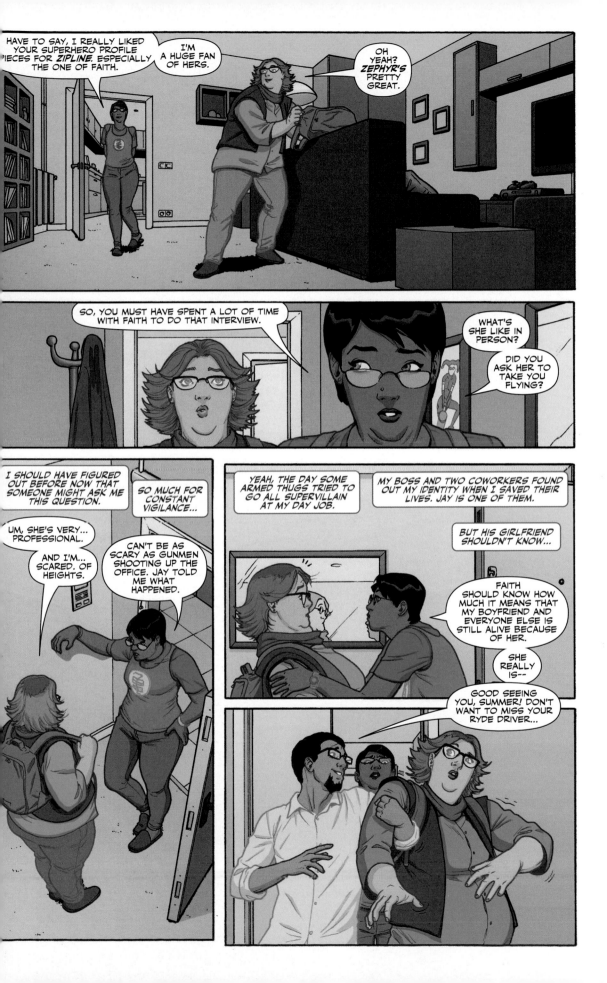

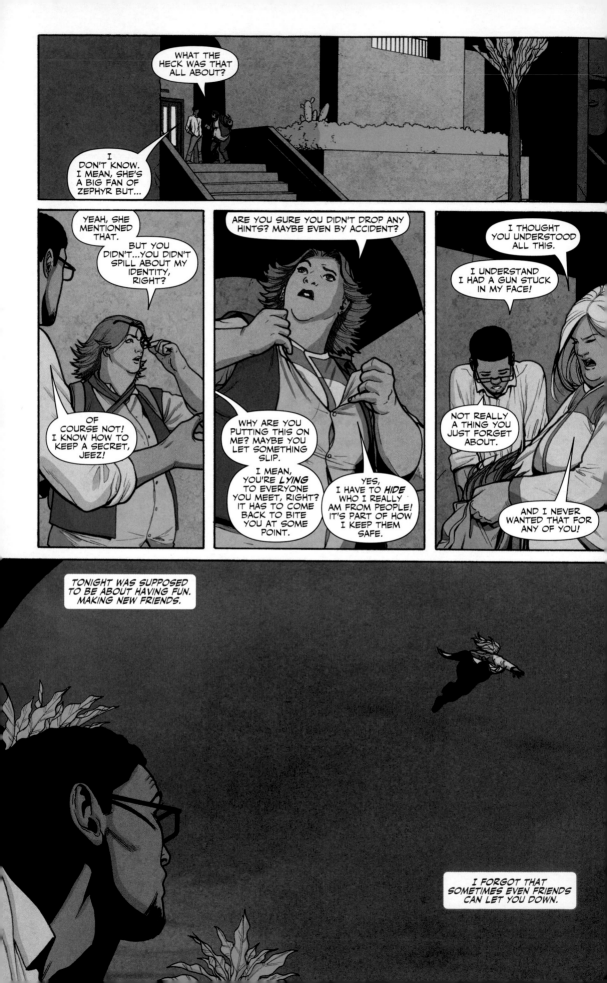

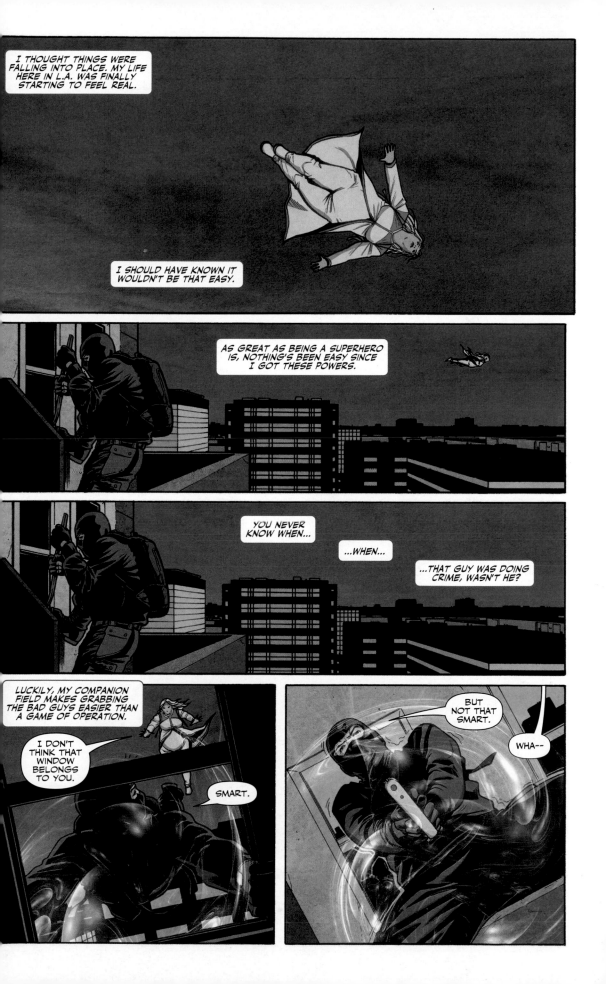

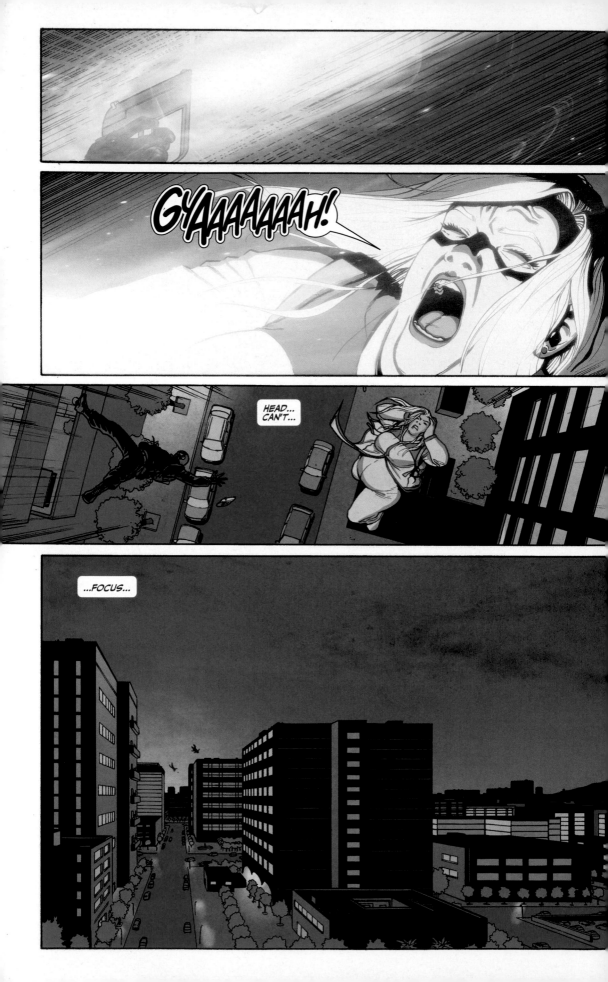

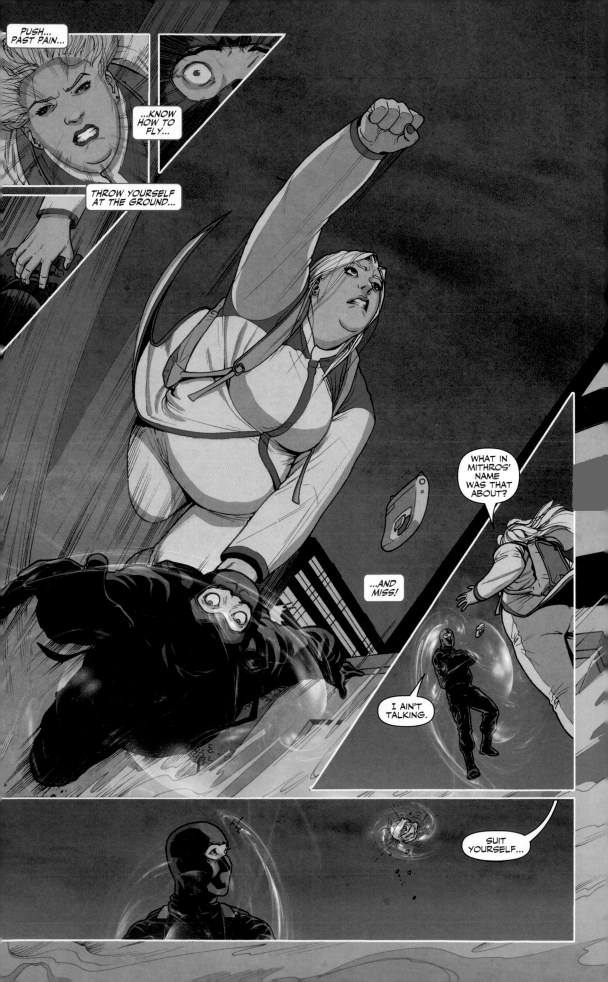

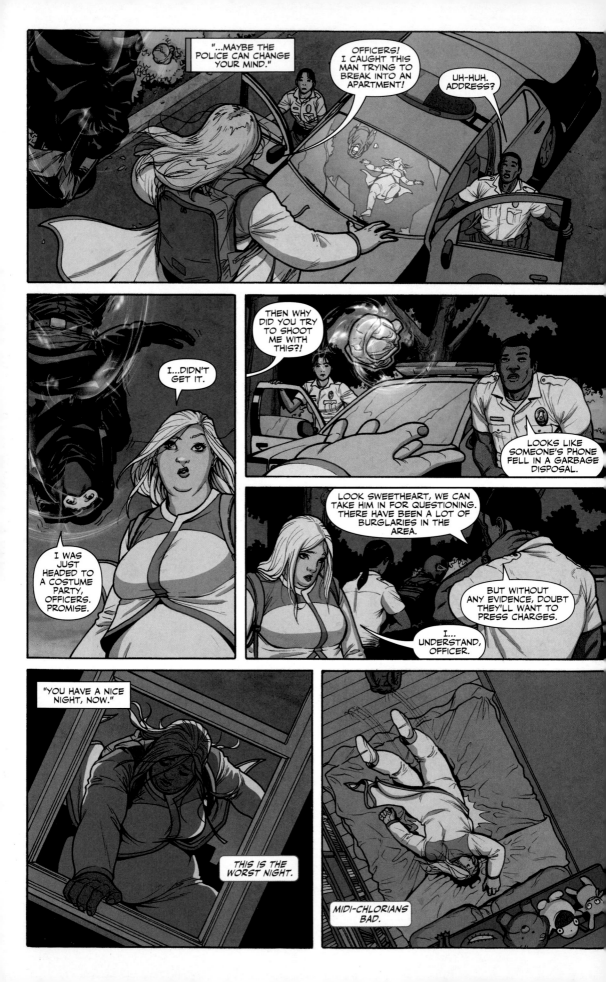

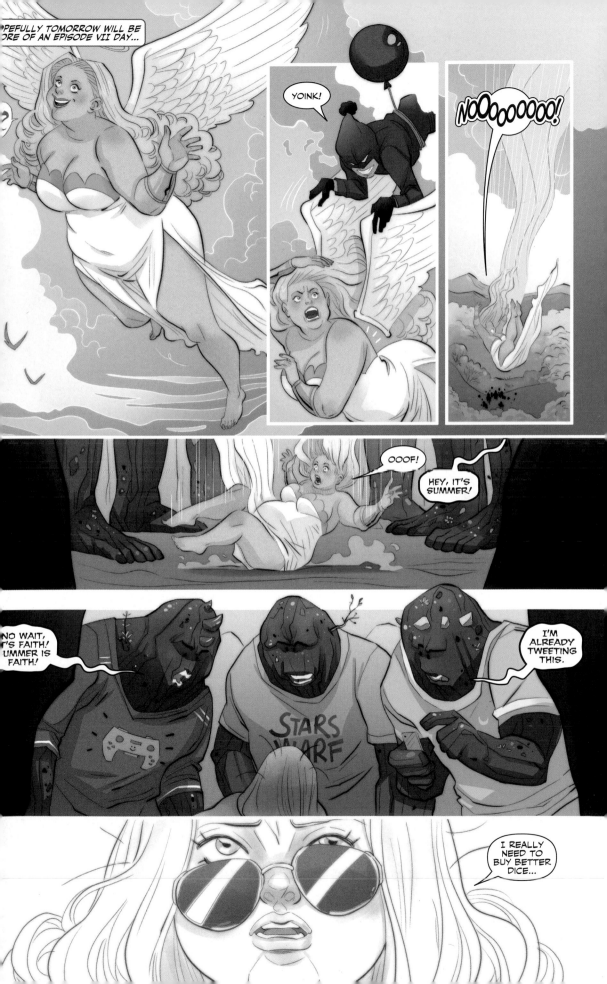

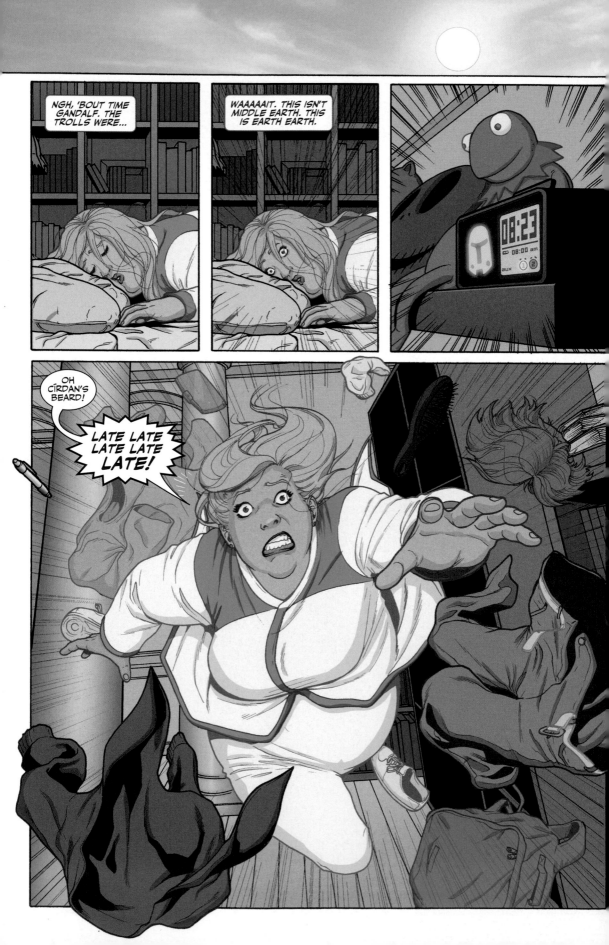

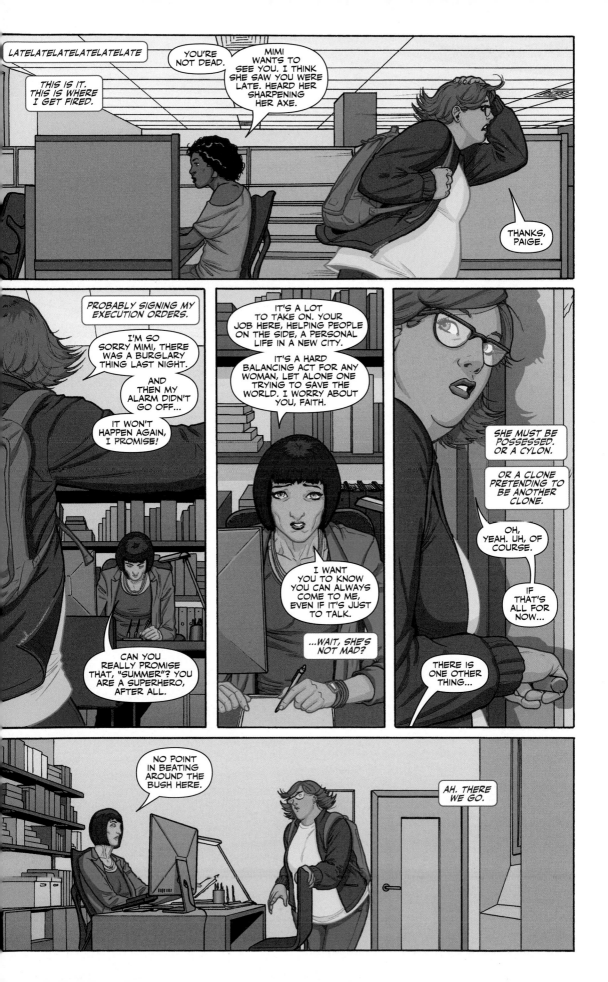

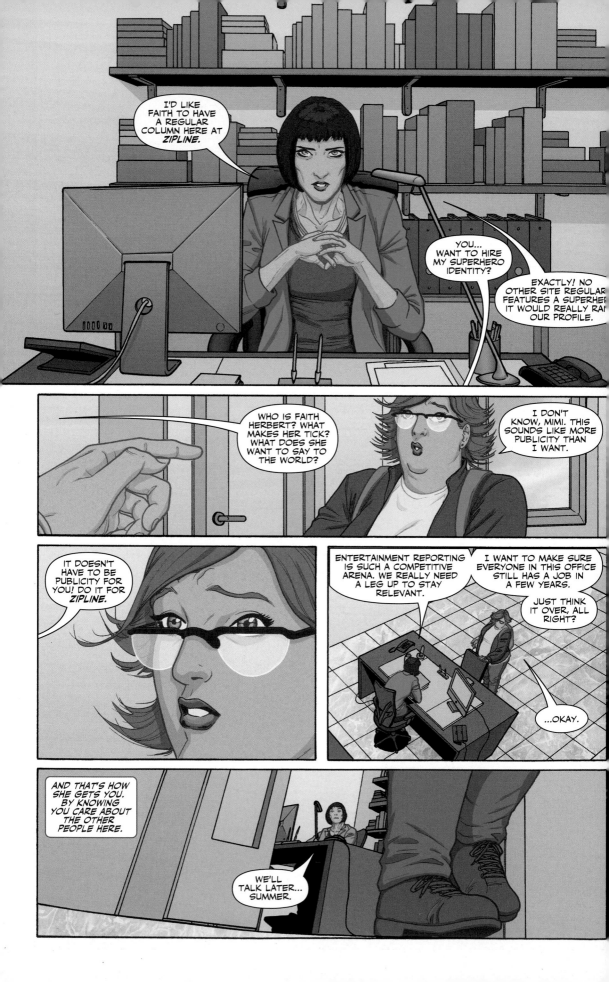

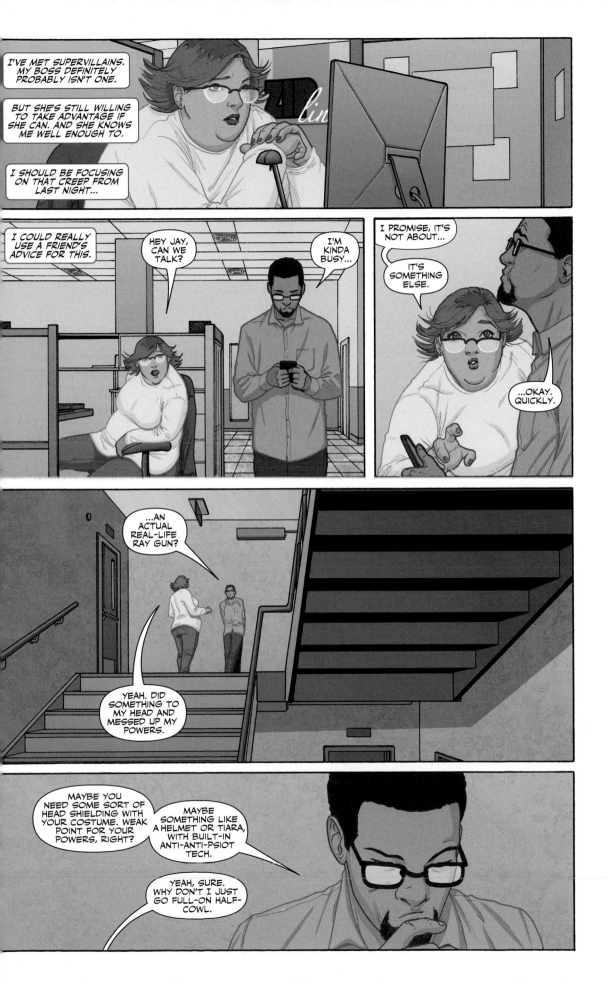

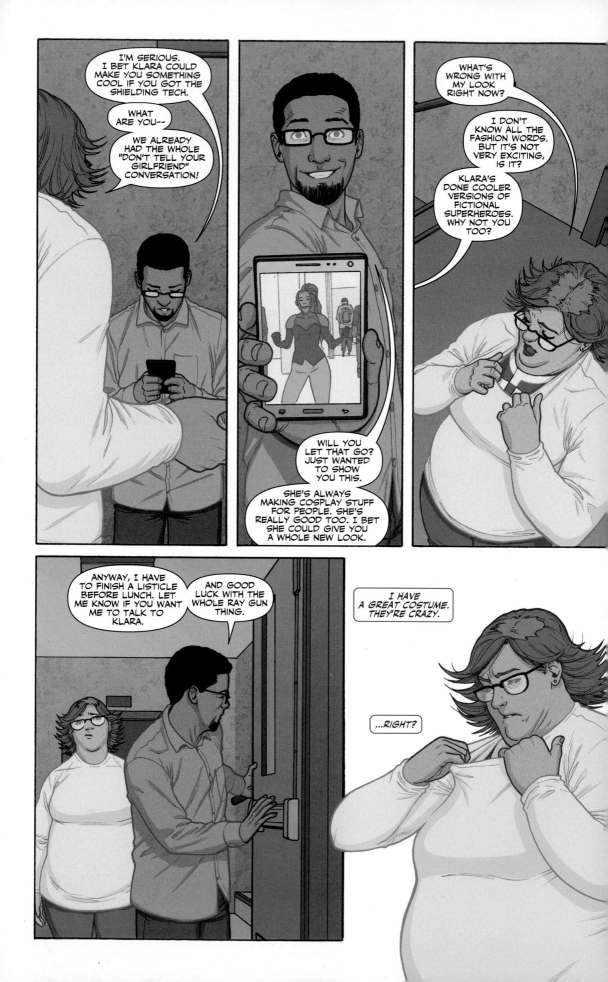

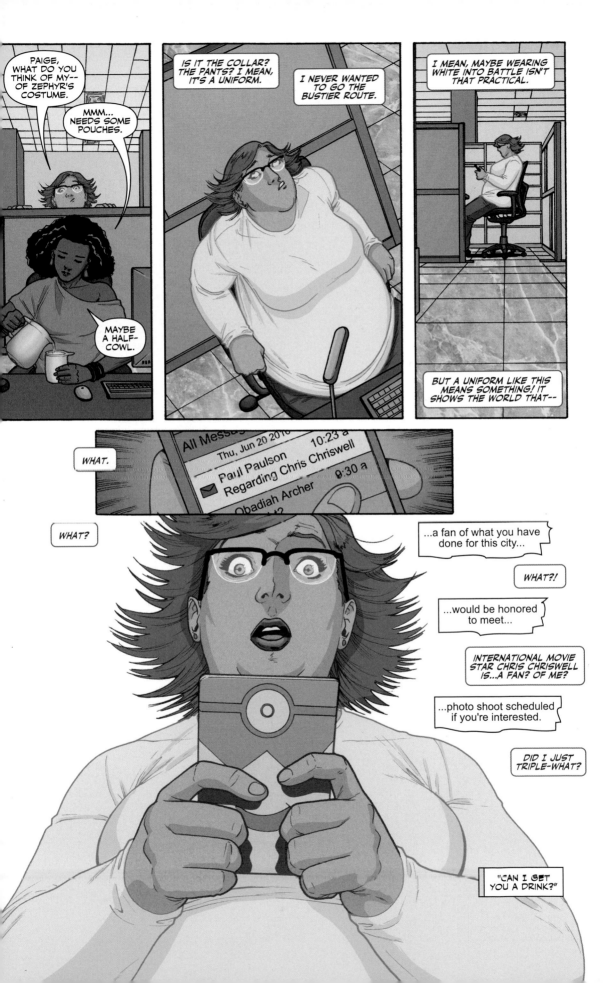

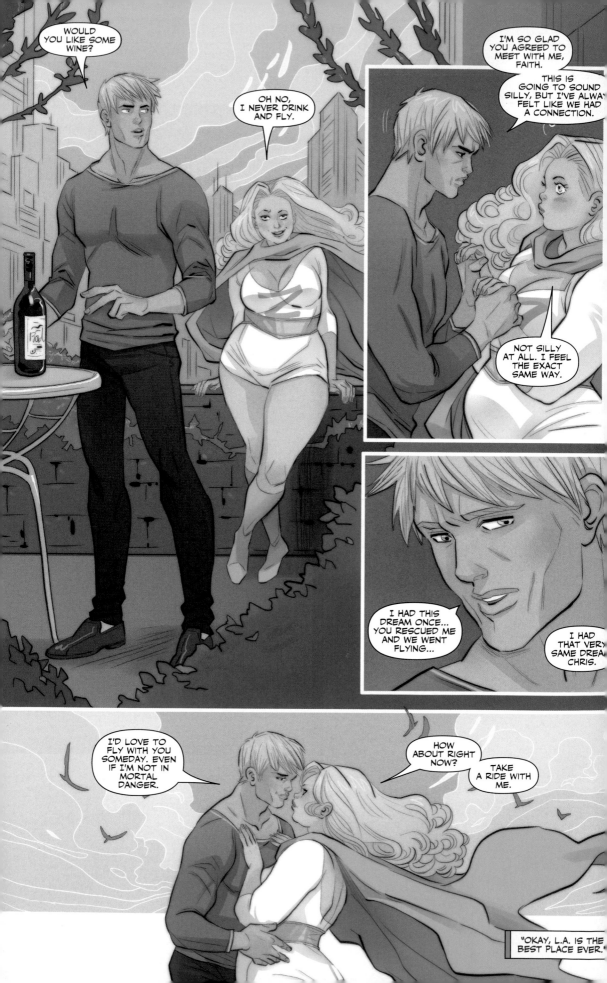

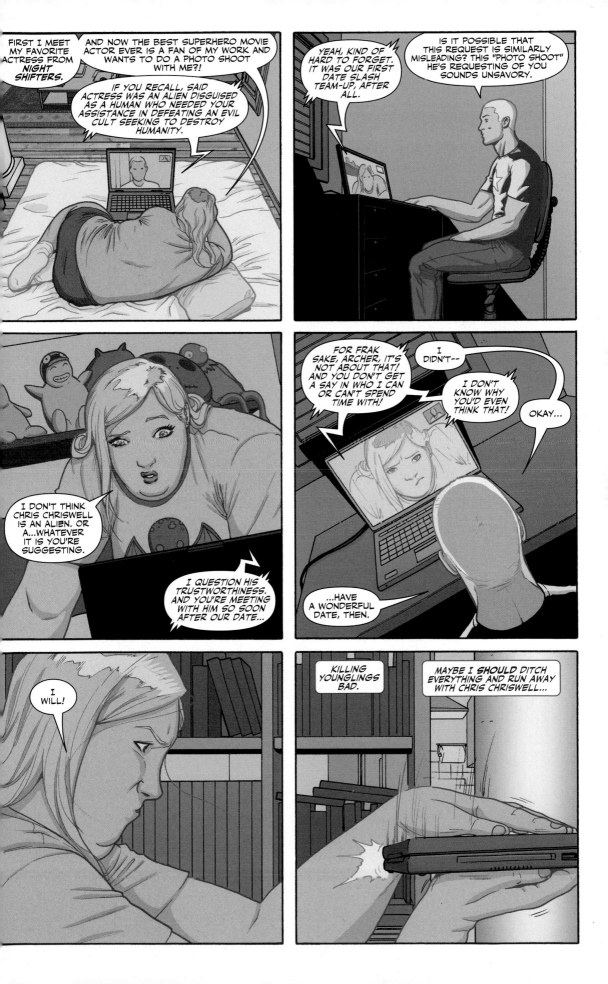

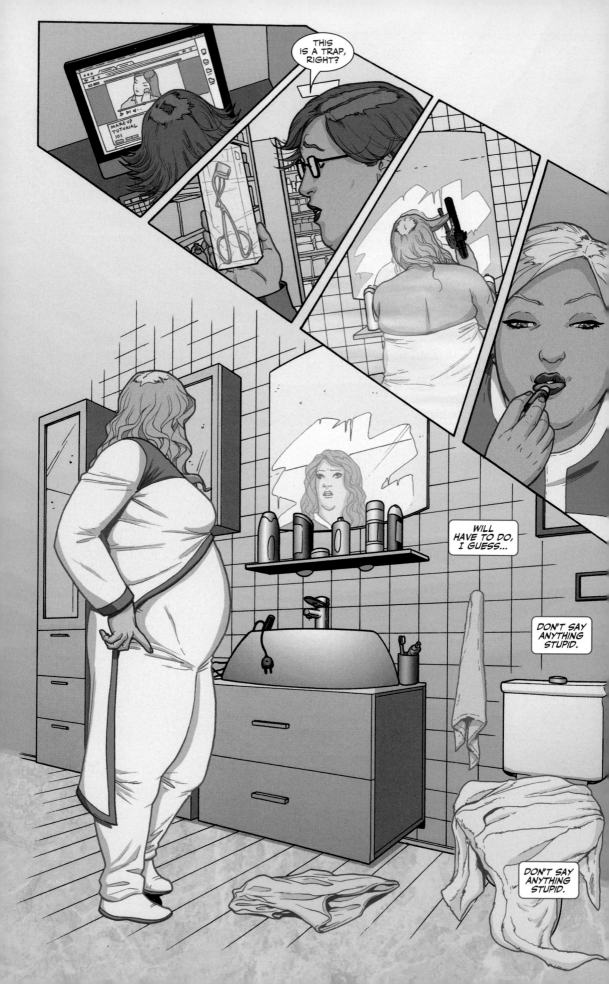

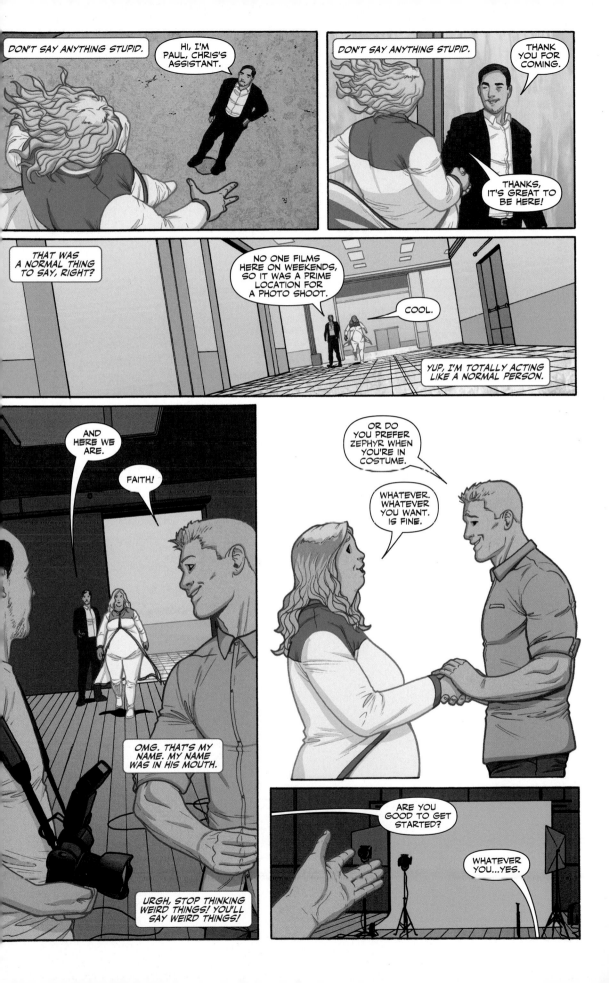

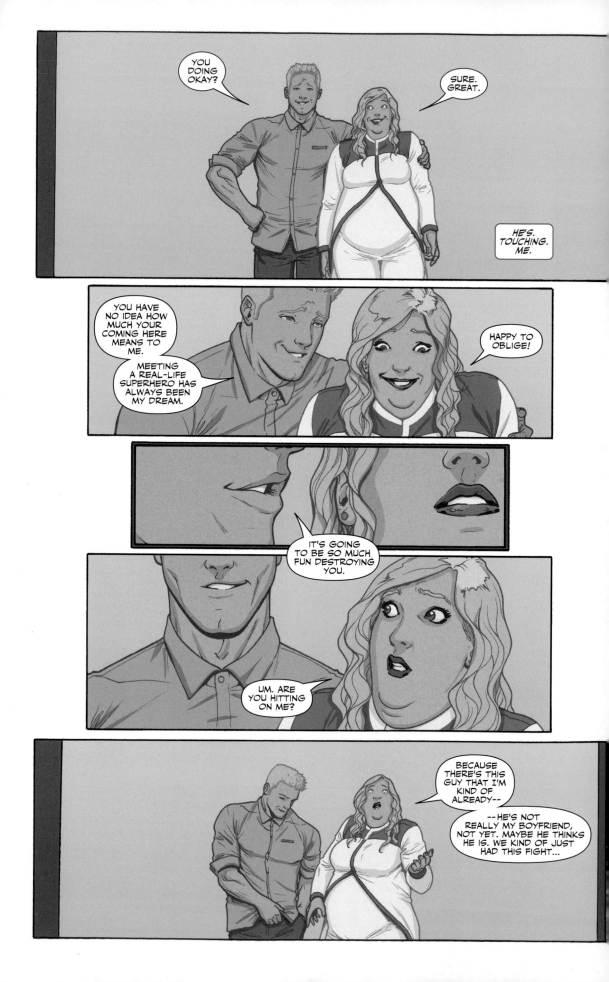

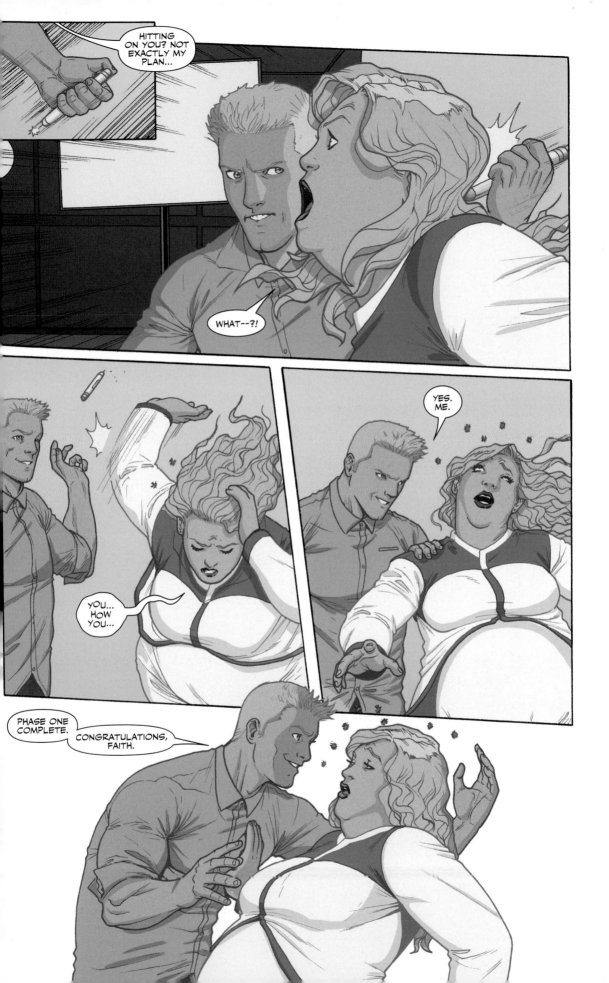

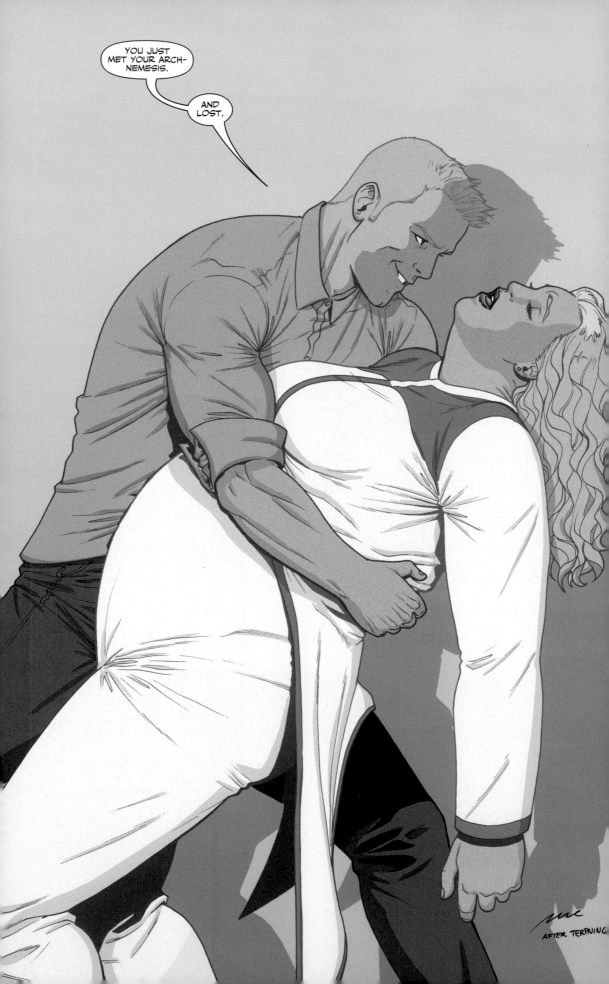

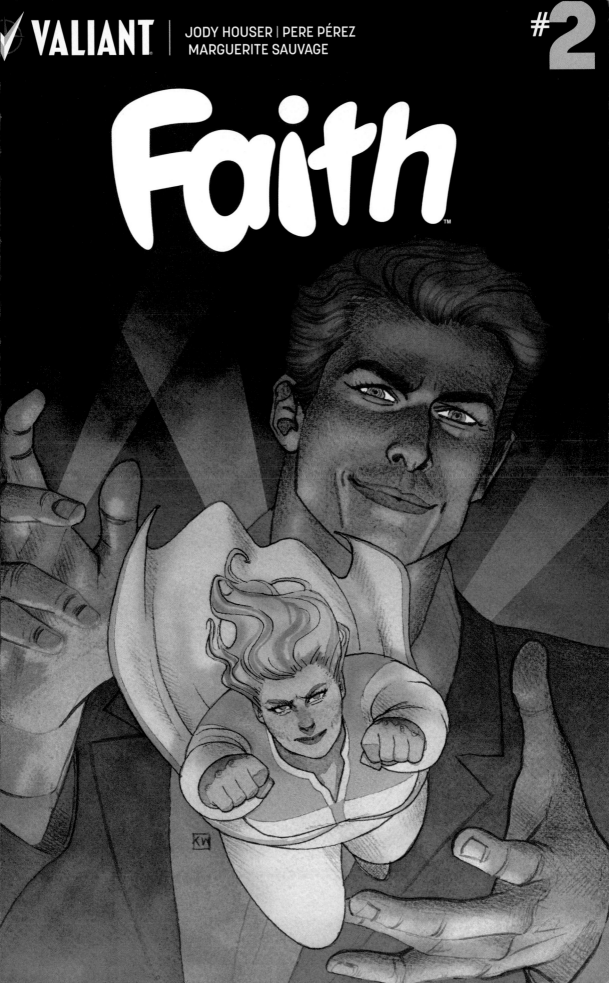

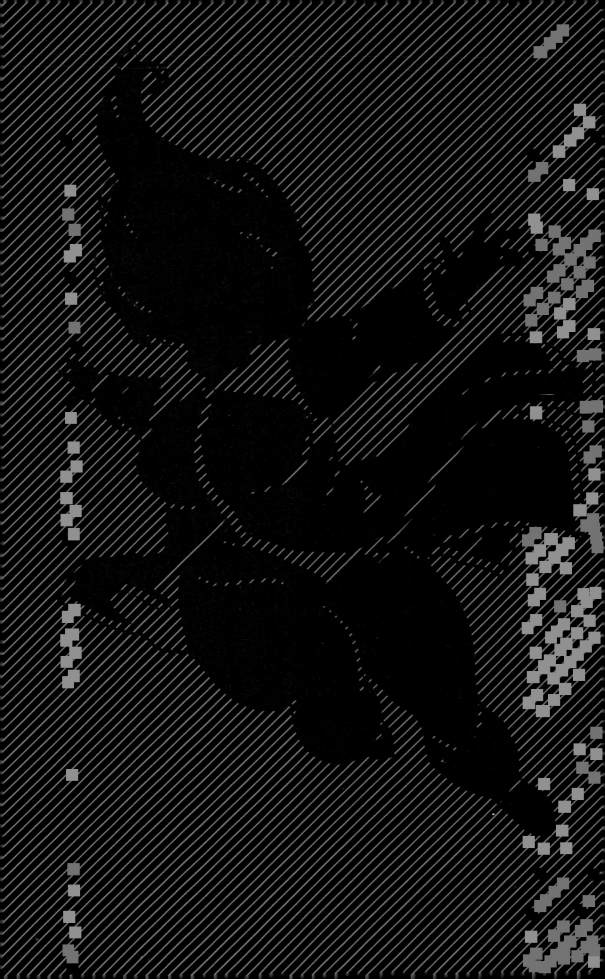

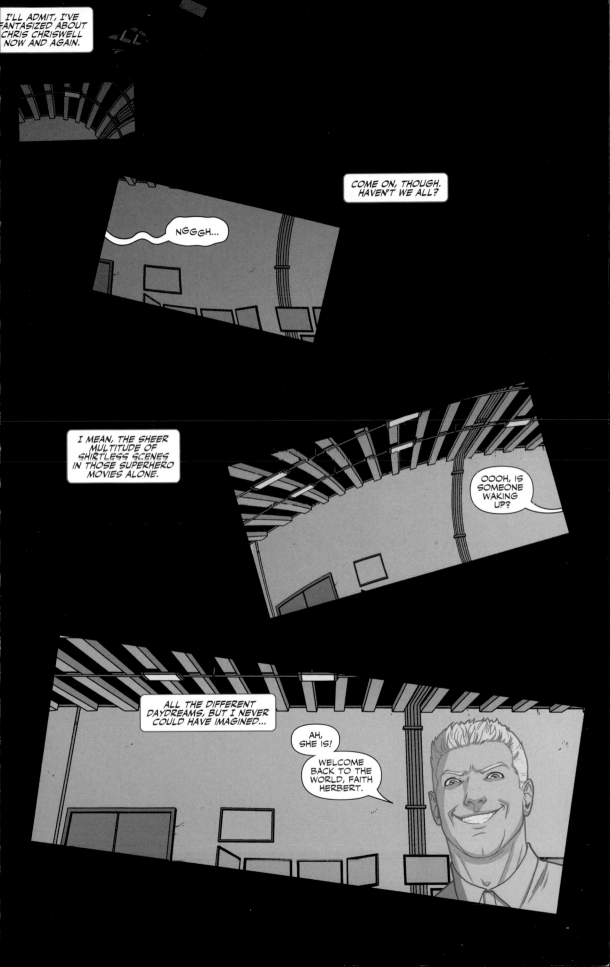

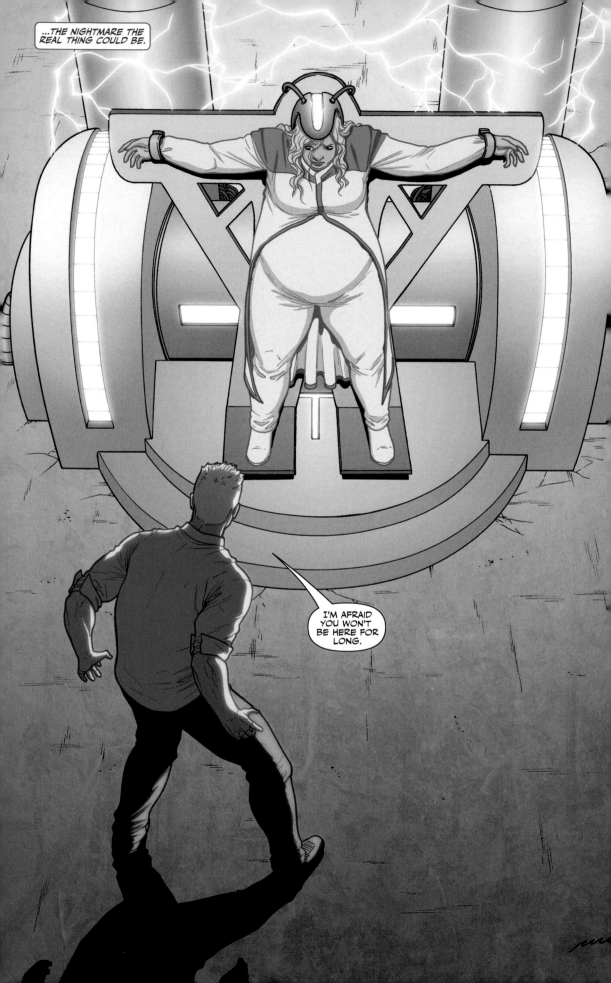

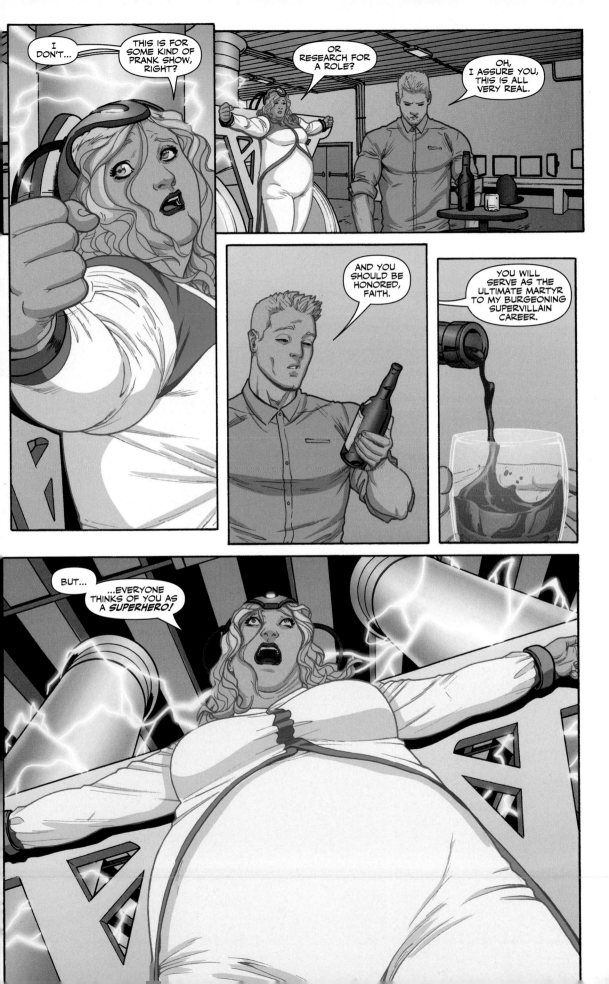

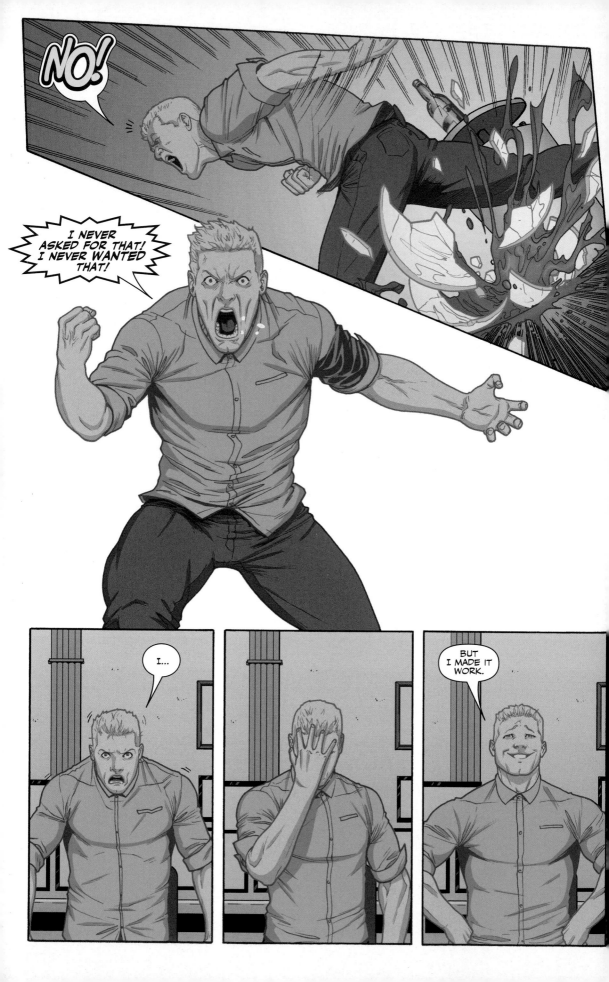

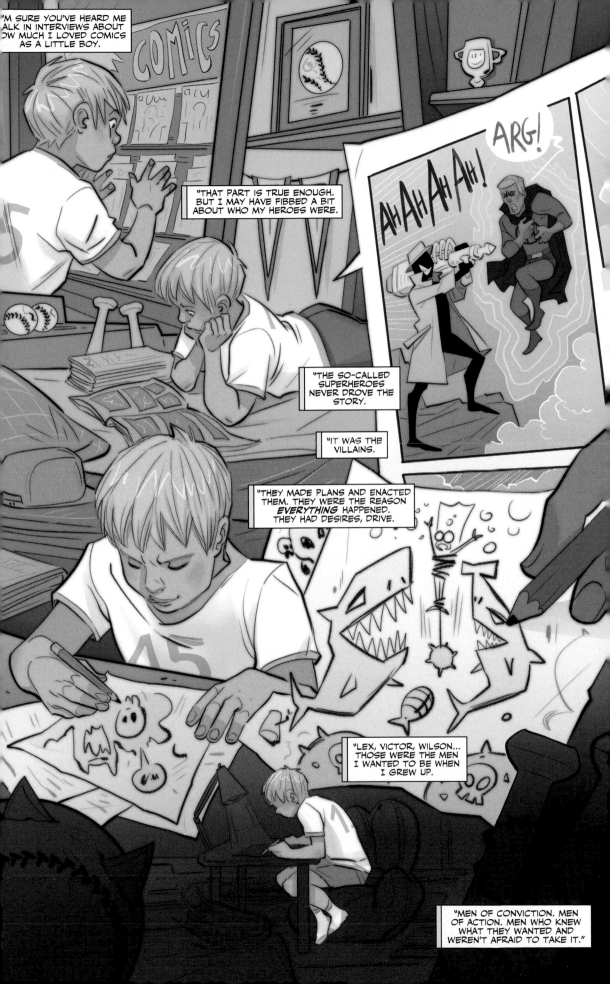

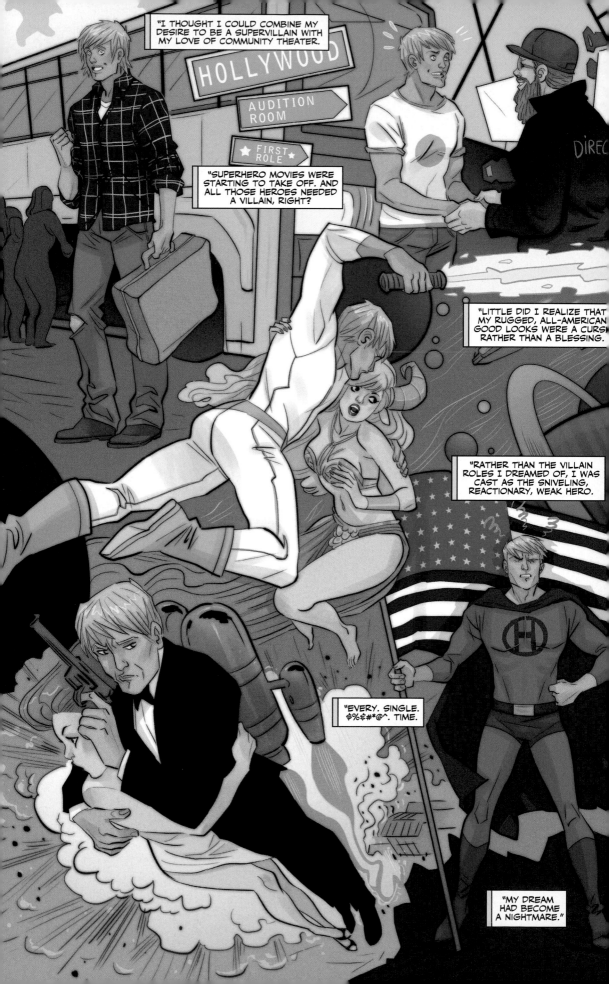

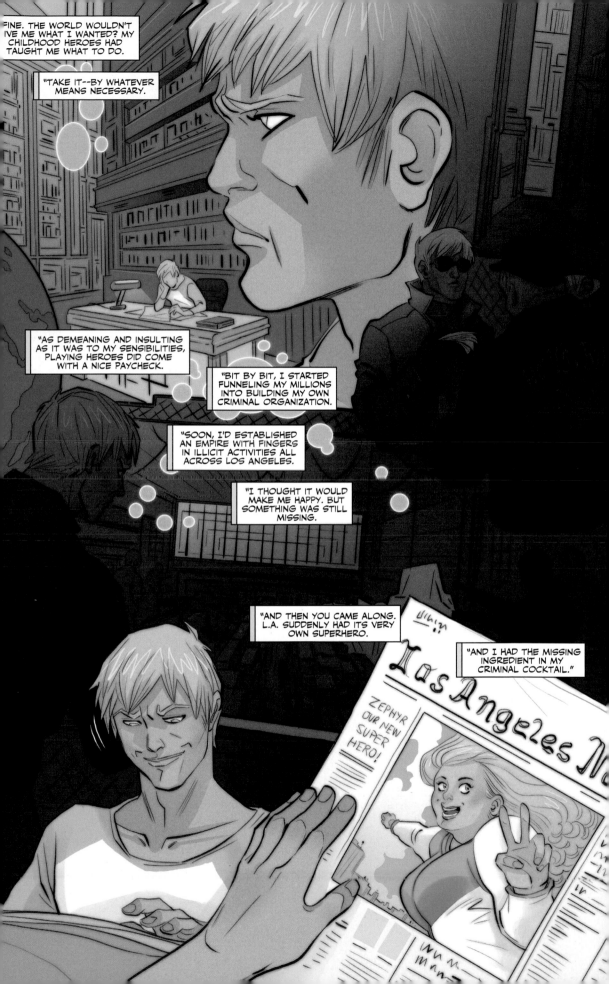

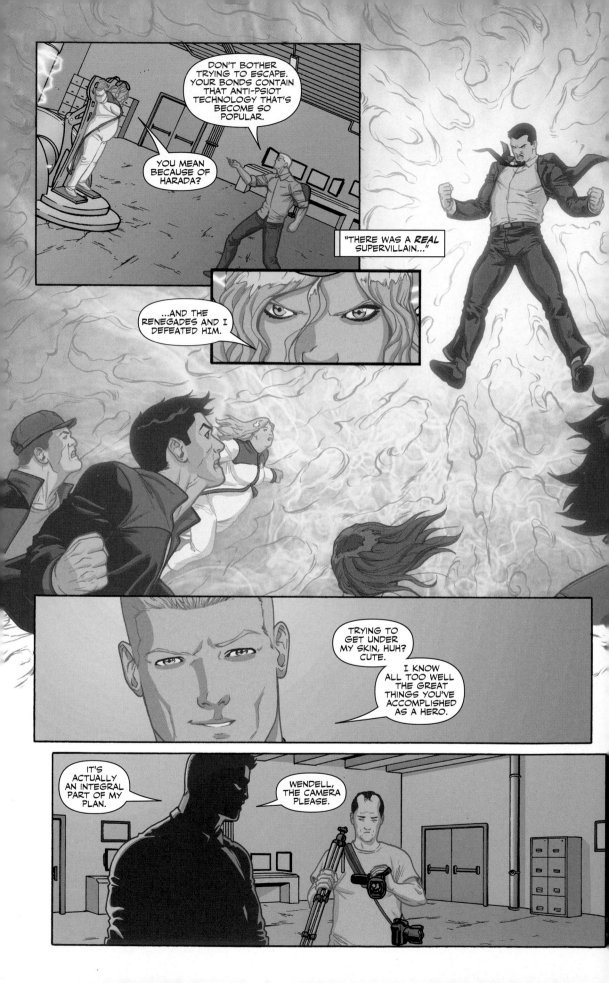

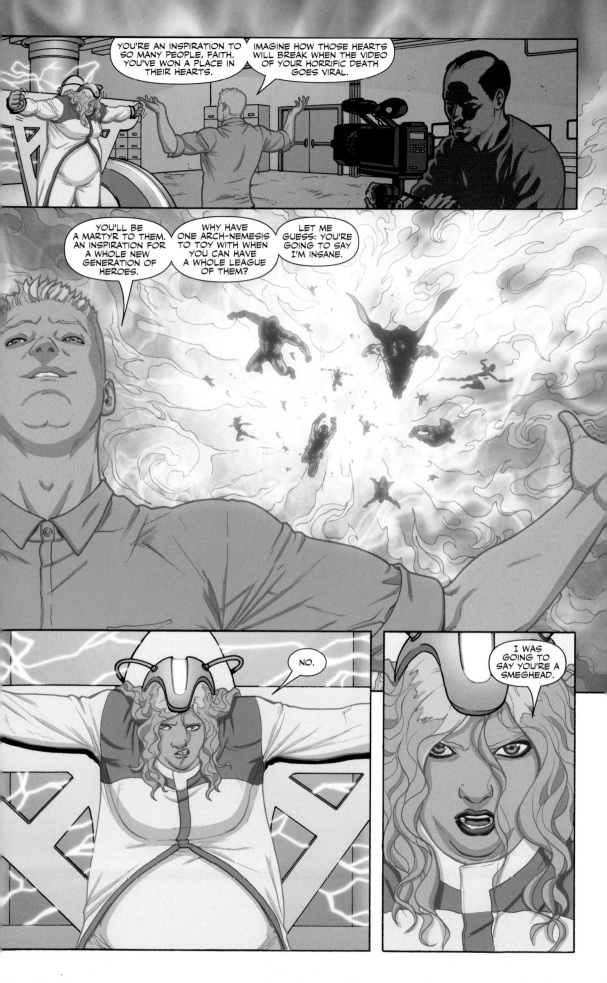

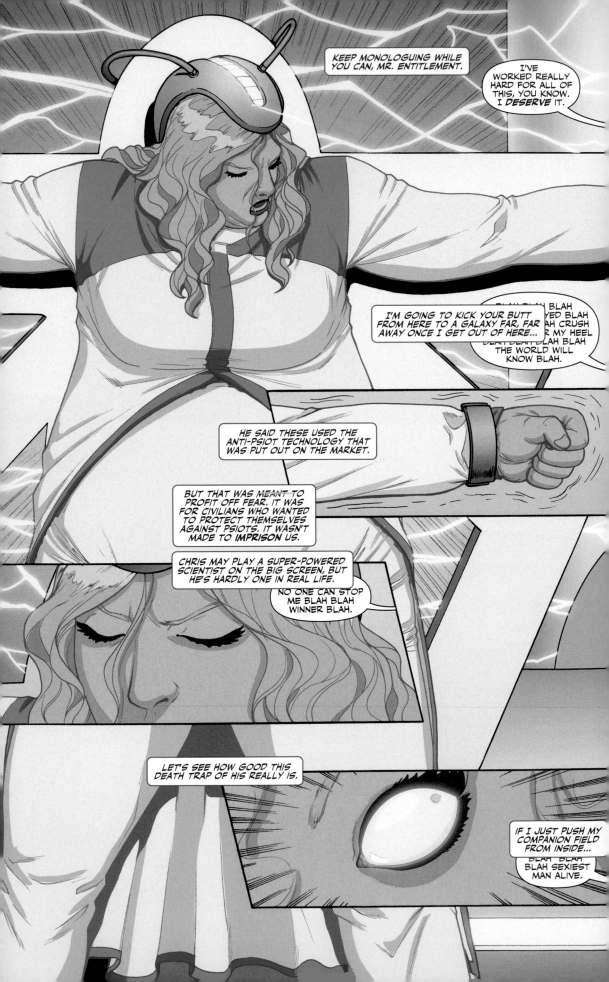

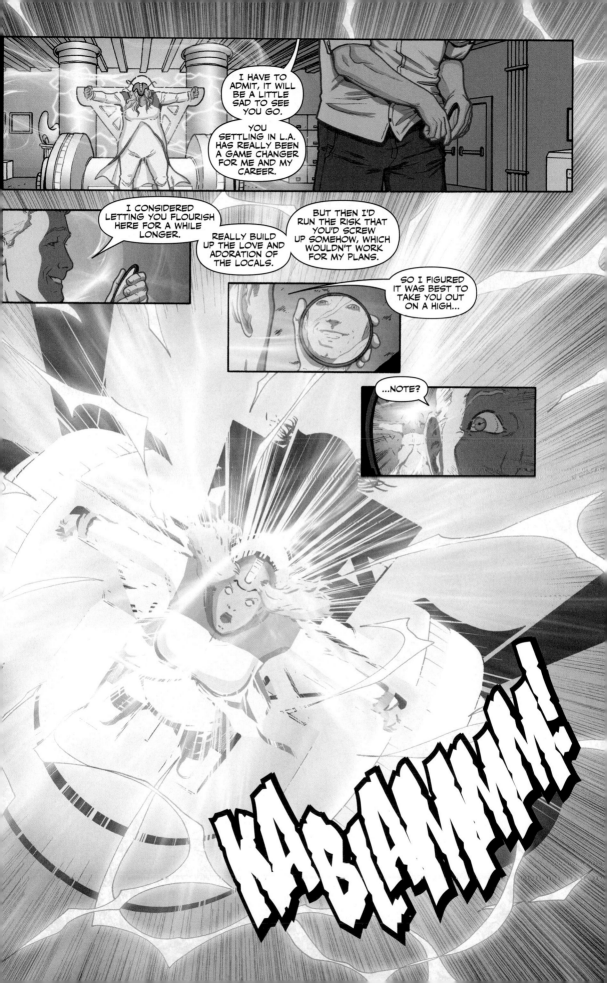

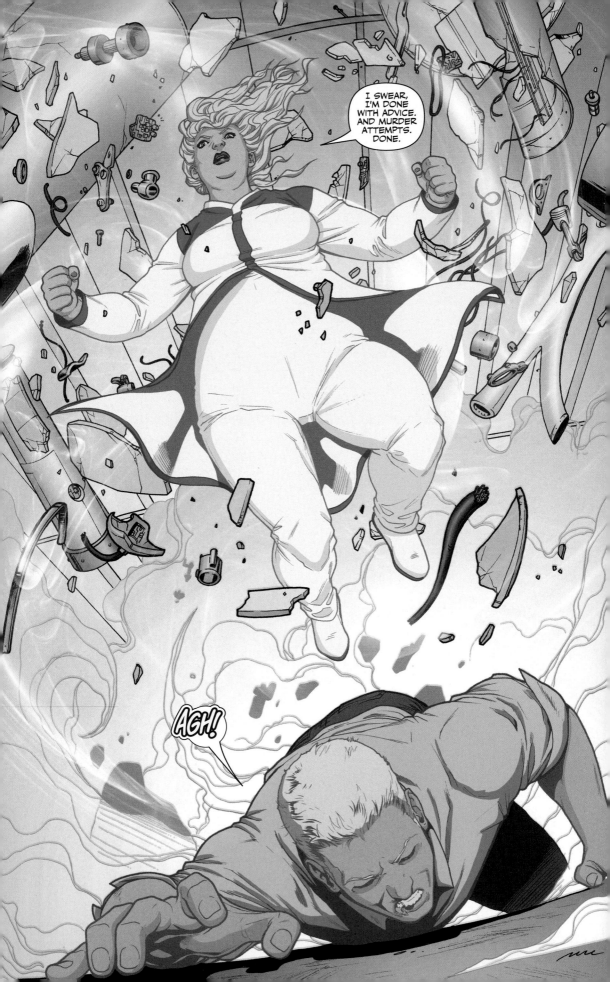

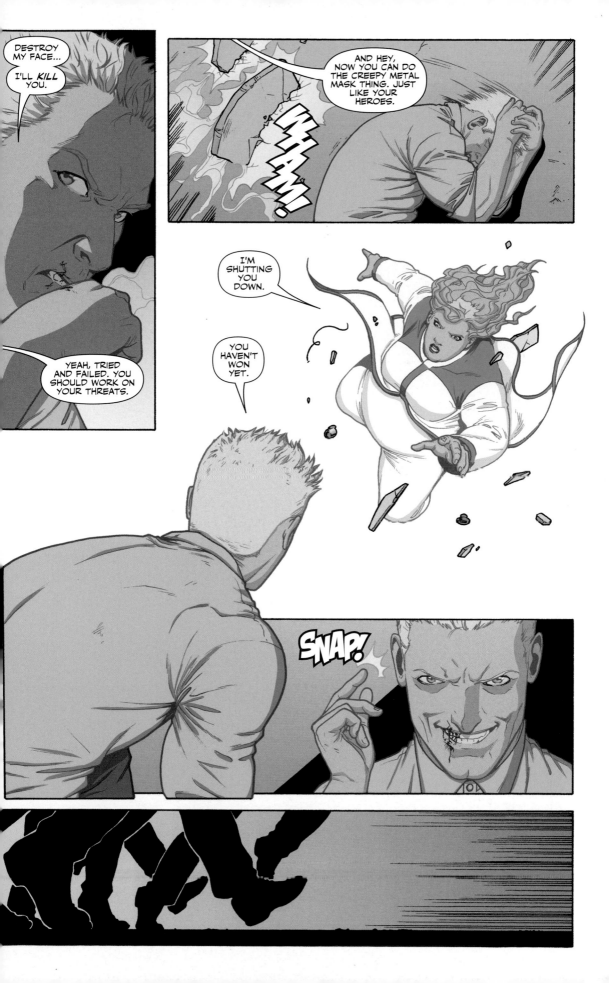

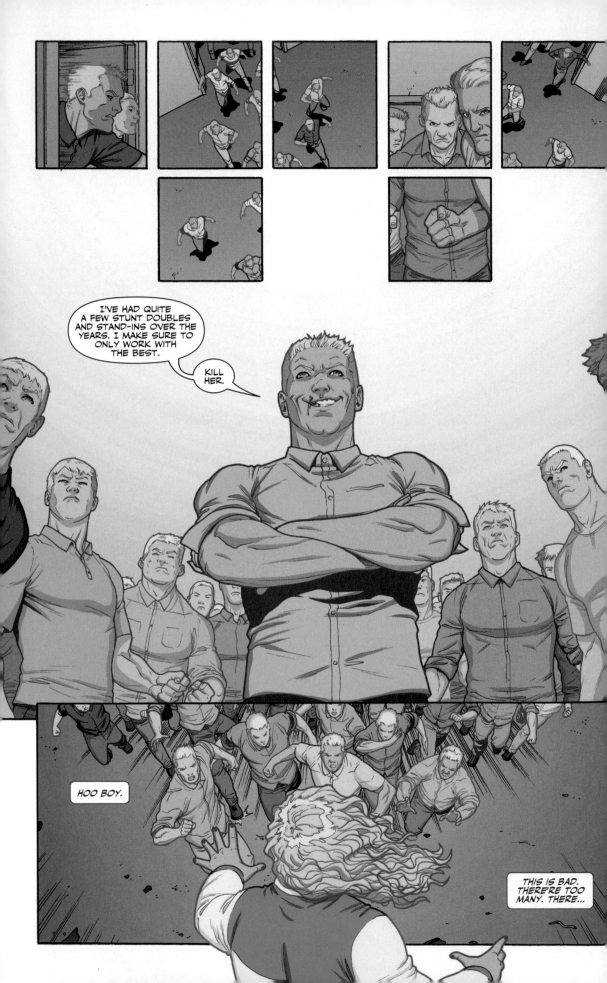

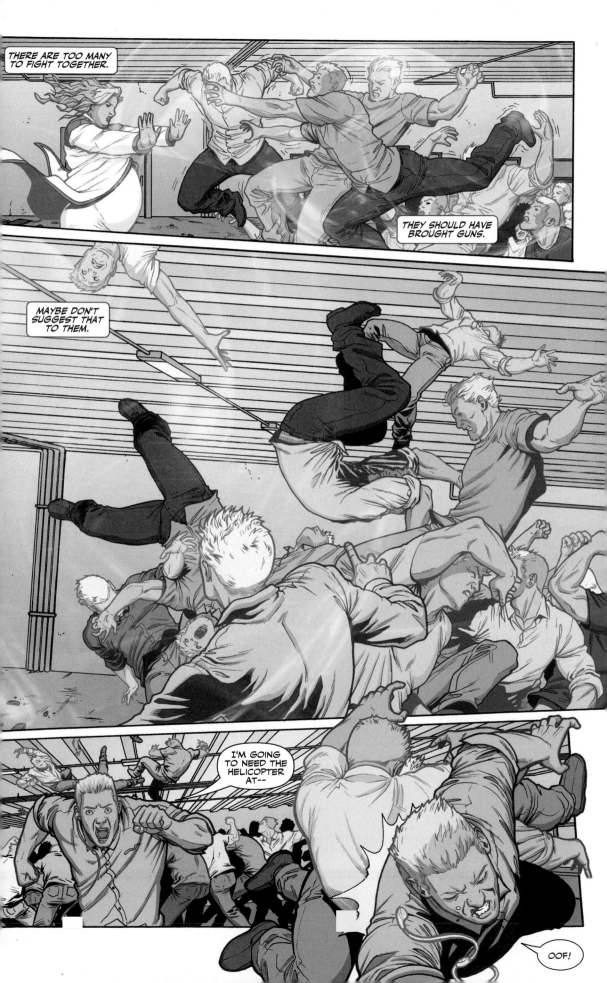

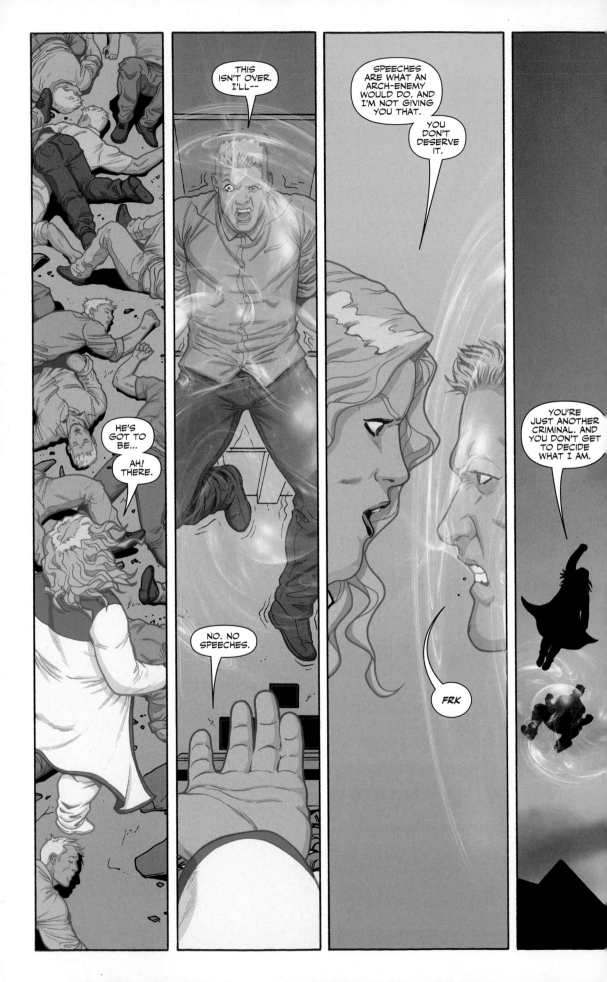

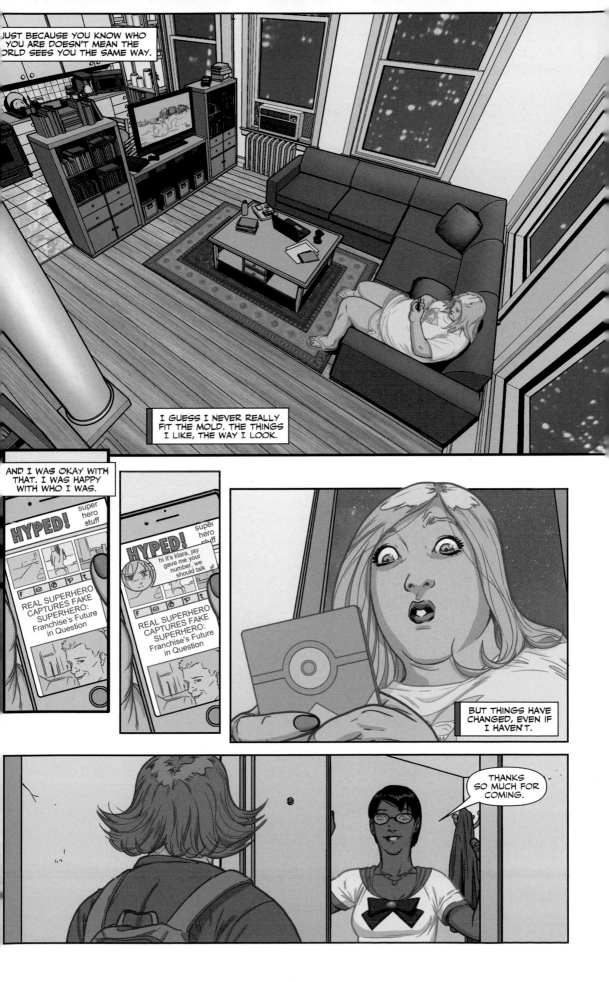

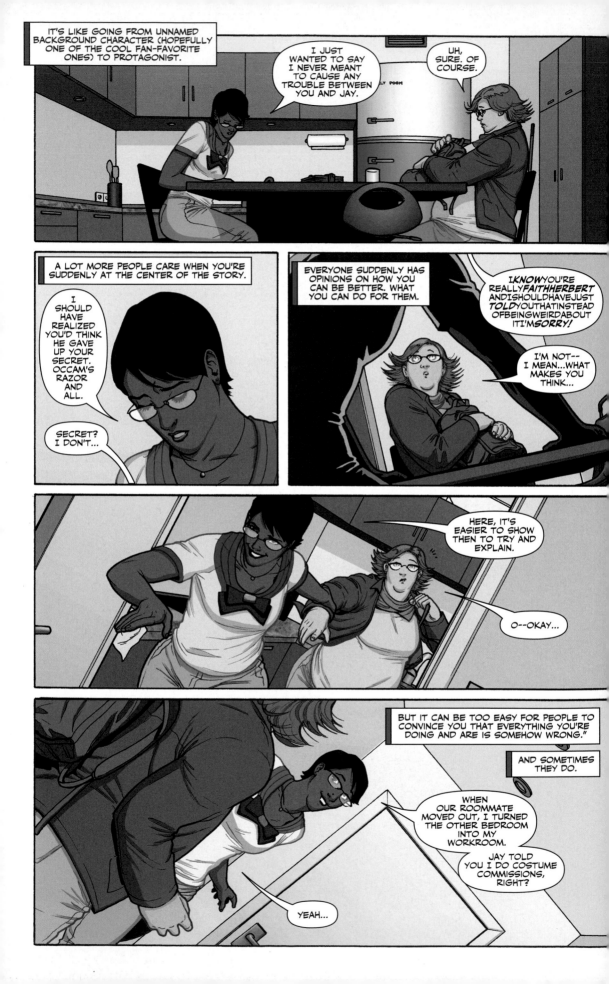

IT'S LIKE GOING FROM UNNAMED BACKGROUND CHARACTER (HOPEFULLY ONE OF THE COOL FAN-FAVORITE ONES) TO PROTAGONIST.

I JUST WANTED TO SAY I NEVER MEANT TO CAUSE ANY TROUBLE BETWEEN YOU AND JAY.

UH, SURE. OF COURSE.

A LOT MORE PEOPLE CARE WHEN YOU'RE SUDDENLY AT THE CENTER OF THE STORY.

I SHOULD HAVE REALIZED YOU'D THINK HE GAVE UP YOUR SECRET. OCCAM'S RAZOR AND ALL.

SECRET? I DON'T...

EVERYONE SUDDENLY HAS OPINIONS ON HOW YOU CAN BE BETTER. WHAT YOU CAN DO FOR THEM.

I *KNOW* YOU'RE REALLY *FAITH HERBERT* AND I SHOULD HAVE JUST *TOLD* YOU THAT INSTEAD OF BEING WEIRD ABOUT IT I'M *SORRY!*

I'M NOT-- I MEAN...WHAT MAKES YOU THINK...

HERE, IT'S EASIER TO SHOW THEN TO TRY AND EXPLAIN.

O--OKAY...

BUT IT CAN BE TOO EASY FOR PEOPLE TO CONVINCE YOU THAT EVERYTHING YOU'RE DOING AND ARE IS SOMEHOW WRONG."

AND SOMETIMES THEY DO.

WHEN OUR ROOMMATE MOVED OUT, I TURNED THE OTHER BEDROOM INTO MY WORKROOM.

JAY TOLD YOU I DO COSTUME COMMISSIONS, RIGHT?

YEAH...

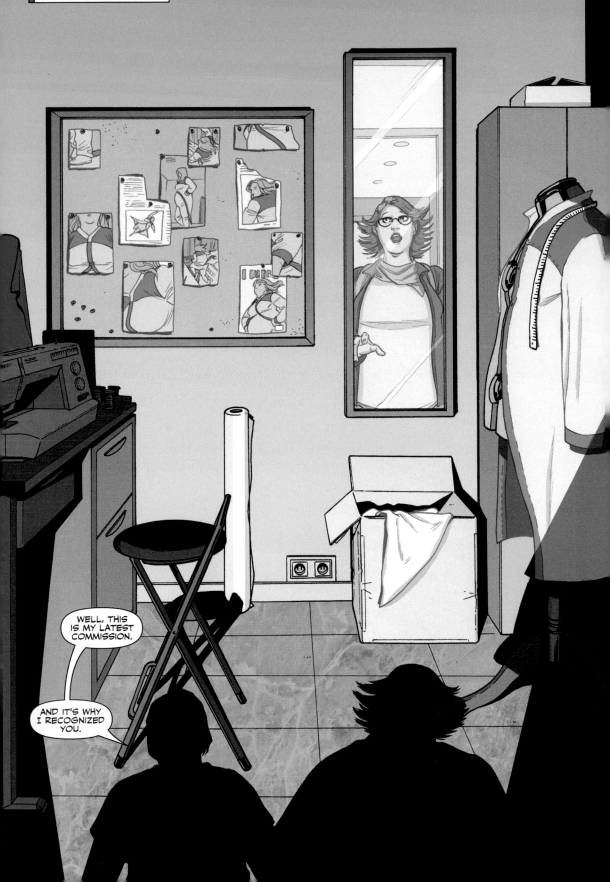

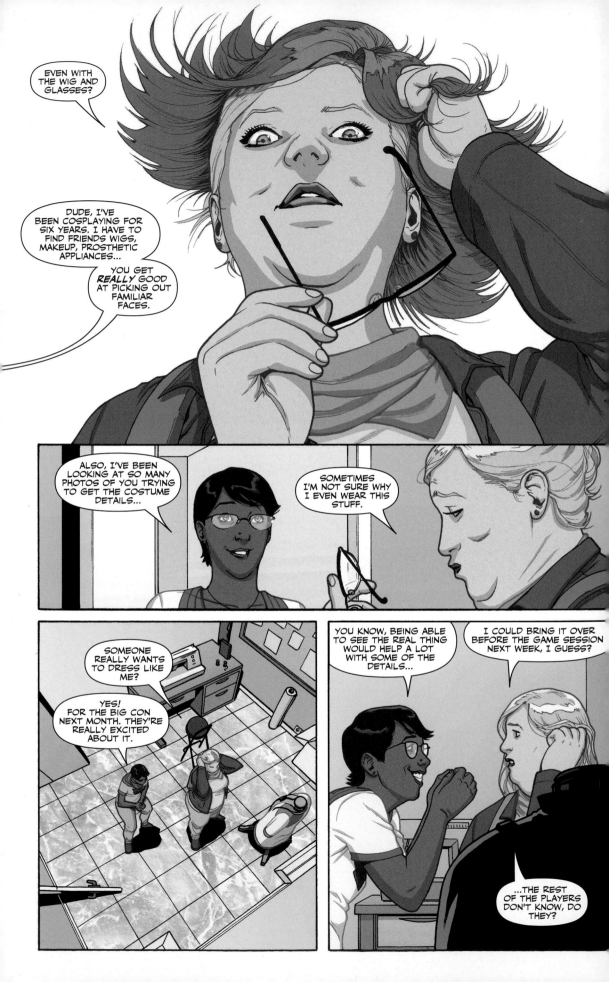

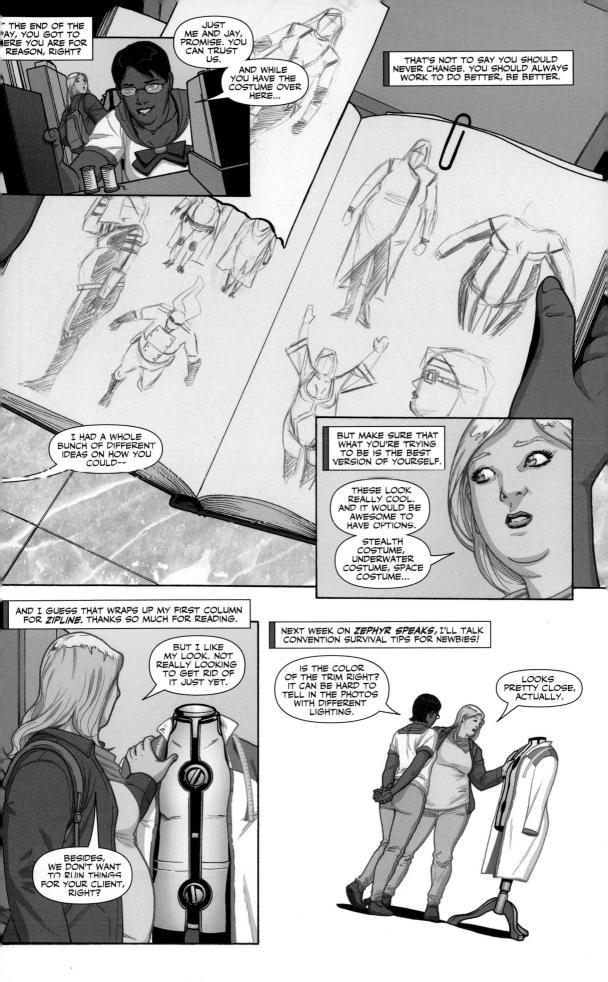

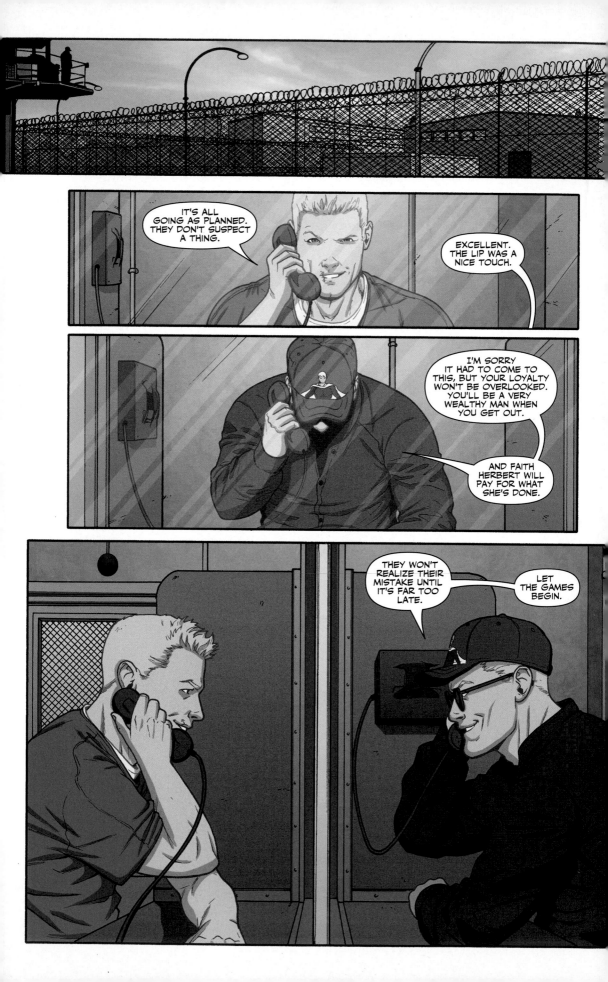

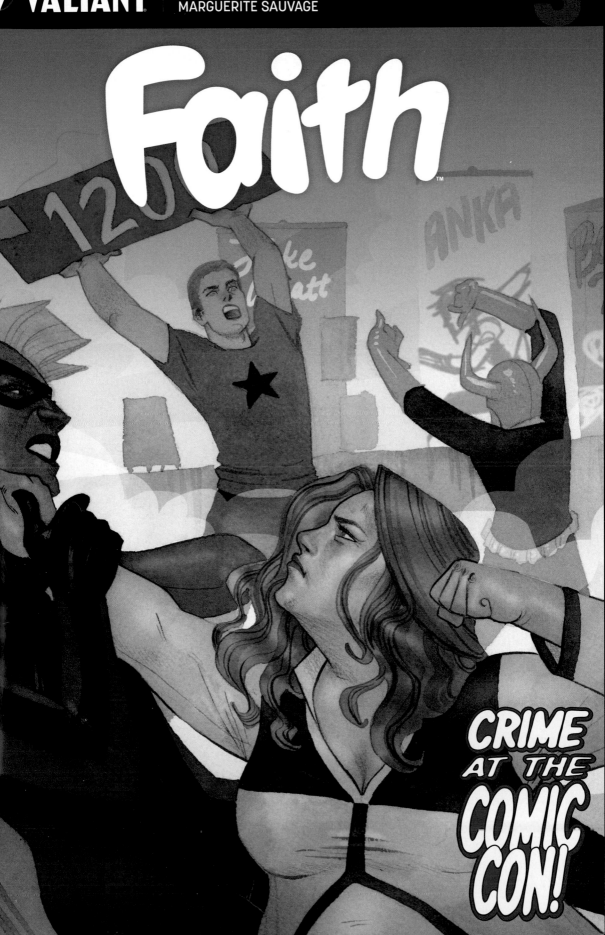

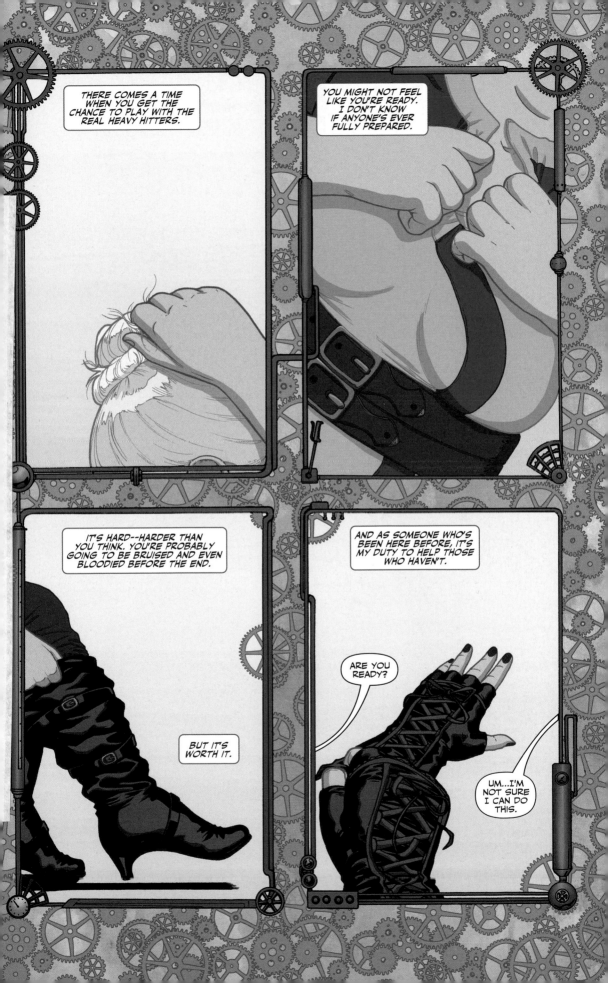

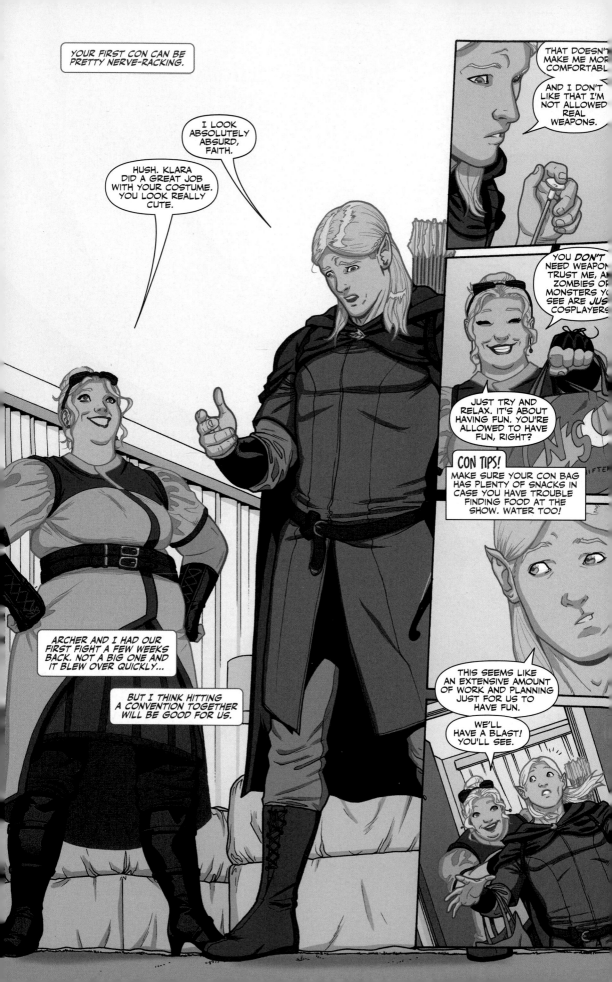

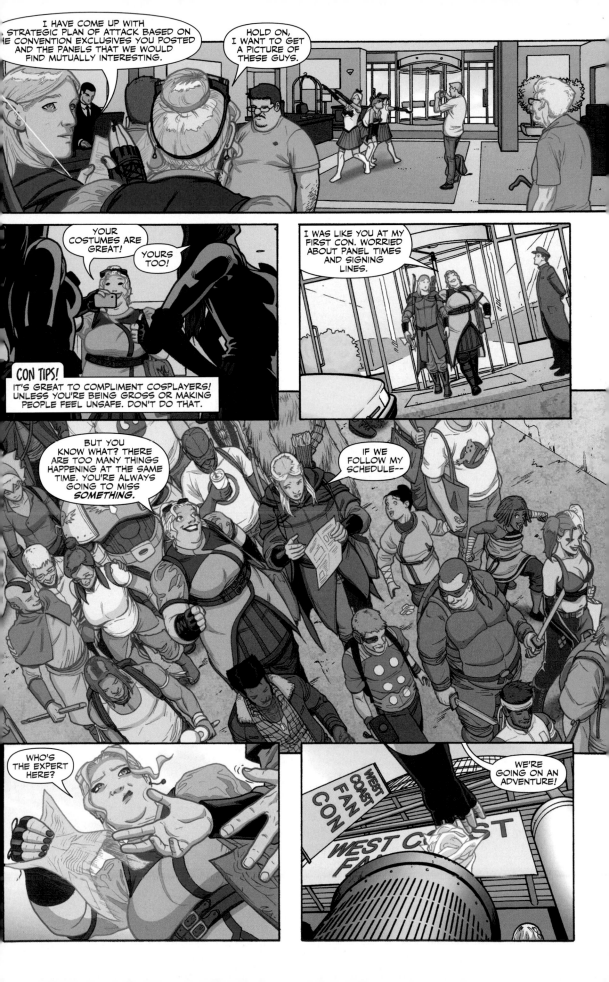

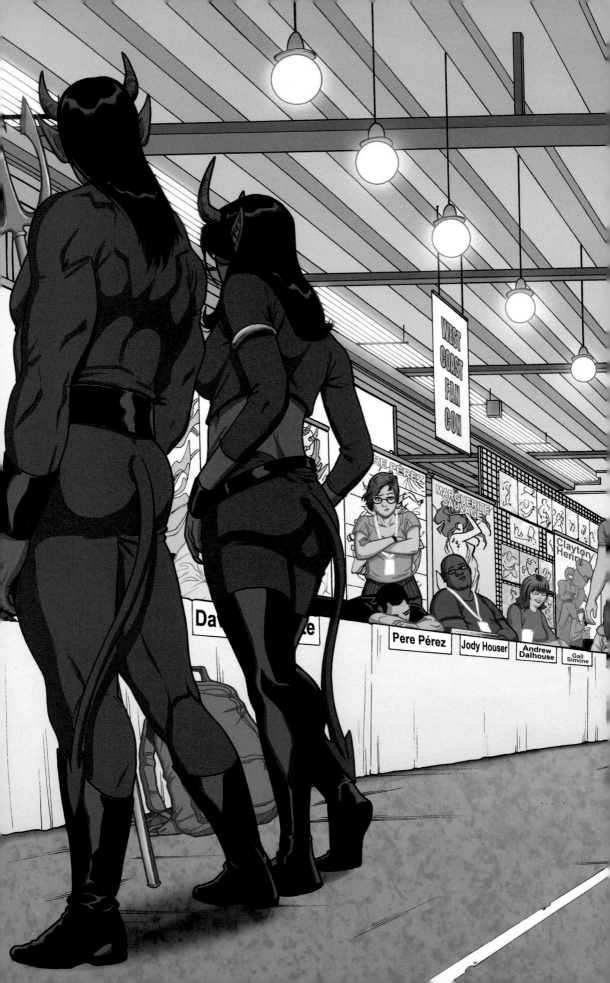

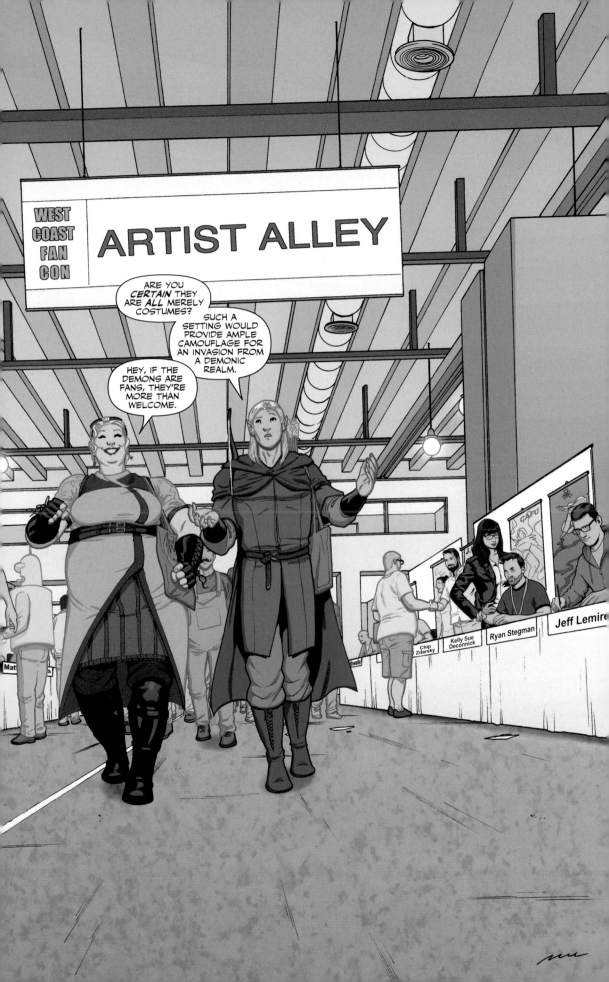

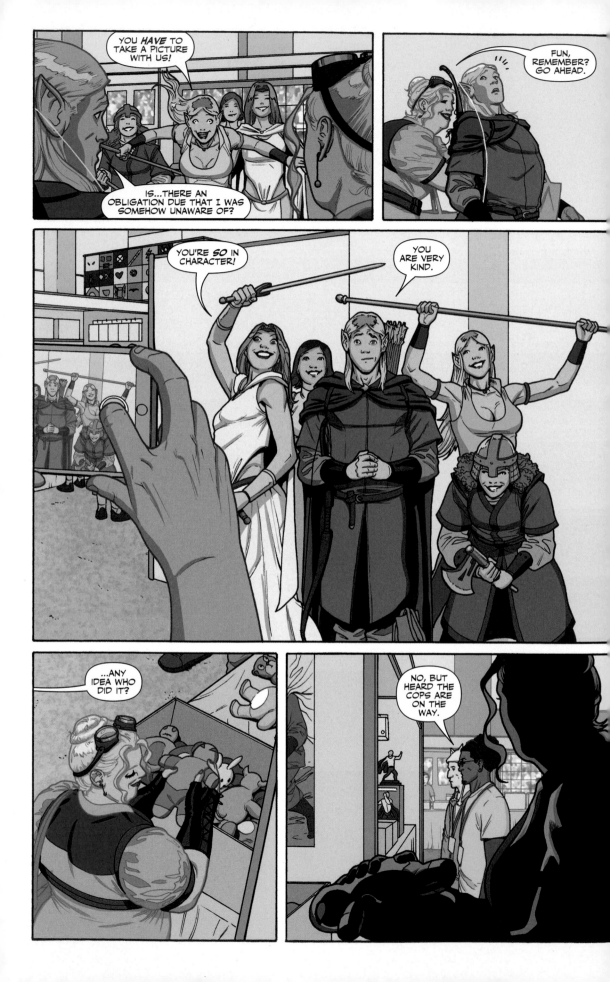

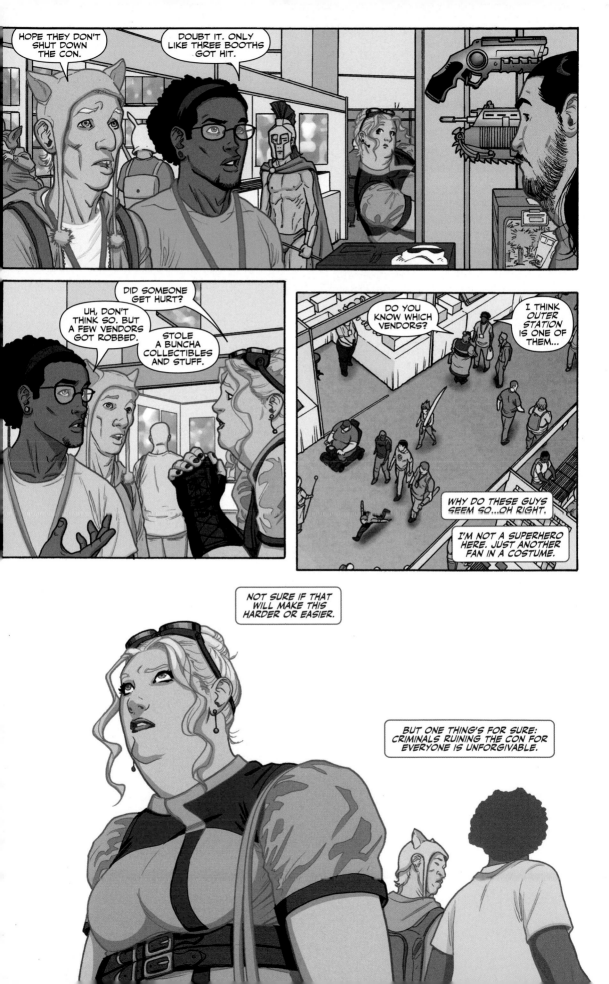

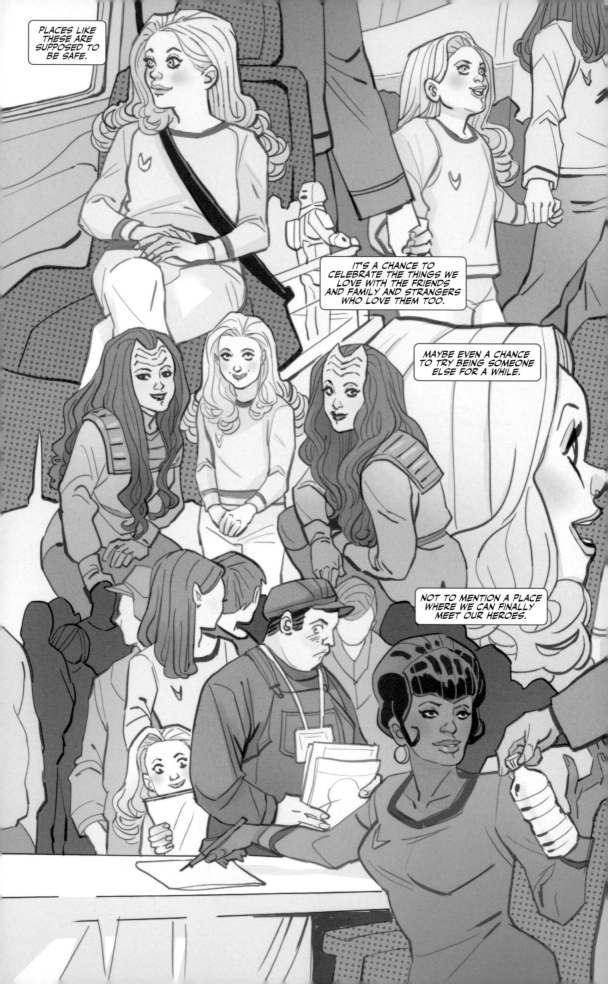

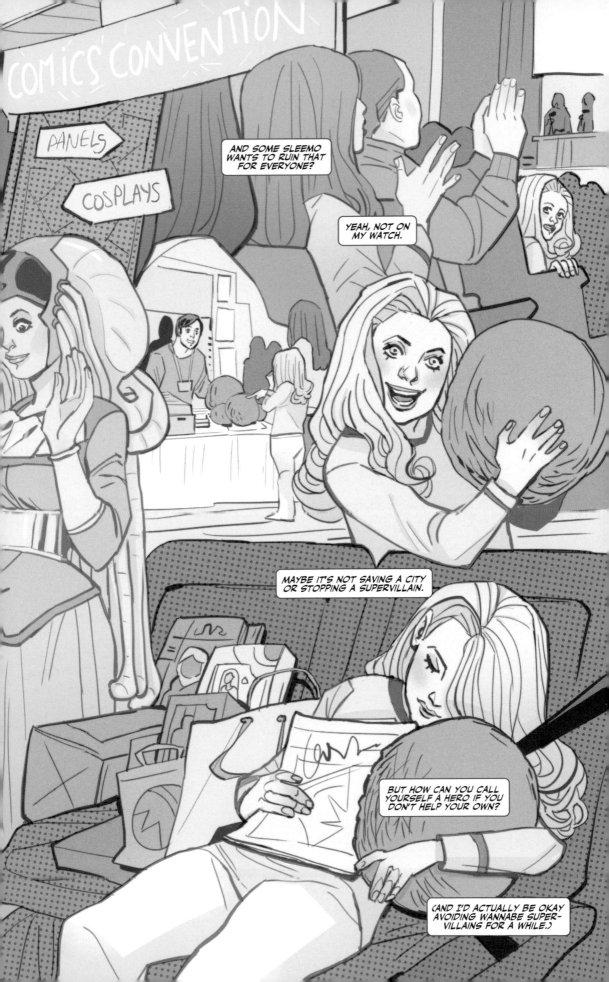

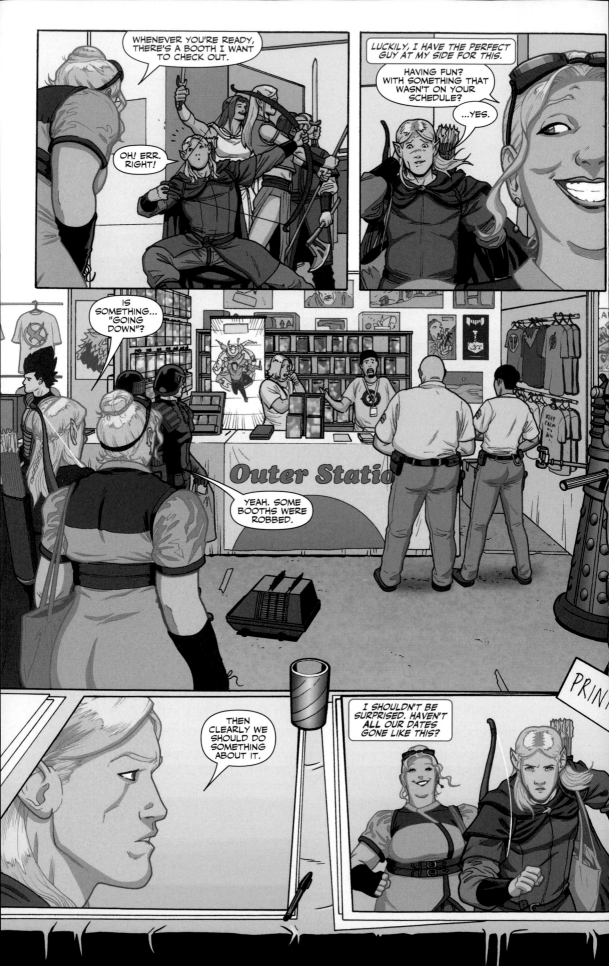

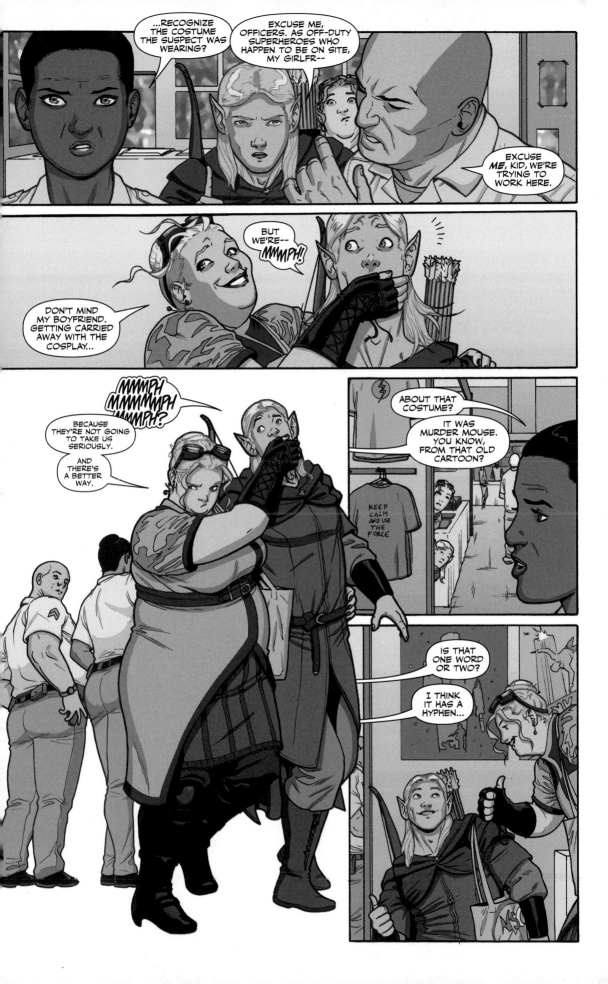

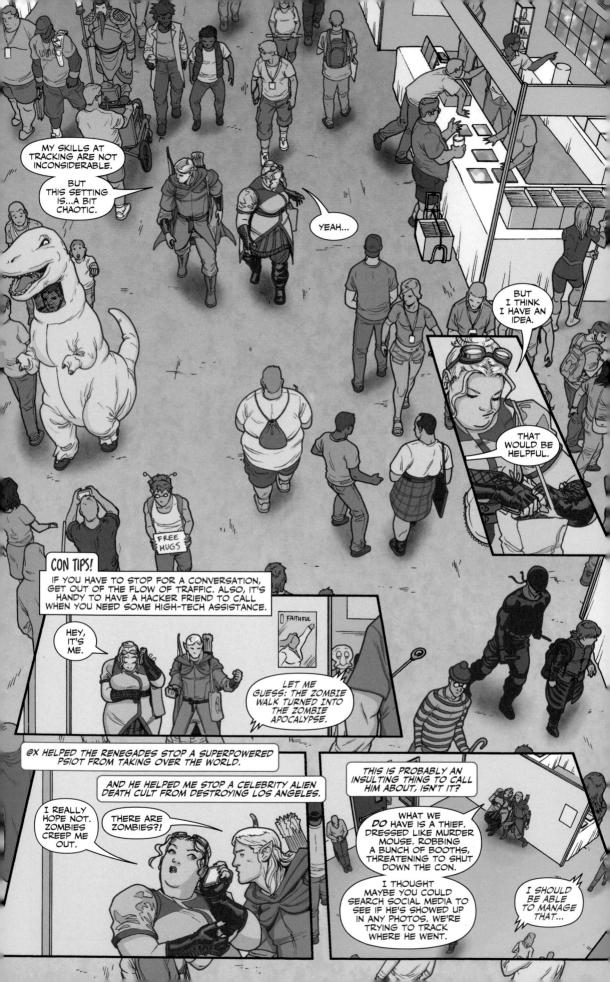

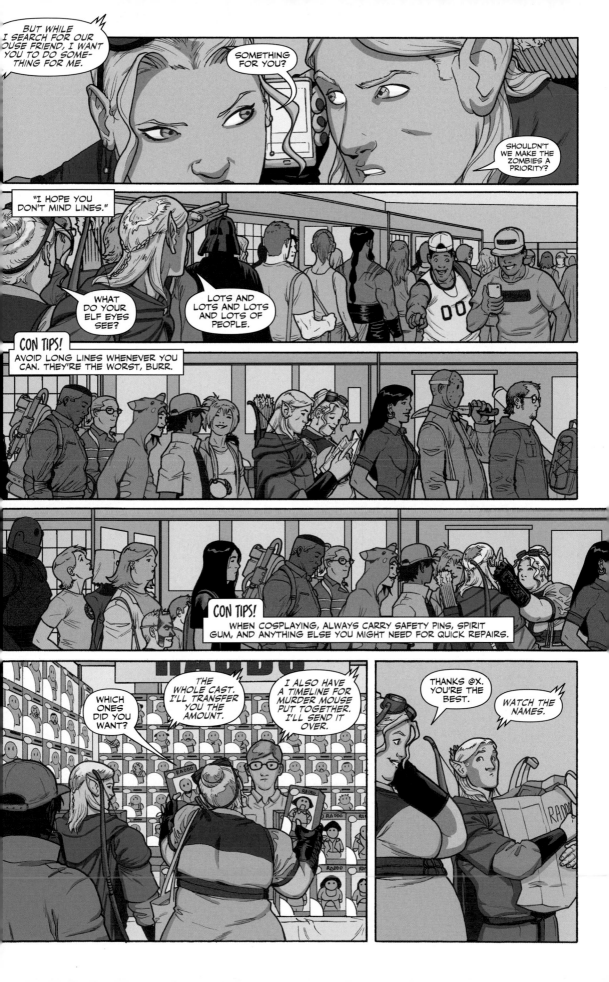

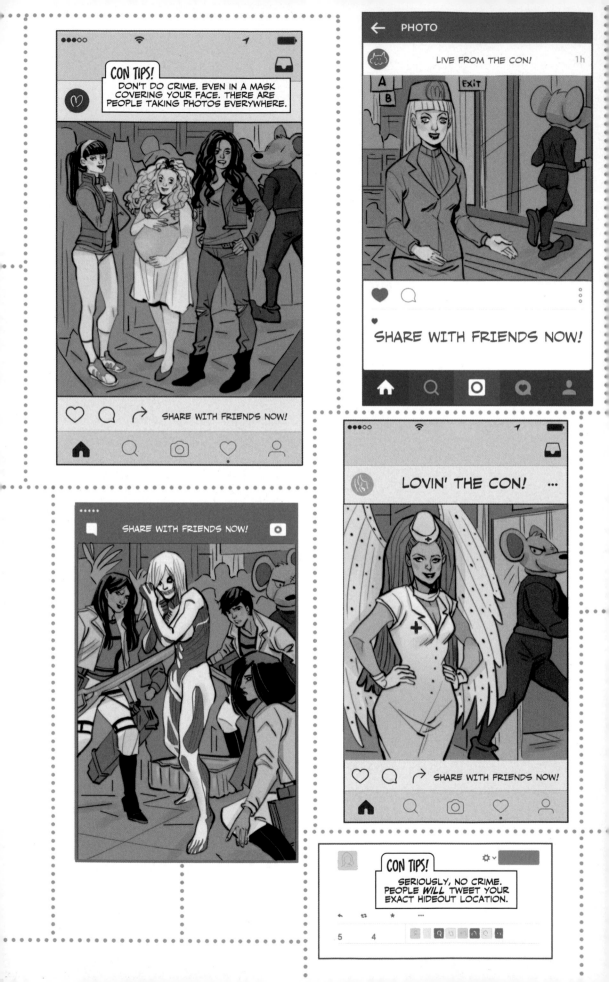

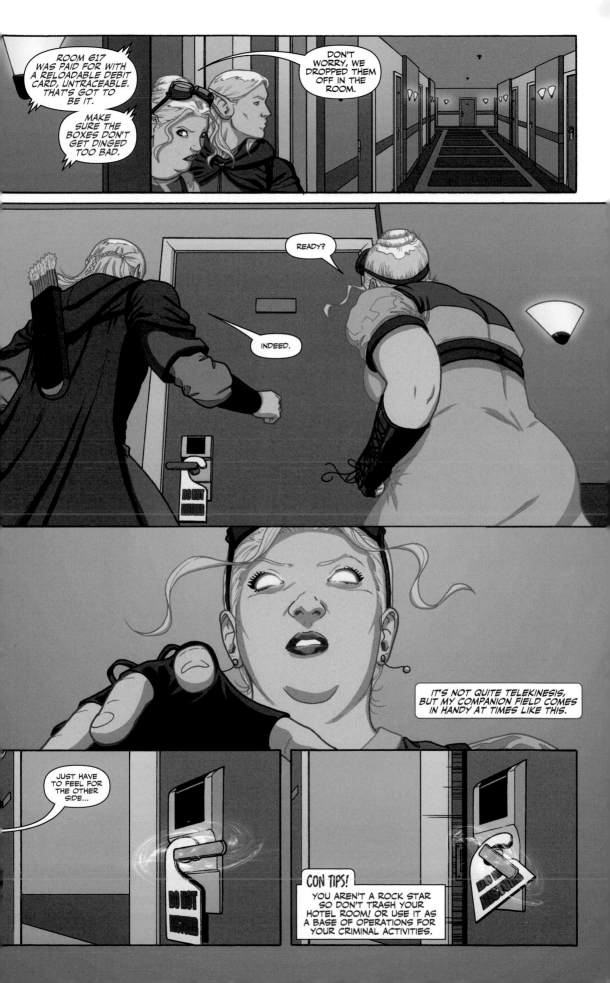

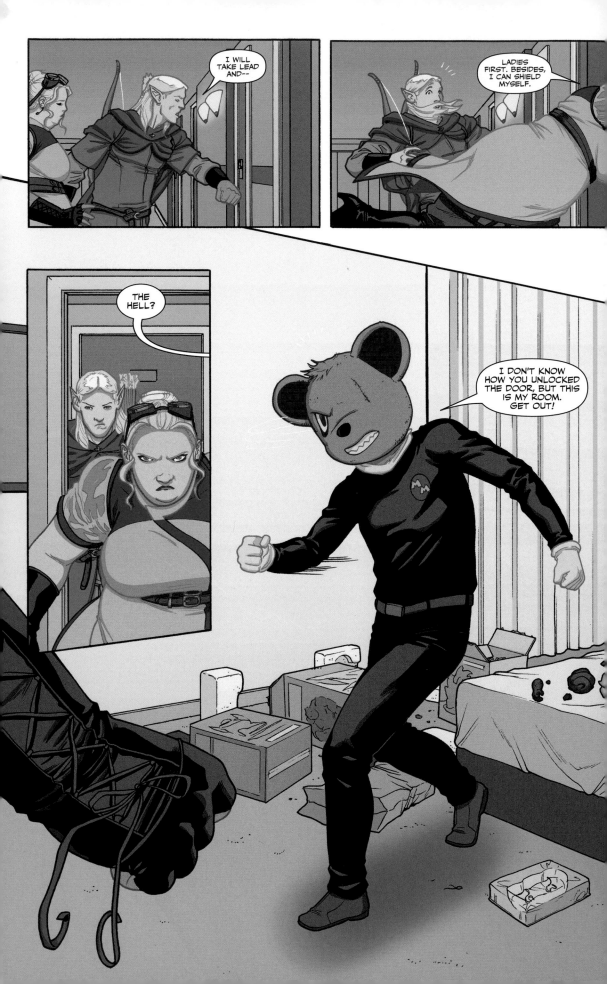

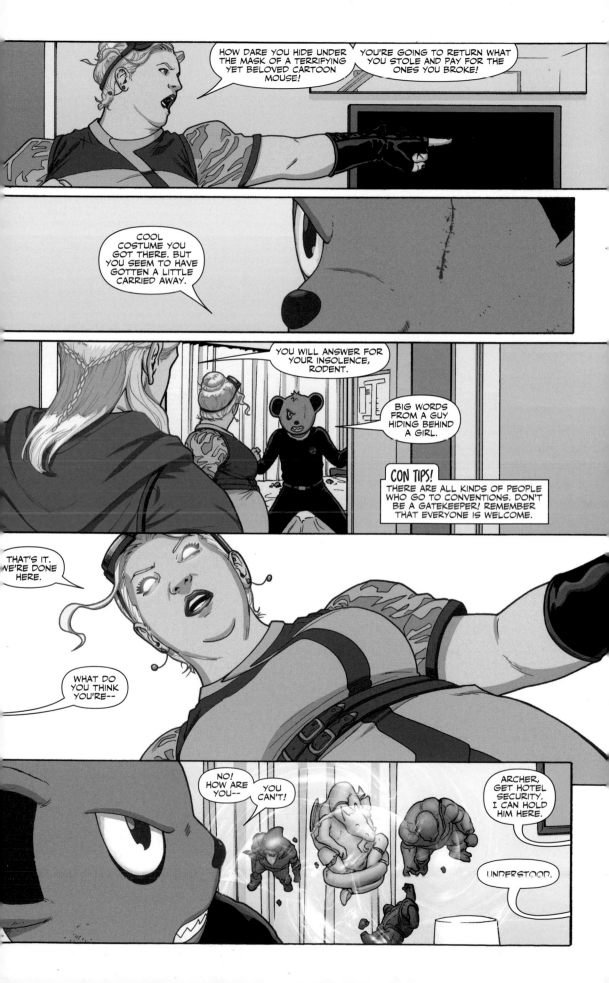

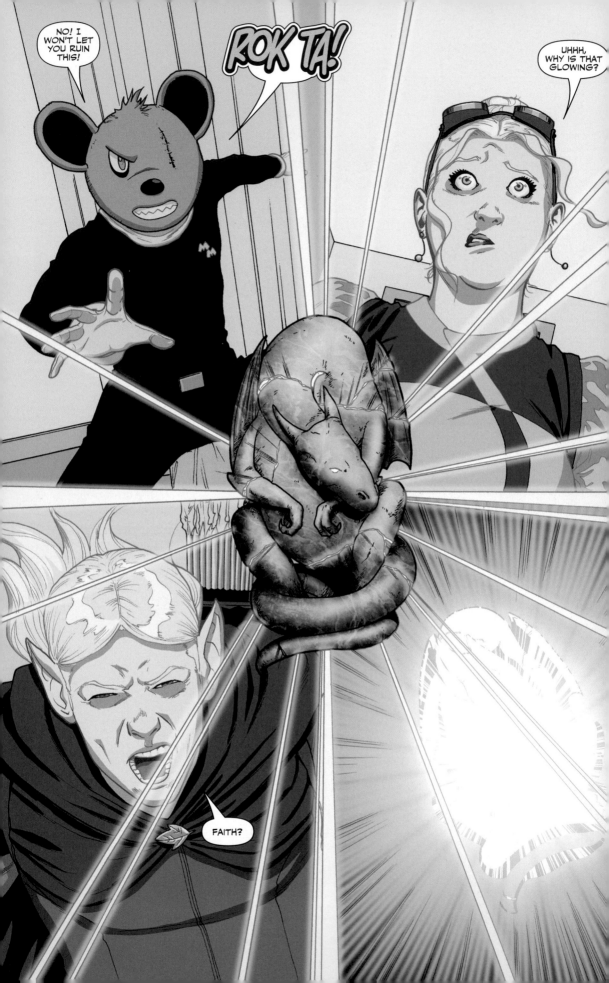

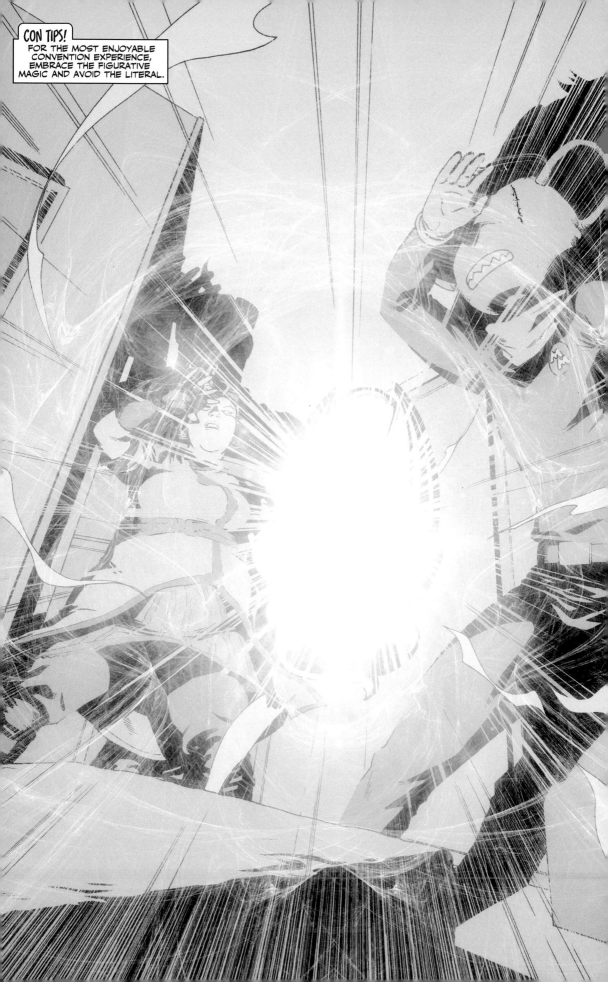

CON TIPS!
FOR THE MOST ENJOYABLE
CONVENTION EXPERIENCE,
EMBRACE THE FIGURATIVE
MAGIC AND AVOID THE LITERAL.

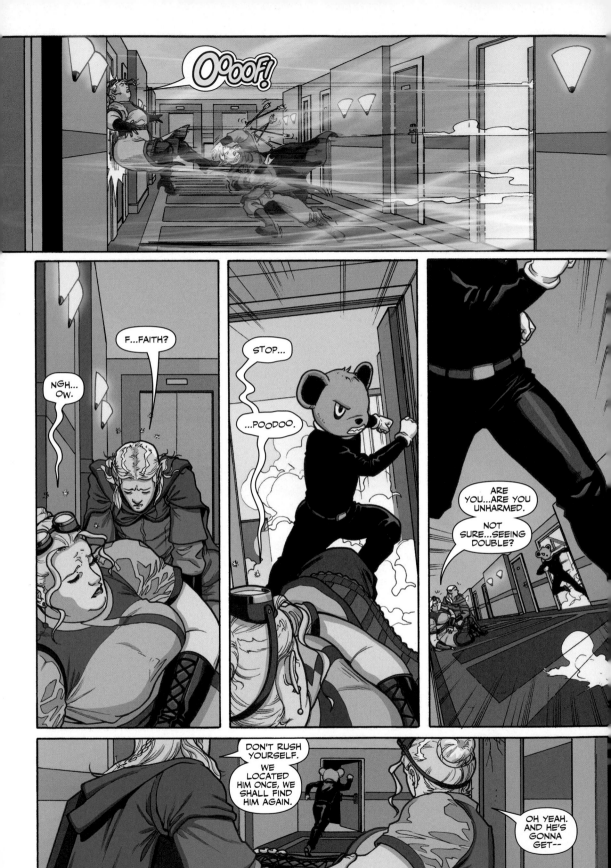

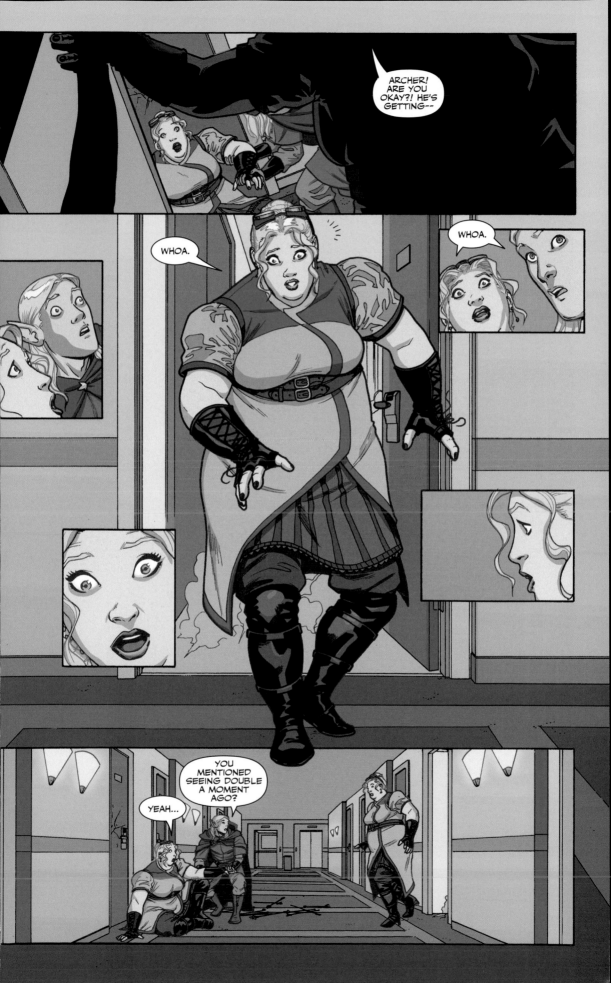

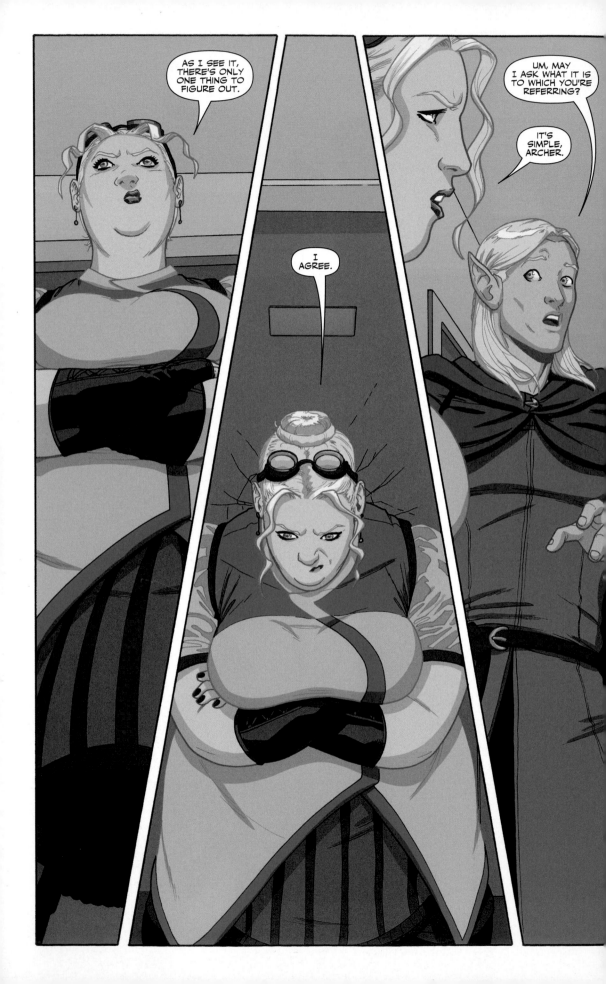

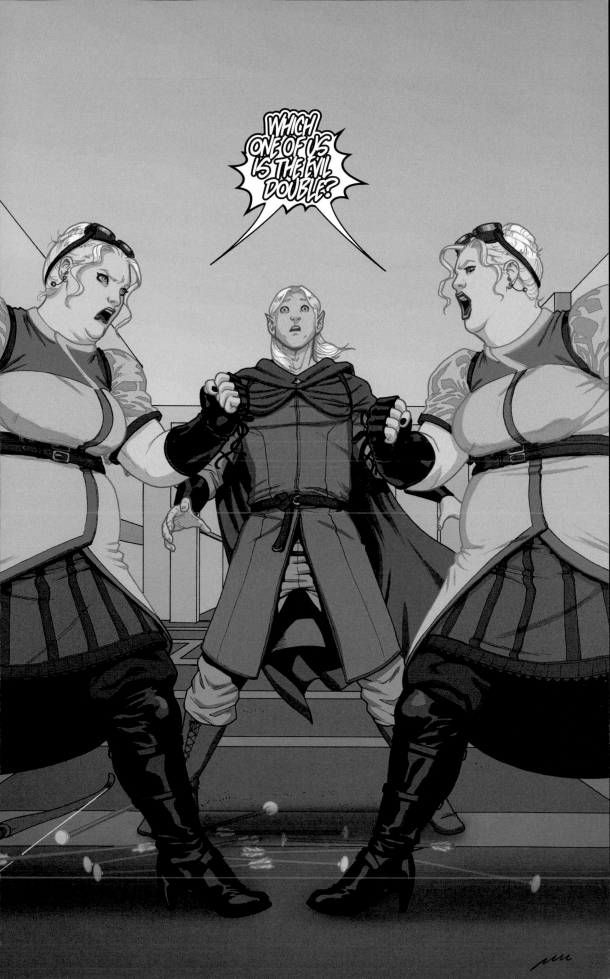

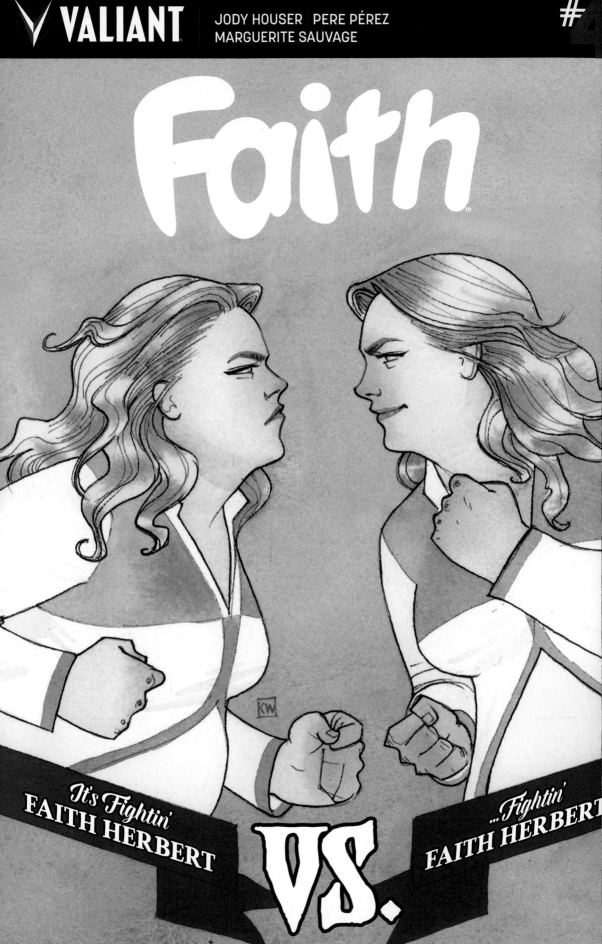

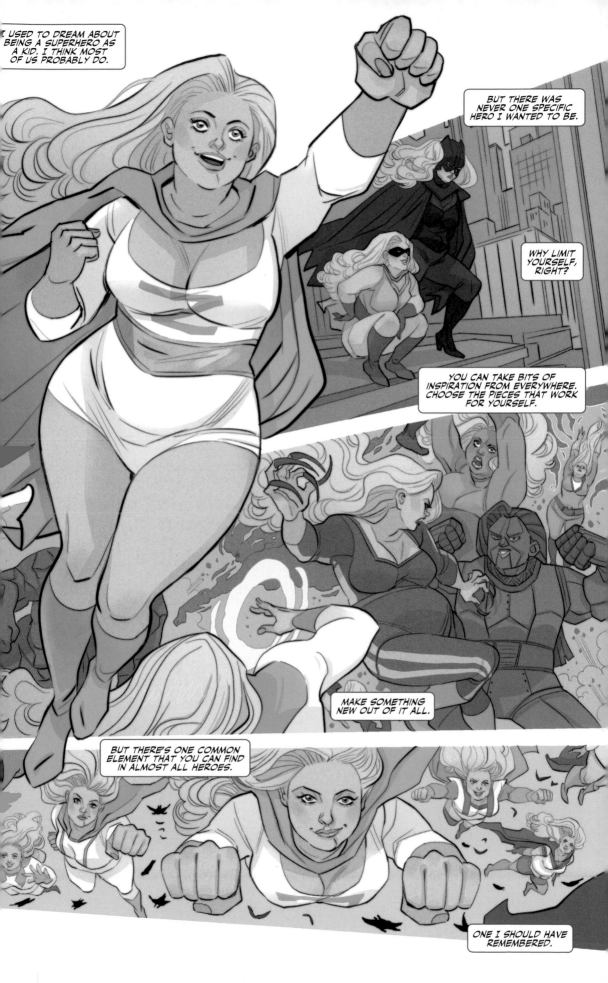

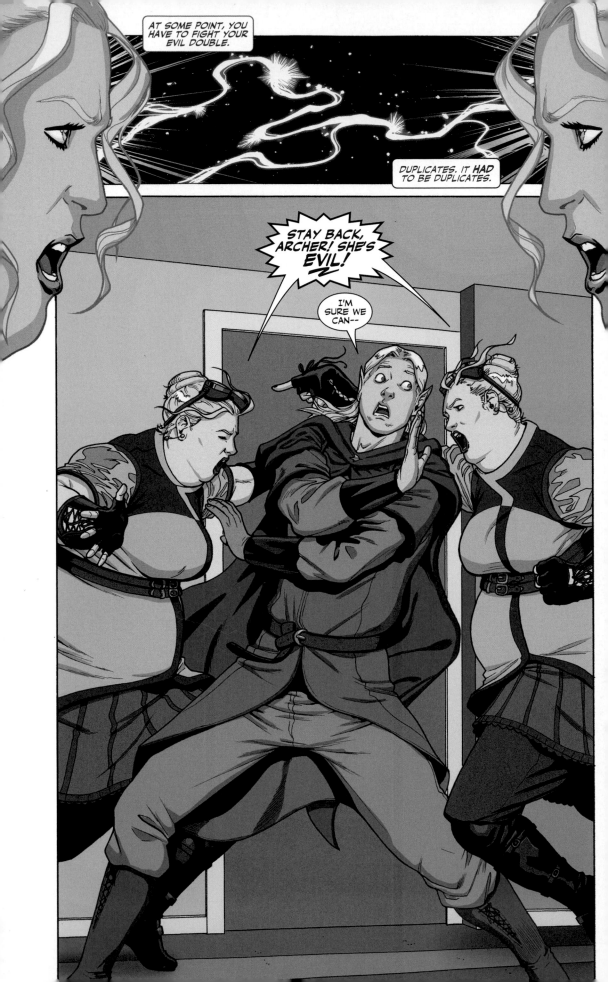

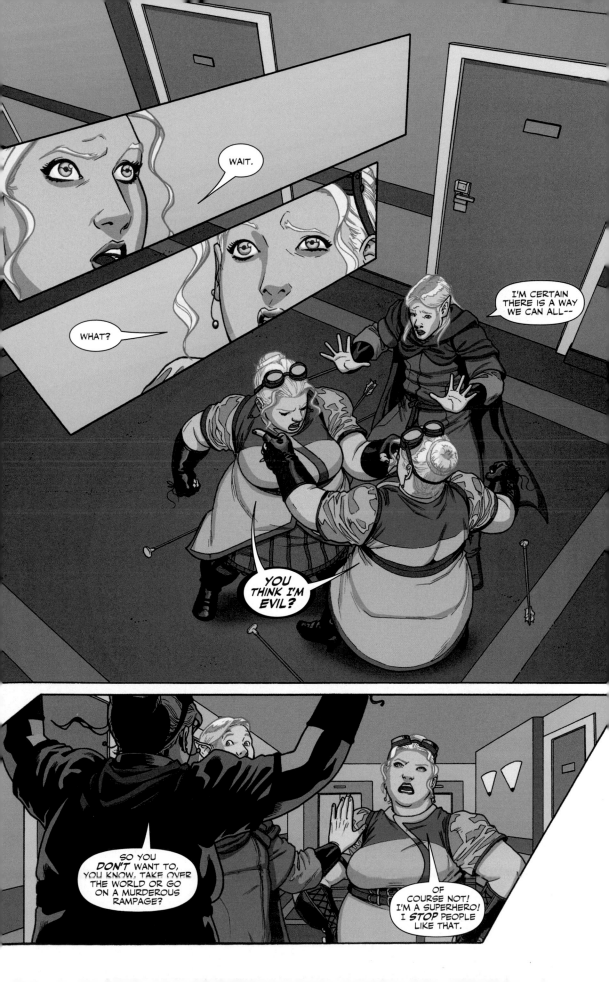

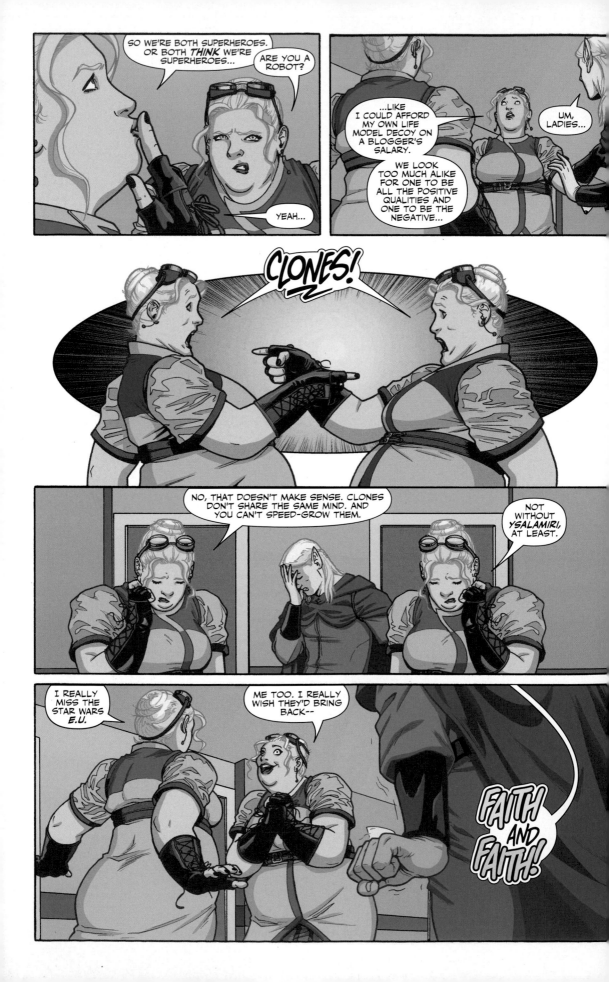

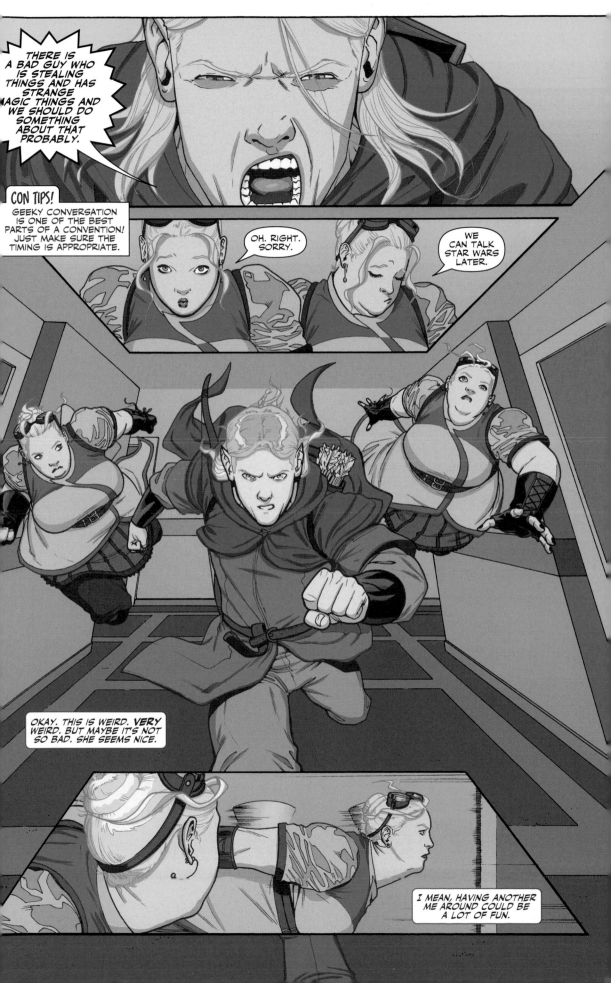

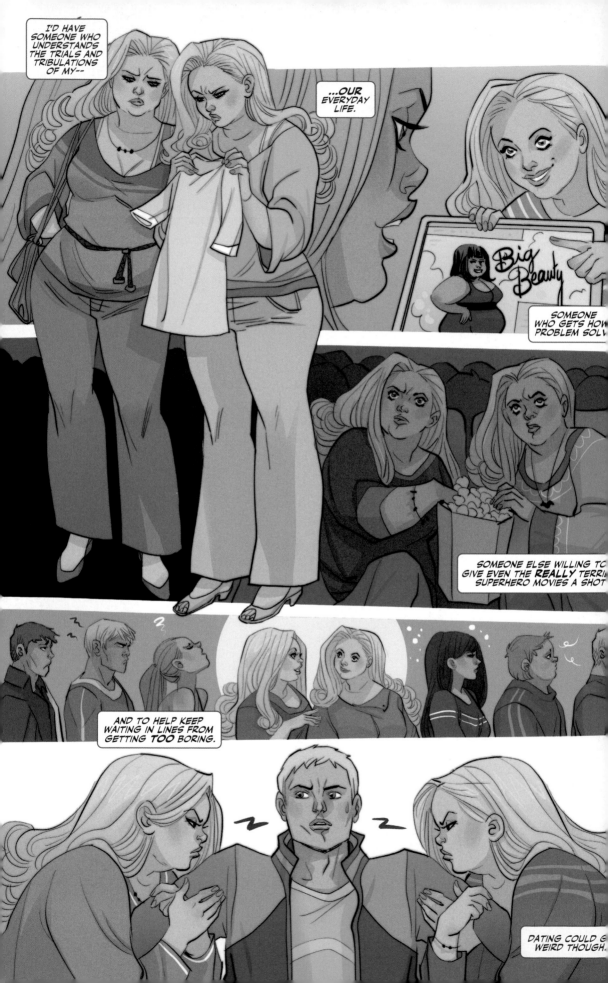

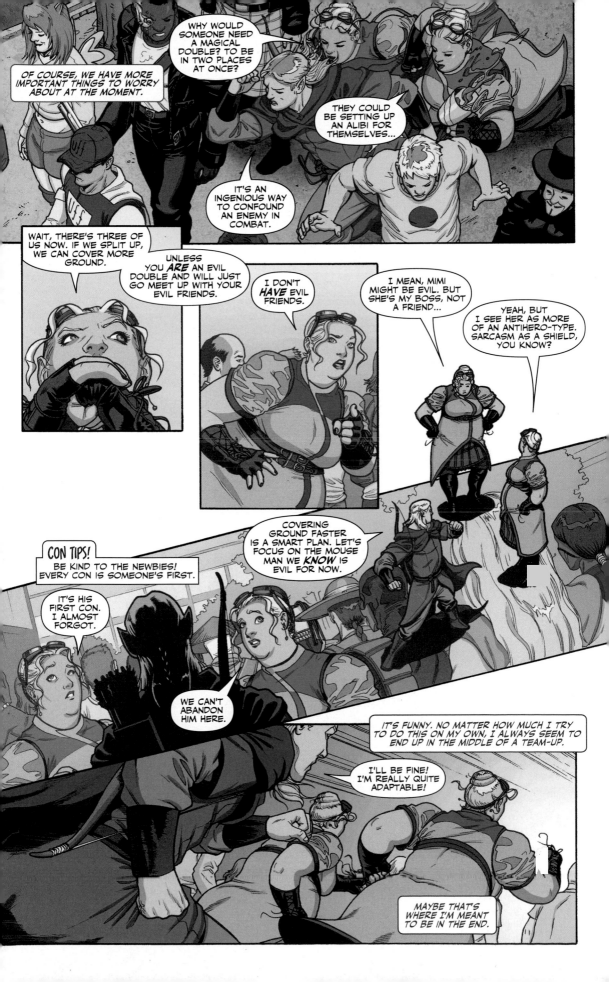

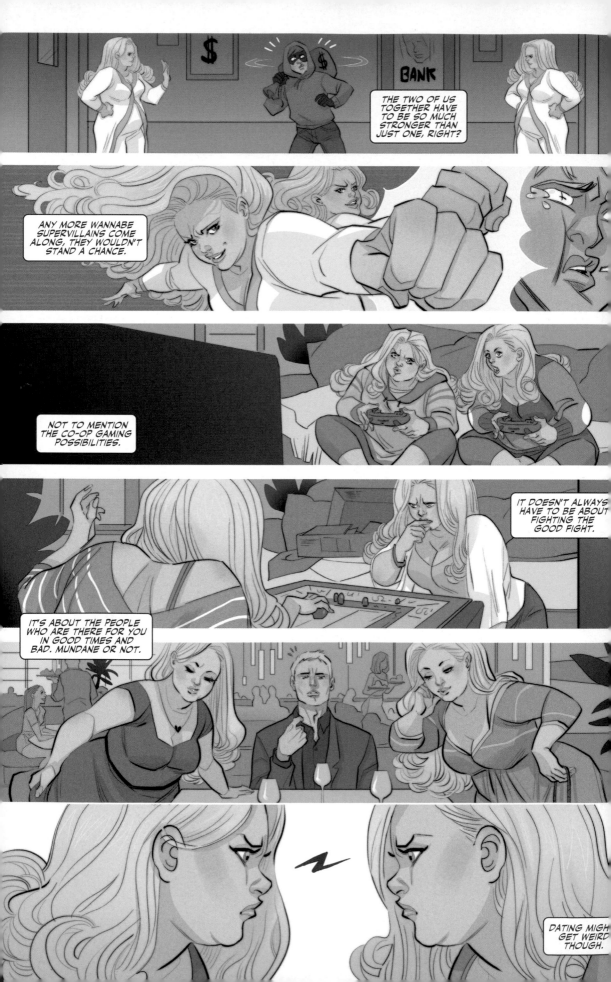

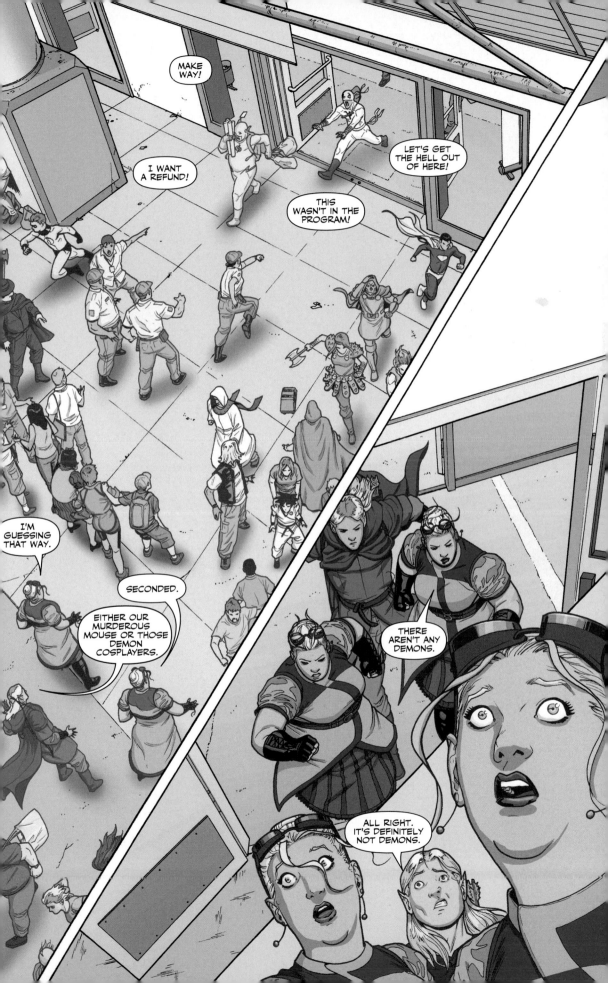

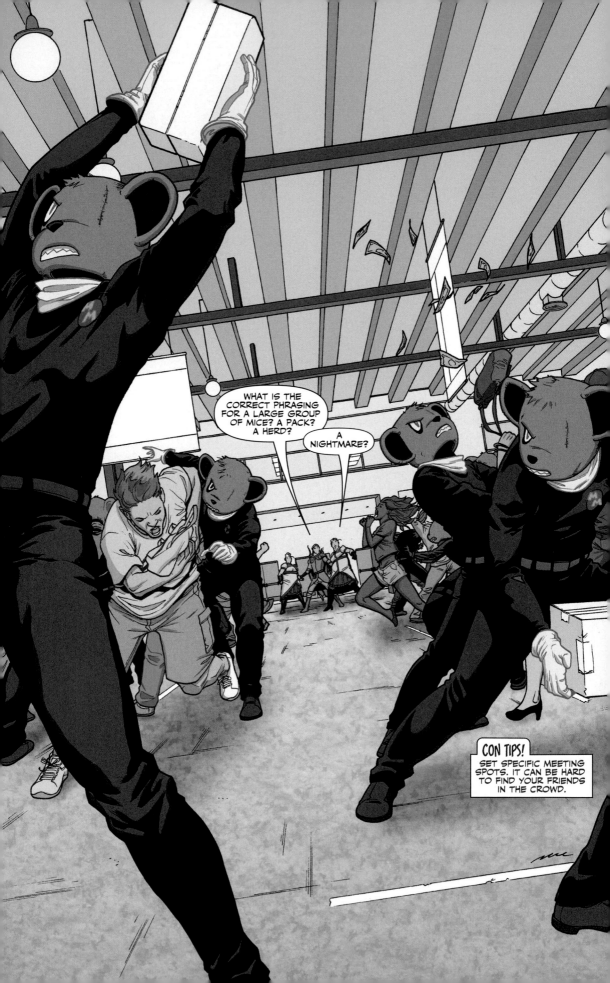

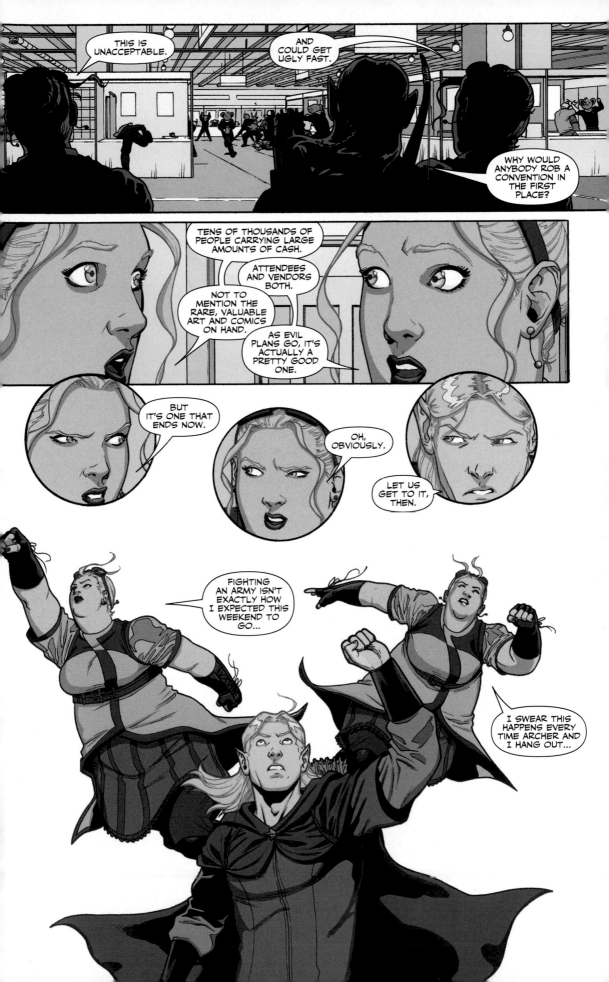

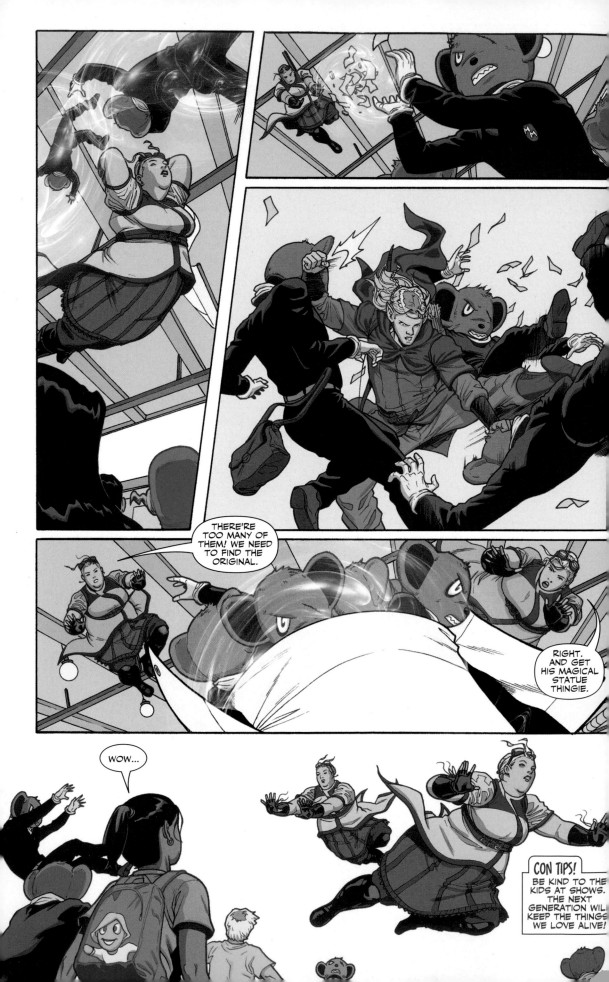

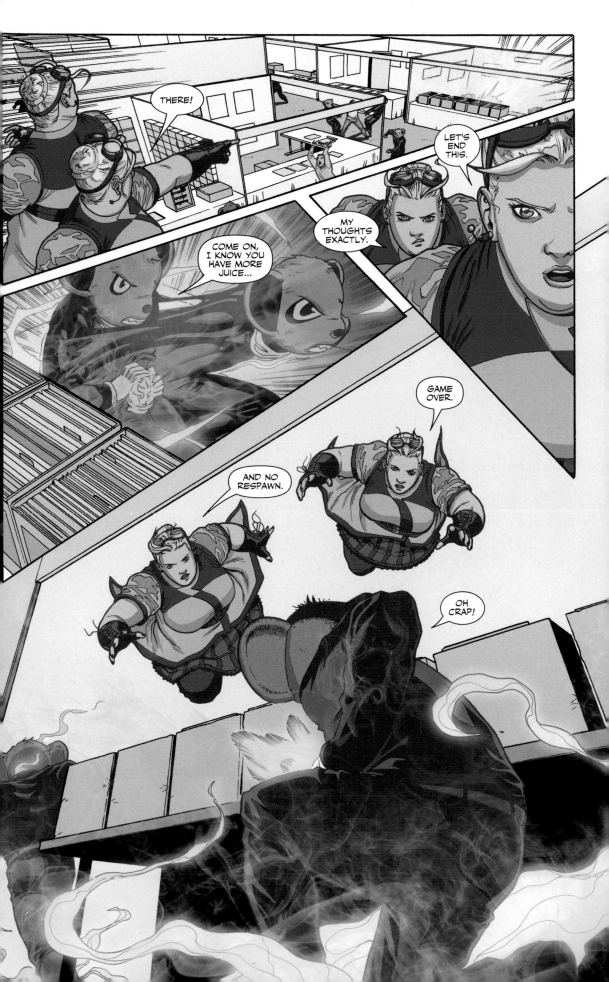

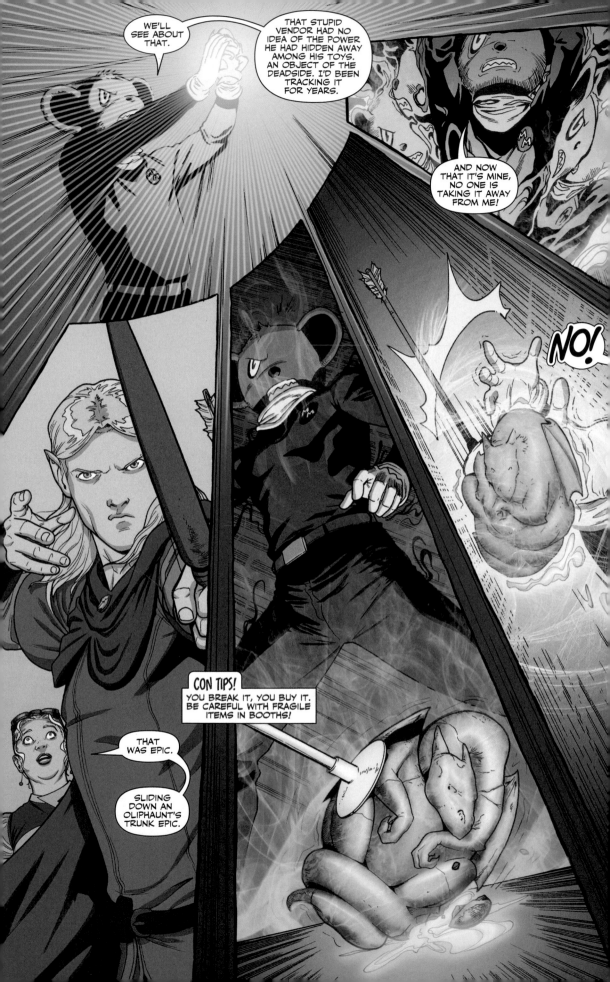

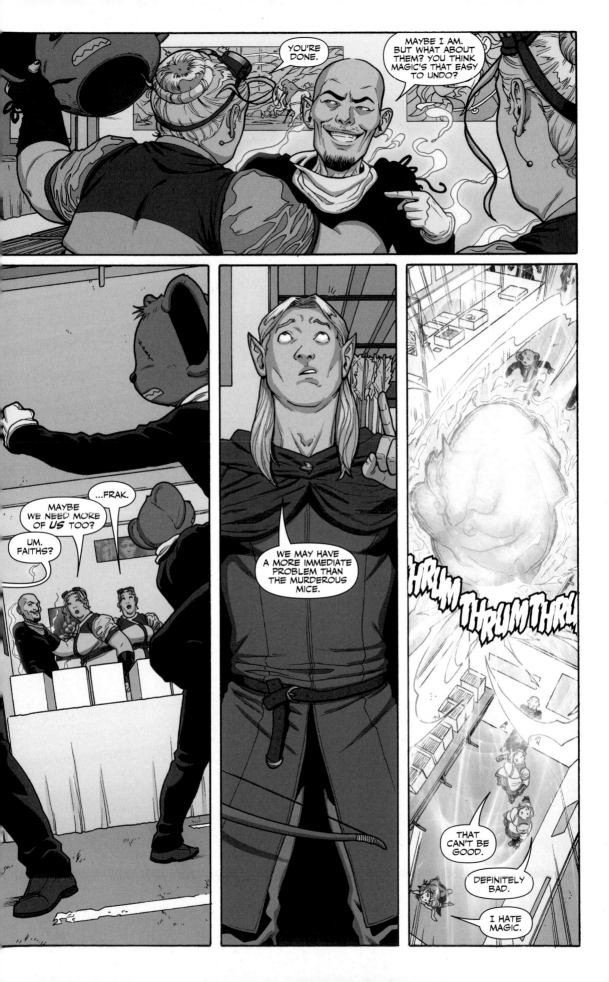

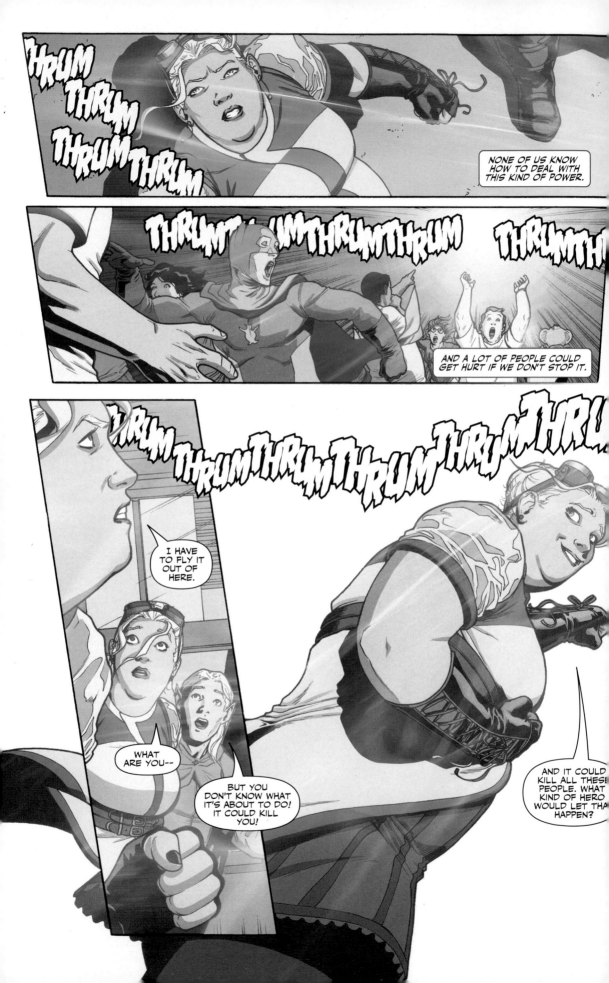

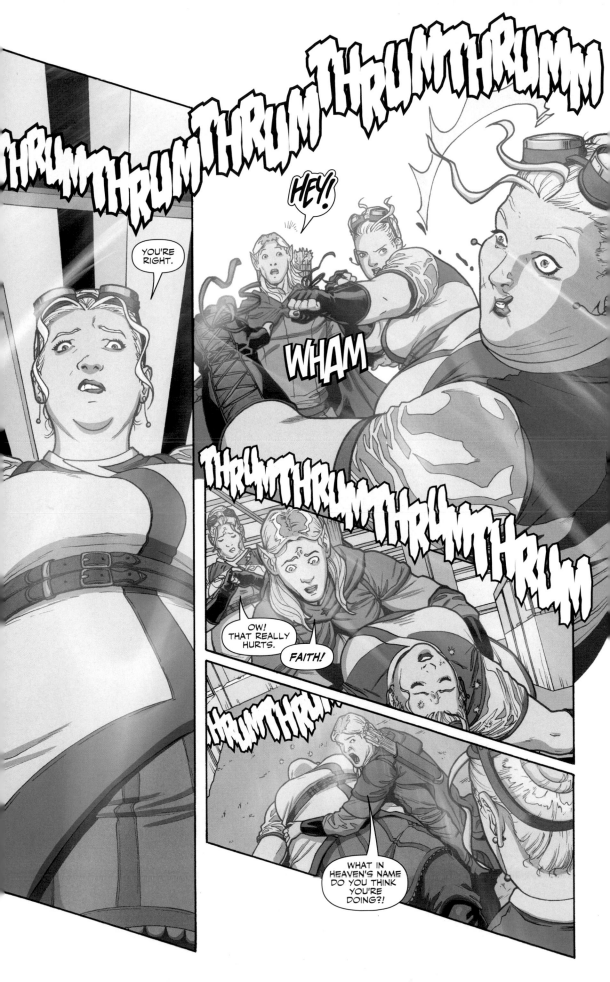

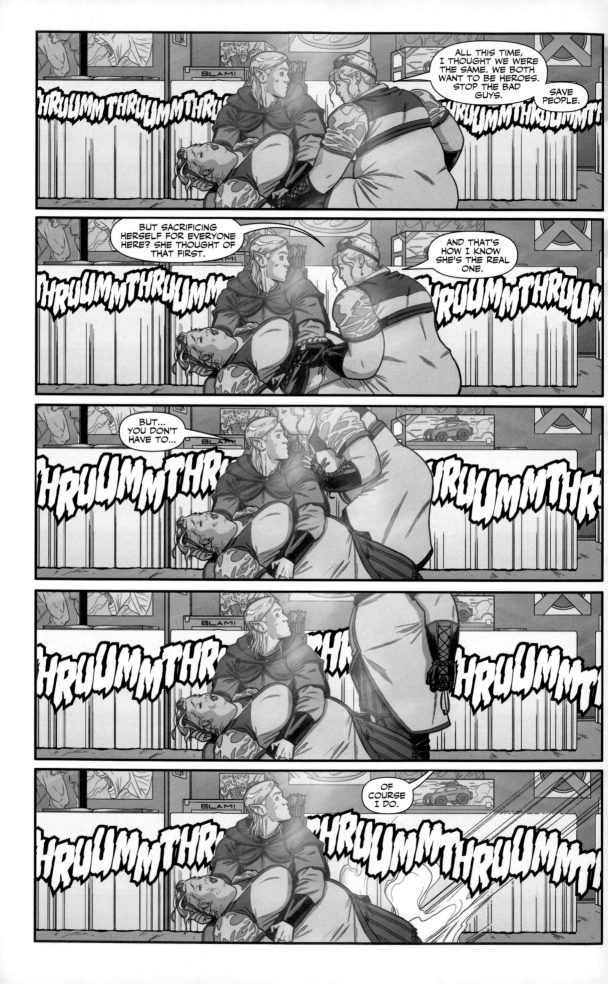

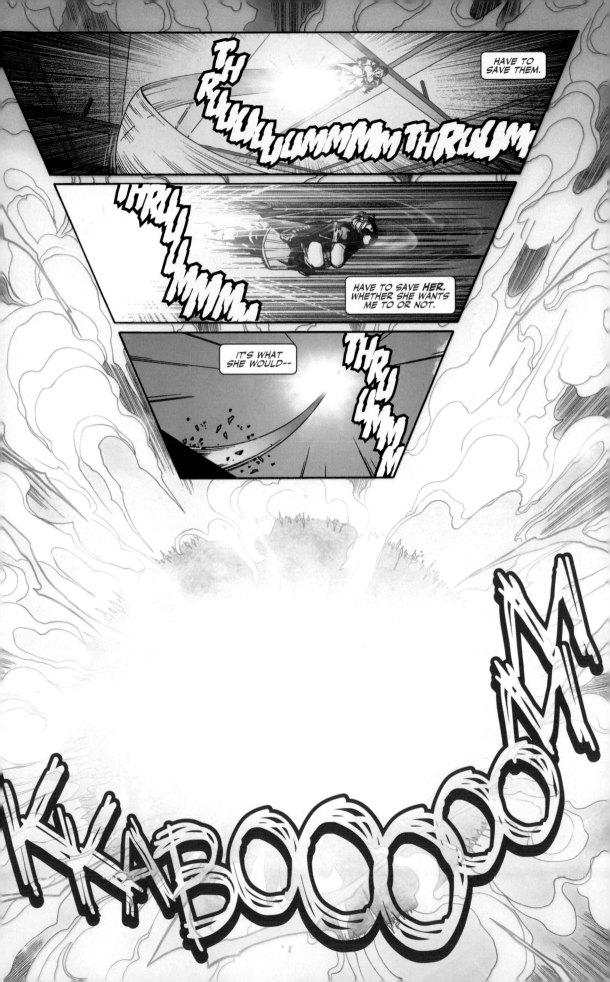

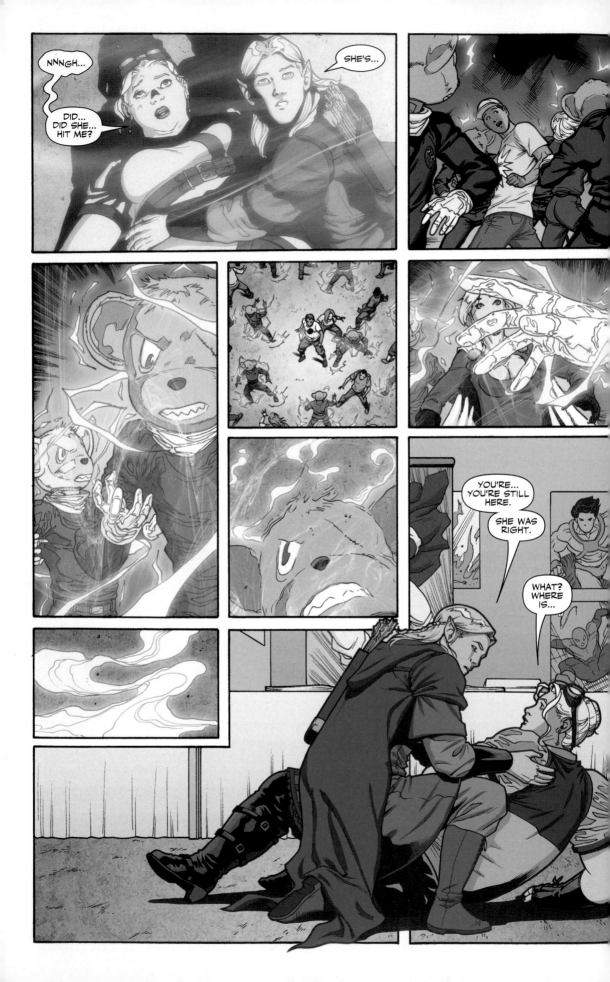

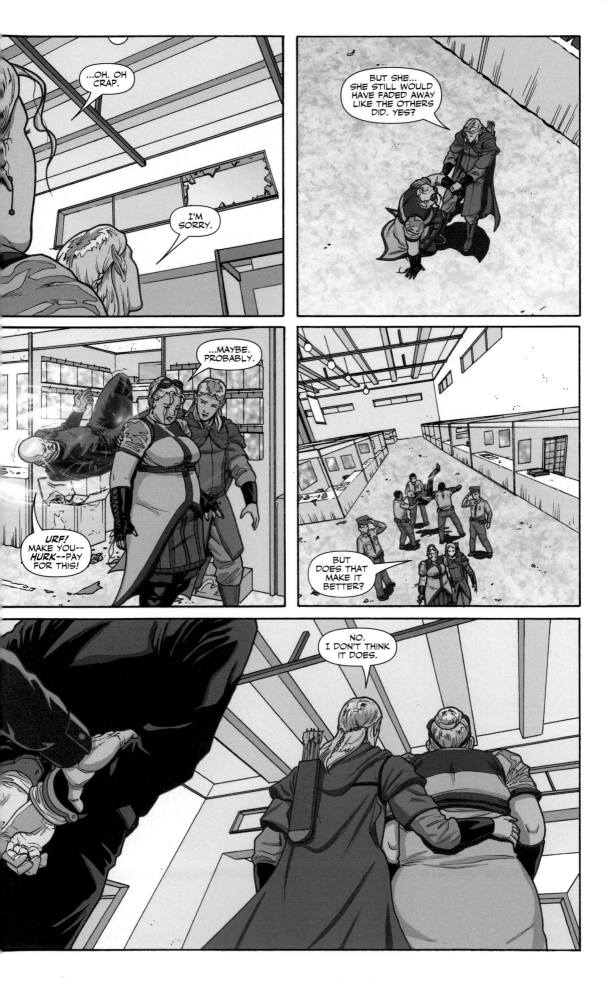

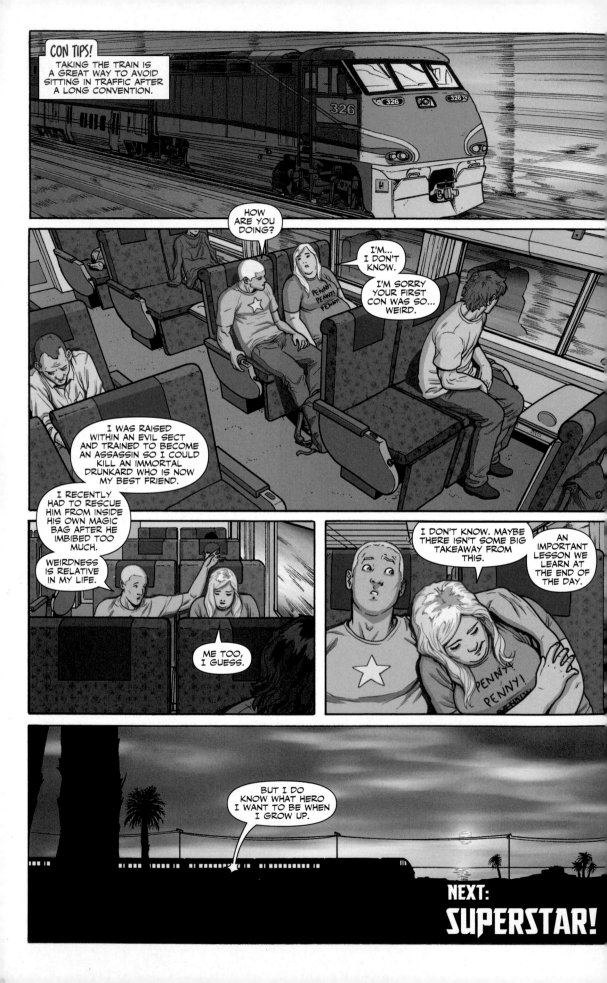

CON TIPS! TAKING THE TRAIN IS A GREAT WAY TO AVOID SITTING IN TRAFFIC AFTER A LONG CONVENTION.

HOW ARE YOU DOING?

I'M... I DON'T KNOW.

I'M SORRY YOUR FIRST CON WAS SO... WEIRD.

I WAS RAISED WITHIN AN EVIL SECT AND TRAINED TO BECOME AN ASSASSIN SO I COULD KILL AN IMMORTAL DRUNKARD WHO IS NOW MY BEST FRIEND.

I RECENTLY HAD TO RESCUE HIM FROM INSIDE HIS OWN MAGIC BAG AFTER HE IMBIBED TOO MUCH.

WEIRDNESS IS RELATIVE IN MY LIFE.

ME TOO, I GUESS.

I DON'T KNOW. MAYBE THERE ISN'T SOME BIG TAKEAWAY FROM THIS.

AN IMPORTANT LESSON WE LEARN AT THE END OF THE DAY.

BUT I DO KNOW WHAT HERO I WANT TO BE WHEN I GROW UP.

NEXT: **SUPERSTAR!**

FAITH #1 COVER D
Art by EMANUELA LUPACCHINO with BRAD SIMPSON

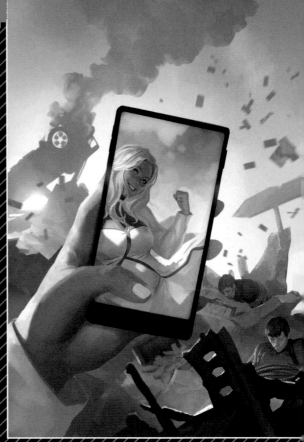

FAITH #4 VARIANT COVER
Art by CLAYTON HENRY with BRIAN REBER

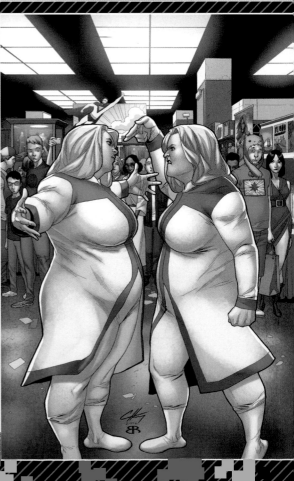

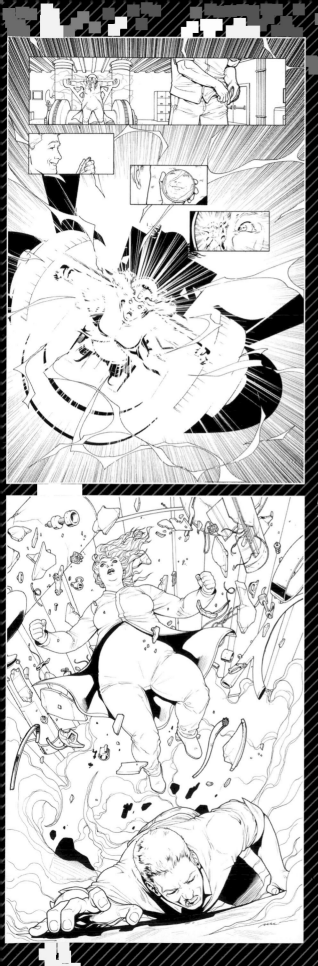

FAITH #1, p. 11
Art by PERE PÉREZ

FAITH #1, p. 12
Art by PERE PÉREZ

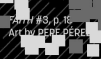

FAITH #3, p. 23
Art by PERE PÉREZ

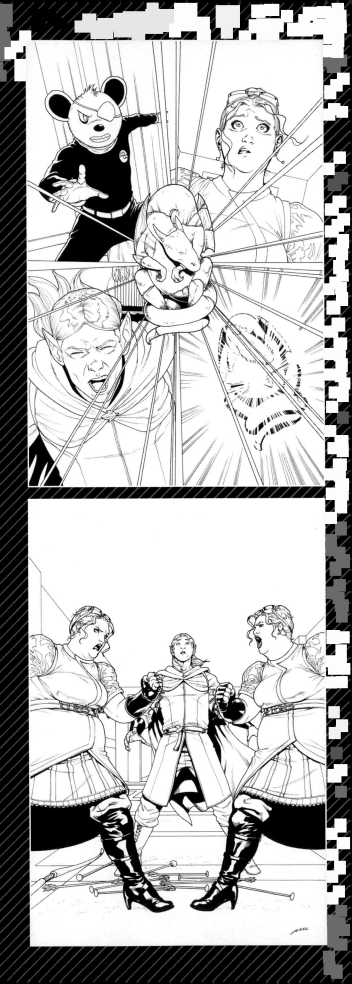

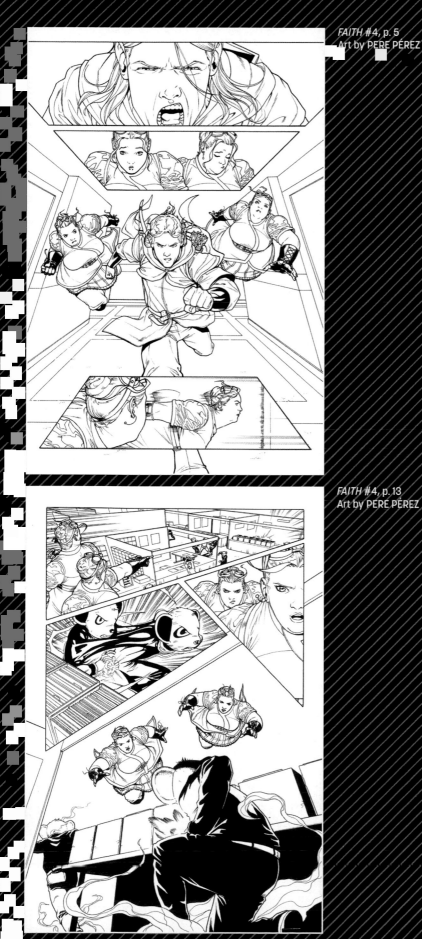

FAITH #4, p. 5
Art by PERE PÉREZ

FAITH #4, p. 13
Art by PERE PÉREZ

EXPLORE THE VALIANT UNIVERSE

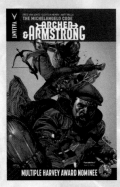
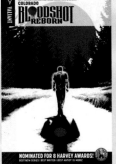
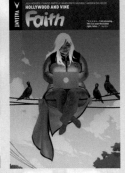
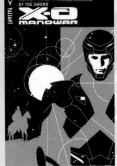
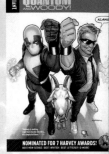

4001 A.D.

4001 A.D.
ISBN: 9781682151433

4001 A.D.: Beyond New Japan
ISBN: 9781682151464

Rai Vol 4: 4001 A.D.
ISBN: 9781682151471

A&A: THE ADVENTURES OF ARCHER AND ARMSTRONG

Volume 1: In the Bag
ISBN: 9781682151495

ARCHER & ARMSTRONG

Volume 1: The Michelangelo Code
ISBN: 9780979640988

Volume 2: Wrath of the Eternal Warrior
ISBN: 9781939346049

Volume 3: Far Faraway
ISBN: 9781939346148

Volume 4: Sect Civil War
ISBN: 9781939346254

Volume 5: Mission: Improbable
ISBN: 9781939346353

Volume 6: American Wasteland
ISBN: 9781939346421

Volume 7: The One Percent and Other Tales
ISBN: 9781939346537

ARMOR HUNTERS

Armor Hunters
ISBN: 9781939346452

Armor Hunters: Bloodshot
ISBN: 9781939346469

Armor Hunters: Harbinger
ISBN: 9781939346506

Unity Vol. 3: Armor Hunters
ISBN: 9781939346445

X-O Manowar Vol. 7: Armor Hunters
ISBN: 9781939346476

BLOODSHOT

Volume 1: Setting the World on Fire
ISBN: 9780979640964

Volume 2: The Rise and the Fall
ISBN: 9781939346032

Volume 3: Harbinger Wars
ISBN: 9781939346124

Volume 4: H.A.R.D. Corps
ISBN: 9781939346193

Volume 5: Get Some!
ISBN: 9781939346315

Volume 6: The Glitch and Other Tales
ISBN: 9781939346711

BLOODSHOT REBORN

Volume 1: Colorado
ISBN: 9781939346674

Volume 2: The Hunt
ISBN: 9781939346827

Volume 3: The Analog Man
ISBN: 9781682151334

BOOK OF DEATH

Book of Death
ISBN: 9781939346971

Book of Death: The Fall of the Valiant Universe
ISBN: 9781939346988

DEAD DROP

ISBN: 9781939346858

THE DEATH-DEFYING DOCTOR MIRAGE

Volume 1
ISBN: 9781939346490

Volume 2: Second Lives
ISBN: 9781682151297

THE DELINQUENTS

ISBN: 9781939346513

DIVINITY

Volume 1
ISBN: 9781939346766

Volume 2
ISBN: 9781682151518

ETERNAL WARRIOR

Volume 1: Sword of the Wild
ISBN: 9781939346209

Volume 2: Eternal Emperor
ISBN: 9781939346292

Volume 3: Days of Steel
ISBN: 9781939346742

WRATH OF THE ETERNAL WARRIOR

Volume 1: Risen
ISBN: 9781682151235

Volumel 2: Labyrinth
ISBN: 9781682151594

FAITH

Faith Vol 1: Hollywood and Vine
ISBN: 9781682151402

Faith Vol 2: California Scheming
ISBN: 9781682151631

HARBINGER

Volume 1: Omega Rising
ISBN: 9780979640957

Volume 2: Renegades
ISBN: 9781939346025

Volume 3: Harbinger Wars
ISBN: 9781939346117

Volume 4: Perfect Day
ISBN: 9781939346155

Volume 5: Death of a Renegade
ISBN: 9781939346339

Volume 6: Omegas
ISBN: 9781939346384

HARBINGER WARS

Harbinger Wars
ISBN: 9781939346094

Bloodshot Vol. 3: Harbinger Wars
ISBN: 9781939346124

Harbinger Vol. 3: Harbinger Wars
ISBN: 9781939346117

EXPLORE THE VALIANT UNIVERSE

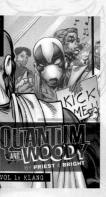
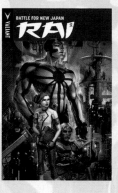
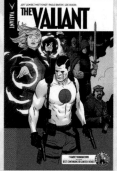
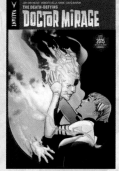
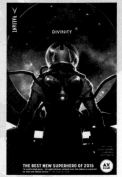

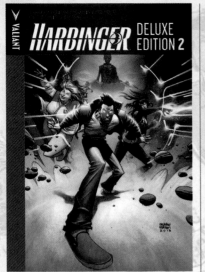

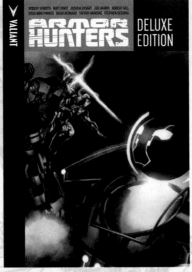

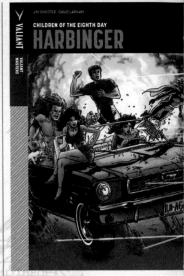

Omnibuses

Archer & Armstrong:
The Complete Classic Omnibus
ISBN: 9781939346872
Collecting ARCHER & ARMSTRONG (1992) #0-26,
ETERNAL WARRIOR (1992) #25 along with ARCHER
& ARMSTRONG: THE FORMATION OF THE SECT.

Quantum and Woody:
The Complete Classic Omnibus
ISBN: 9781939346360
Collecting QUANTUM AND WOODY (1997) #0, 1-21
and #32, THE GOAT: H.A.E.D.U.S. #1,
and X-O MANOWAR (1996) #16

X-O Manowar Classic Omnibus Vol. 1
ISBN: 9781939346308
Collecting X-O MANOWAR (1992) #0-30,
ARMORINES #0, X-O DATABASE #1, as well
as material from SECRETS OF THE
VALIANT UNIVERSE #1

Deluxe Editions

Archer & Armstrong Deluxe Edition Book 1
ISBN: 9781939346223
Collecting ARCHER & ARMSTRONG #0-13

Archer & Armstrong Deluxe Edition Book 2
ISBN: 9781939346957
Collecting ARCHER & ARMSTRONG #14-25,
ARCHER & ARMSTRONG: ARCHER #0 and BLOOD-
SHOT AND H.A.R.D. CORPS #20-21.

Armor Hunters Deluxe Edition
ISBN: 9781939346728
Collecting Armor Hunters #1-4, Armor Hunters:
Aftermath #1, Armor Hunters: Bloodshot #1-3,
Armor Hunters: Harbinger #1-3, Unity #8-11, and
X-O MANOWAR #23-29

Bloodshot Deluxe Edition Book 1
ISBN: 9781939346216
Collecting BLOODSHOT #1-13

Bloodshot Deluxe Edition Book 2
ISBN: 9781939346810
Collecting BLOODSHOT AND H.A.R.D. CORPS #14-23,
BLOODSHOT #24-25, BLOODSHOT #0, BLOOD-
SHOT AND H.A.R.D. CORPS: H.A.R.D. CORPS #0,
along with ARCHER & ARMSTRONG #18-19

Book of Death Deluxe Edition

ISBN: 9781682151150
Collecting BOOK OF DEATH #1-4, BOOK OF DEATH:
THE FALL OF BLOODSHOT #1, BOOK OF DEATH: THE
FALL OF NINJAK #1, BOOK OF DEATH: THE FALL OF
HARBINGER #1, and BOOK OF DEATH: THE FALL OF
X-O MANOWAR #1.

Divinity Deluxe Edition
ISBN: 97819393460993
Collecting DIVNITY #1-4

Harbinger Deluxe Edition Book 1
ISBN: 9781939346131
Collecting HARBINGER #0-14

Harbinger Deluxe Edition Book 2
ISBN: 9781939346773
Collecting HARBINGER #15-25, HARBINGER: OME-
GAS #1-3, and HARBINGER: BLEEDING MONK #0

Harbinger Wars Deluxe Edition
ISBN: 9781939346322
Collecting HARBINGER WARS #1-4, HARBINGER
#11-14, and BLOODSHOT #10-13

Ivar, Timewalker Deluxe Edition Book 1
ISBN: 9781682151198
Collecting IVAR, TIMEWALKER #1-12

Quantum and Woody Deluxe Edition Book 1
ISBN: 9781939346681
Collecting QUANTUM AND WOODY #1-12 and
QUANTUM AND WOODY: THE GOAT #0

Q2: The Return of Quantum and
Woody Deluxe Edition
ISBN: 9781939346568
Collecting Q2: THE RETURN OF QUANTUM
AND WOODY #1-5

Rai Deluxe Edition Book 1
ISBN: 9781682151174
Collecting RAI #1-12, along with material from RAI
#1 PLUS EDITION and RAI #5 PLUS EDITION

Shadowman Deluxe Edition Book 1
ISBN: 9781939346438
Collecting SHADOWMAN #0-10

Shadowman Deluxe Edition Book 2
ISBN: 9781682151075
Collecting SHADOWMAN #11-16, SHADOWMAN
#13X, SHADOWMAN: END TIMES #1-3 and PUNK
MAMBO #0

Unity Deluxe Edition Book 1
ISBN: 9781939346575

Collecting UNITY #0-14

The Valiant Deluxe Edition
ISBN: 9781939346086
Collecting THE VALIANT #1-4

X-O Manowar Deluxe Edition Book 1
ISBN: 9781939346100
Collecting X-O MANOWAR #1-14

X-O Manowar Deluxe Edition Book 2
ISBN: 9781939346520
Collecting X-O MANOWAR #15-22, and UNITY #1-

X-O Manowar Deluxe Edition Book 3
ISBN: 9781682151310
Collecting X-O MANOWAR #23-29 and ARMOR
HUNTERS #1-4.

Valiant Masters

Bloodshot Vol. 1 - Blood of the Machine
ISBN: 9780979640933

H.A.R.D. Corps Vol. 1 - Search and Destroy
ISBN: 9781939346285

Harbinger Vol. 1 - Children of the Eighth Day
ISBN: 9781939346483

Ninjak Vol. 1 - Black Water
ISBN: 9780979640971

Rai Vol. 1 - From Honor to Strength
ISBN: 9781939346070

Shadowman Vol. 1 - Spirits Within
ISBN: 9781939346018

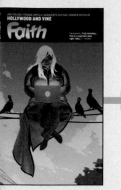

Faith Vol. 1:
Hollywood and Vine

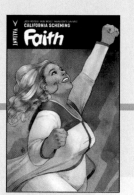

Faith Vol. 2:
California Scheming

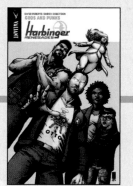

Harbinger Renegades Vol. 1:
Gods and Punks
(OPTIONAL)

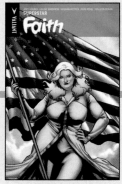

Faith Vol. 3:
Superstar

Read the origin and earliest adventures of the sky-soaring Zephyr!

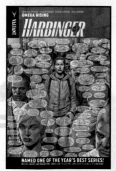

Harbinger Vol. 1:
Omega Rising

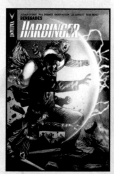

Harbinger Vol. 2:
Renegades

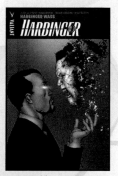

Harbinger Vol. 3:
Harbinger Wars

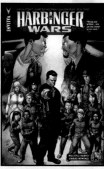

Harbinger Wars

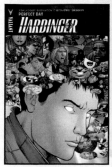

Harbinger Vol. 4:
Perfect Day

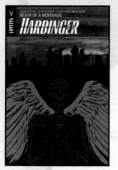

Harbinger Vol. 5:
Death of a Renegade

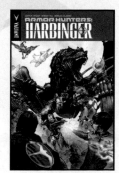

Armor Hunters:
Harbinger

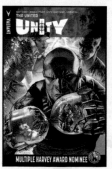

Unity Vol. 4:
The United

Faith

VOLUME THREE: SUPERSTAR

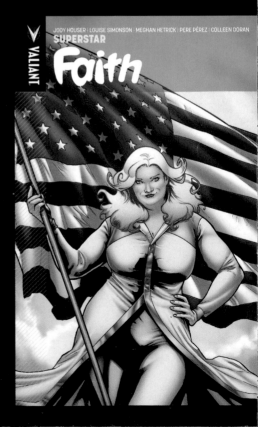

FIGHT AND FLIGHT!

As Los Angeles' high-flying protector, Faith has inspired the dreams of an entire metropolis... Now get ready to meet its worst nightmare! When an escaped psiot prisoner starts tearing through the streets, Faith must stop her fiery rampage before all hell breaks loose! But this isn't just any ordinary threat... Not only can this empowered escapee drain the energy of everything in sight, she's one of L.A.'s most controversial pop stars to boot!

Valiant's chart-topping superhero is about to add a major new player to her frenemies list, courtesy of breakout writer Jody Houser (*Mother Panic*) and acclaimed artists Meghan Hetrick (*Red Thorn*) and Marguerite Sauvage (*DC Comics Bombshells*)! Plus: legendary writer Louise Simonson and Harvey Award-nominated artist Pere Pérez present history in the making as they bring together the leading female hero in comics today with the first female nominee from a major political party for a presidential milestone like no other!

TRADE PAPERBACK
ISBN: 978-1-68215-199-0